Biological Data Analysis

The Practical Approach Series

Affinity Chromatography
Anaerobic Microbiology
Animal Cell Culture (2nd Edition)
Animal Virus Pathogenesis
Antibodies I and II
Biochemical Toxicology
Biological Data Analysis
Biological Membranes
Biomechanics—Materials
Biomechanics—Structures and Systems
Biosensors
Carbohydrate Analysis
Cell–Cell Interactions
Cell Growth and Division
Cellular Calcium
Cellular Neurobiology
Centrifugation (2nd Edition)
Clinical Immunology
Computers in Microbiology
Crystallization of Nucleic Acids and Proteins
Cytokines
The Cytoskeleton
Diagnostic Molecular Pathology I and II
Directed Mutagenesis
DNA Cloning I, II, and III
Drosophila
Electron Microscopy in Biology
Electron Microscopy in Molecular Biology
Electrophysiology
Enzyme Assays
Essential Molecular Biology I and II
Eukaryotic Gene Transcription
Experimental Neuroanatomy
Fermentation
Flow Cytometry
Gel Electrophoresis of Nucleic Acids (2nd Edition)
Gel Electrophoresis of Proteins (2nd Edition)
Genome Analysis
Growth Factors
Haemopoiesis
Histocompatibility Testing
HPLC of Macromolecules
HPLC of Small Molecules
Human Cytogenetics I and II (2nd Edition)
Human Genetic Diseases
Immobilised Cells and Enzymes

In Situ Hybridization
Iodinated Density Gradient Media
Light Microscopy in Biology
Lipid Analysis
Lipid Modification of Proteins
Lipoprotein Analysis
Liposomes
Lymphocytes
Mammalian Cell Biotechnology
Mammalian Development
Medical Bacteriology
Medical Mycology
Microcomputers in Biochemistry
Microcomputers in Biology
Microcomputers in Physiology
Mitochondria
Molecular Genetic Analysis of Populations
Molecular Neurobiology
Molecular Plant Pathology I and II
Monitoring Neuronal Activity
Mutagenicity Testing
Neural Transplantation
Neurochemistry
Neuronal Cell Lines
Nucleic Acid and Protein Sequence Analysis
Nucleic Acid Hybridisation
Nucleic Acids Sequencing
Oligonucleotides and Analogues
Oligonucleotide Synthesis
PCR
Peptide Hormone Action
Peptide Hormone Secretion
Photosynthesis: Energy Transduction
Plant Cell Culture
Plant Molecular Biology
Plasmids
Pollination Ecology
Postimplantation Mammalian Embryos
Preparative Centrifugation
Prostaglandins and Related Substances
Protein Architecture
Protein Engineering
Protein Function
Protein Purification Applications
Protein Purification Methods
Protein Sequencing
Protein Structure
Protein Targeting
Proteolytic Enzymes
Radioisotopes in Biology
Receptor Biochemistry
Receptor–Effector Coupling
Receptor–Ligand Interactions
Ribosomes and Protein Synthesis
RNA Processing
Signal Transduction
Solid Phase Peptide Synthesis
Spectrophotometry and Spectrofluorimetry
Steroid Hormones
Teratocarcinomas and Embryonic Stem Cells
Transcription Factors
Transcription and Translation
Tumour Immunobiology
Virology
Yeast

Biological Data Analysis

A Practical Approach

Edited by

JOHN C. FRY

School of Pure and Applied Biology,
University of Wales College of Cardiff

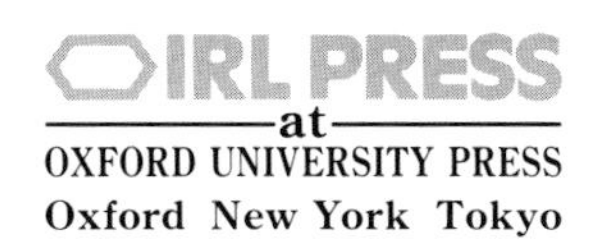

Oxford University Press, Walton Street, Oxford OX2 6DP
Oxford New York Toronto
Delhi Bombay Calcutta Madras Karachi
Kuala Lumpur Singapore Hong Kong Tokyo
Nairobi Dar es Salaam Cape Town
Melbourne Auckland Madrid
and associated companies in
Berlin Ibadan

Oxford is a trade mark of Oxford University Press

A Practical Approach is a registered trade mark
of the Chancellor, Masters, and Scholars of the University of Oxford
trading as Oxford University Press

Published in the United States
by Oxford University Press Inc., New York

A catalogue record for this book is available from the British Library

Library of Congress Cataloging in Publication Data
Biological data analysis : a practical approach / edited by John C. Fry.
(The Practical approach series)
Includes bibliographical references and index.
1. Biometry. 2. Biology—Data processing. I. Fry, John C. II. Series.
QH323.5.B46 1993 574'.015195—dc20 92–27977

ISBN 0–19–963340–1 (hbk.)
ISBN 0–19–963339–8 (pbk.)

Typeset by Footnote Graphics, Warminster, Wilts
Printed in Great Britain by Information Press Ltd, Eynsham, Oxon

Preface

This book has emerged as a logical extension to a course on Biological Data Analysis, for final-year undergraduates and Masters degree students, which I have been involved with in Cardiff, since the mid-1970s. This course itself grew from another which taught biology postgraduates and staff how to use computers to carry out statistical analysis. The basic approach adopted is to discuss how specially selected data sets or modelling problems can be analysed and the results interpreted. Many examples of the computer commands needed from a wide range of computer packages and programs are given, along with example output; so readers can test the analytical procedures described with the particular package they have available. I intend that this will be done first with the examples provided with the book, before readers move on to analyse their own data. I would encourage discussion with mathematicians about points of difficulty.

This volume aims to allow biologists to carry out accurate statistical analysis and modelling with the minimum chance of making mistakes. Error-free statistical analysis is important, as otherwise results and data obtained with considerable effort will be misinterpreted. Most biologists find it hard to plan the correct path through a statistical analysis. This text strives to make such a task easier. So all the statistical chapters include sections describing the form that data should take for the analysis being described. The modelling section of the book is intended as a brief introduction to dynamic mathematical modelling, and readers with special interest in this subject would need to read other books. The authors have assumed that all readers will have done an elementary statistics course and already understand a little about distributions, simple descriptive statistics (for example mean and variance) and hypothesis testing. Hence we have aimed at final-year undergraduate students, Masters degree students, postgraduates and professional biologists in industry, research and education. The provision of data sets from many biological disciplines should make the book useful to all types of biologist.

Many people have contributed both directly and indirectly to the final form of this volume. First, I am grateful to the authors who have willingly succumbed to my badgering to write in the overall form in which the chapters appear. In particular I thank Terence Iles for his patient answers to a barrage of statistical questions over about 20 years. I also thank David Staples, my first Ph.D. student, whose disgust at my inability to help him decide which of his results were different from each other led me to start seriously to learn about practical statistics by reading the excellent first edition of *Biometry* by R. R. Sokal and F. J. Rohlf. Thanks are also due to Clecom Ltd. and Minitab Inc. for providing me with a free copy of Minitab release 8.2 with which many of the statistical approaches have been tested. I also thank my wife and family who have tolerated me during the long process of putting this book together. Almost all the authors reported that writing their chapters took much longer than expected. Let us all hope that the effort has been worthwhile. Only you, the readers, can judge! So please, feel free to write to me with suggestions for improvements if you find the book useful.

April 1992
Cardiff

J.C.F.

Contents

Contributors

DAVID W. BOWKER
School of Pure and Applied Biology, University of Wales College of Cardiff, PO Box 915, Cardiff CF1 3TL, UK.

P. D. BRIDGE
International Mycological Institute, Bakeham Lane, Englefield Green, Egham, Surrey TW20 9TY, UK.

F. D. J. DUNSTAN
School of Mathematics, University of Wales College of Cardiff, PO Box 916, Cardiff CF2 4AG, UK.

JOHN C. FRY
School of Pure and Applied Biology, University of Wales College of Cardiff, PO Box 915, Cardiff CF1 3TL, UK.

TERENCE C. ILES
School of Mathematics, University of Wales College of Cardiff, PO Box 916, Cardiff CF2 4AG, UK.

P. F. RANDERSON
School of Pure and Applied Biology, University of Wales College of Cardiff, PO Box 915, Cardiff CF1 3TL, UK.

RICHARD G. WIEGERT
Department of Zoology, University of Georgia, Athens, Georgia 30602, USA.

Symbols and abbreviations used in Part 1

The chapter(s) in which the symbol or abbreviation is first introduced is given after the definitions. Where a symbol is used more than once it is also defined more than once in this list. Some of the symbols and abbreviations given here also occur with descriptive subscripts not in this list; they are defined locally.

A, B, C,	factors in factorial experiments (Chapter 2)
ANOVA	analysis of variance (Chapters 1, 2, and 3)
AR	autoregressive process in time series analysis (Chapter 7)
ARIMA	autoregressive, integrated moving average model (Chapter 7)
ARMA	autoregressive moving average model (Chapter 7)
a, b, c	number of levels of factors A, B, C respectively in ANOVA (Chapter 2)
α, β	overall effects of factors A, B, in linear model for ANOVA (Chapter 2)
α	normally accepted probability (Chapter 3)
α	significance level of test, also used in confidence coefficient (Chapter 4)
$\alpha\beta$	interaction effect of crossed factors A and B in linear model for ANOVA (Chapter 2)
a	total number of groups in a one-way ANOVA or in factor A of a factorial anova (Chapters 1 and 2)
acf	autocorrelation function (Chapter 7)
β	true slope (Chapter 3)
β	seasonal constant in an ARIMA time series model (*Chapter 7*)
$\beta(\alpha)$	hierarchical effect of factor B within factor A in linear model for ANOVA of nested model (Chapter 2)
β_0	true intercept (Chapter 3)
$\beta_{0 \ldots k}$	partial regression coefficient, the multiplier for the jth predictor variable x_j in a multiple regression equation (Chapters 4 and 7)
B	backshift operator: $\mathrm{B}x_t = x_{t-1}$ (Chapter 7)
b	calculated slope; b, b_2, . . . , b_n are calculated slopes for multiple predictor variables (x_1, x_2, . . . , x_n) (Chapters 3)
b_0	calculated intercept (Chapters 3 and 4)

$b_{0...k}$	estimate of β from a set of multiple or polynomial regression data (Chapters 3 and 4)
C	Cochran's C statistic for homogeneity of variances (Chapters 1 and 2)
C	letter value (Chapter 1)
C	Sorensen (Czekanowski) coefficient; C_{jh} in Q-mode, C_{ik} in R-mode (Chapter 5)
CF	correction factor (Chapter 2)
CI_F	confidence interval based on F (Chapter 3)
CI_L	lower confidence interval (Chapter 3)
CI_t	confidence interval based on t (Chapter 3)
CI_U	upper confidence interval (Chapter 3)
C_p	Mallows' C_p (Chapters 3 and 4)
c	number of confidence intervals calculated simultaneously (Chapter 4)
c	amplitude of a sine wave (Chapter 7)
c	constant in an ARMA model in time series analysis (Chapter 7)
$c(0)$	variance of a time series (Chapter 7)
χ^2	chi-squared test statistic (Chapter 2)
c_i, d_i	weights in linear contrasts (Chapter 2)
$\cos \eta$	angular distance coefficient (Chapter 6)
Δ_AB	Euclidean distance between individuals A and B (Chapter 6)
D	intermediate statistic for calculating confidence interval for $\hat{x}$ (Chapter 3)
D	number of seasonal differences in a seasonal ARIMA model (Chapter 7)
D	letter value (Chapter 1)
D	Cook's D (Chapters 3 and 4)
D	Euclidean or Pythagorean distance; D_{jh} (interstand distance) in Q-mode, D_{ik} in R-mode (Chapter 5)
D	Manhattan or city-block distance between two individuals (Chapter 6)
DCA	detrended correspondence analysis (Chapter 5)
DF	discriminant function (Chapter 5)
D_p	pattern difference coefficient for association (Chapter 6)
D_TAB	total difference between individuals A and B (Chapter 6)
D_VAB	difference in vigour between individuals A and B (Chapter 6)
DW	calculated Durbin–Watson statistic (Chapter 3)
d	number of differences taken in an ARIMA(p,d.q) model (Chapter 7)
d_AB	taxonomic distance between individuals A and B (Chapter 6)
df	degrees of freedom (Chapters 1–4)
d_L	lower value for tabulated Durbin–Watson statistic (Chapter 3)
d_U	upper value for tabulated Durbin–Watson statistic (Chapter 3)

ε	true error term in linear model for ANOVA and regression (Chapters 2, 3, and 4)
ε_t	tth term in a white noise series (Chapter 7)
E	eighth (letter value) (Chapter 1)
E[MS]	expected value of mean square (Chapter 2)
e	residuals from regression (Chapter 3)
e_t	residual tth value for a time series (Chapter 7)
F	F-statistic; variance ratio (Chapters 1–4)
FA	factor analysis (Chapter 5)
$F_{\max}$	Hartley's $F_{\max}$ statistic for homogeneity of variances (Chapter 1)
γ_i	adjustment for ith group in one-way ANOVA (Chapter 2)
G	grand total of all data in experiment (Chapter 2)
g	sum of group values; Σx (Chapter 1)
g_i	total for ith group in one-way ANOVA (Chapter 2)
H	hinge (letter value) (Chapter 1)
H	intermediate statistic for calculating confidence interval for $\hat{x}$ (Chapter 3)
h_{ii}	leverage of ith observation (Chapters 3 and 4)
i, j, k	subscripts for levels of factors or replications (Chapter 2)
i	index or subscript for observations (Chapters 4 and 6)
J	intermediate statistic for calculating confidence interval for $\hat{x}$ (Chapter 3)
j,l	index or subscript for predictor variables x_j, x_l (Chapter 4)
φ	phase of a sine wave (Chapter 7)
φ_j	coefficient of the jth term in an autoregressive model (Chapter 7)
K	constant in generalized two-bend transformation (Chapter 3)
k	number of predictor (x) variables in a regression (Chapters 3 and 4)
λ	eigenvalue of correlation matrix of predictor variables (Chapter 4)
$\lambda(k)$	lag window (Chapter 7)
$L_{\mathrm{L}},L_{\mathrm{U}}$	lower and upper letter values (Chapter 3)
LSD	least significant difference (Chapters 1 and 2)
μ	overall mean in linear model for ANOVA (Chapter 2)
M	median (Chapters 1 and 3)
MA	moving average model in time series analysis (Chapter 7)
MDA	multiple discriminant analysis (Chapter 5)
MS	mean square; sum of squares divided by degrees of freedom (Chapters 1–4)
MSD	minimum significant difference (Chapters 1 and 2)
$\mathrm{MS}_{\mathrm{error}}$	within groups mean square from an ANOVA (Chapters 1, 2, and 3)

MS_{group}	between groups mean square from a one-way ANOVA (Chapter 1)
MS_{rerror}	error mean square from regression (Chapters 3 and 4)
m	number of comparisons made (Chapter 3)
m	number of attributes in ordination (Chapter 5)
m	truncation point in a lag window (Chapter 7)
m	truncation point used for calculating spectral estimates of a time series (m is normally between $n/5$ and $n/10$) (Chapter 7)
N	total number of replicates in an ANOVA; Σn (Chapters 1 and 2)
n	number of replicates in a group or cell (Chapters 1 and 2)
n	number of points in regression (Chapter 3)
n	number of individuals or OTUs in ordination or classification (Chapters 5 and 6)
n	length of a time series (Chapter 7)
$\tilde{n}$	harmonic mean of a set of ns (Chapter 2)
n_1	number of individuals used to calculate the proportion killed for a mortality curve (Chapter 3)
OTUs	operational taxonomic units (Chapter 6)
P	order of the seasonal autoregressive component in a seasonal ARIMA model (Chapter 7)
P	probability
PC	principal component (Chapter 5)
PCA	principal components analysis (Chapter 5)
PI_F	prediction interval based on F (Chapter 3)
PI_t	prediction interval based on t (Chapter 3)
p	power for a transformation (Chapters 1–4)
p	number of components in ordination (Chapter 5)
p	order of the autoregressive component of an ARMA model (Chapter 7)
p'	number of constants in multiple regression equation, normally $p' = k + 1$ (Chapters 3 and 4)
pacf	partial autocorrelation function (Chapter 7)
Q	studentized range statistic (Chapters 1 and 2)
Q	order of the seasonal moving average component in a seasonal ARIMA model (Chapter 7)
q	number of predictor variables in subset of predictors in multiple regression (Chapter 4)
q	order of the moving average component of an ARMA model (Chapter 7)
R	multiple correlation coefficient (Chapters 3 and 4)
R^2	coefficient of determination (Chapters 3 and 4)
RA	reciprocal averaging (Chapter 5)
R_i	quantitative range for character i (Chapter 6)

r	product moment or Pearson's correlation coefficient (Chapters 3, 4, and 6)
$r(k)$	autocorrelation function at lag k (Chapter 7)
r_i	raw residual for ith observation (Chapter 4)
$r_{xy}(k)$	cross-correlation function between series $\{x_t\}$ and $\{y_t\}$ at lag k (Chapter 7)
Σ	summation operator
S	covariance; S_{jh} in Q-mode, S_{ik} in R-mode (Chapter 5)
SAHN	sequential, agglomerative, hierarchic non-overlapping method of clustering (Chapter 6)
SCH	value of Schwarz's criterion for an ARIMA model (Chapter 7)
S_G	Gower's similarity coefficient (Chapter 6)
S_{iAB}	character score for the ith characters between individuals A and B (Chapter 6)
S_J	Jaccard coefficient of similarity (Chapter 6)
SS	sum of squares (Chapters 1–4)
SS-STP	sum of squares simultaneous test procedure (Chapter 1)
S_{SM}	simple matching coefficient of similarity (Chapter 6)
SS_Q	sum of squares of individuals (Chapter 5)
SS_R	sum of squares of attributes (Chapter 5)
s	standard deviation (Chapters 1–4)
s	length of a cycle in a seasonal ARIMA model (Chapter 7)
σ	standard deviation of error term ε (Chapter 4)
σ^2	variance of error term ε (Chapters 2 and 4)
σ_e	estimated standard deviation (Chapter 1)
$s_{\hat{y}}$	standard error of $\hat{y}$ from given x value (Chapter 3)
$\hat{s}_y$	standard error of $\hat{y}$ from a new x value (Chapter 3)
$s_{.j}$	individual standard deviation (Chapter 5)
s^2	variance (Chapters 1–4)
s_b	standard error of b (Chapter 3)
s_{b_0}	standard error of b_0 (Chapter 3)
$s_{i.}$	attribute standard deviation (Chapter 5)
θ	constant in an ARMA model in time series analysis (Chapter 7)
θ_i	coefficient of ith term in a moving average model (Chapter 7)
t	number of attributes or characters (equivalent to k (multiple regression) and m (ordination)) (Chapter 6)
t	Student's t-statistic (Chapters 1 and 4)
t	time in time series analysis (Chapter 7)
t_i	studentized deleted residual for ith observation (Chapter 4)
VIF	variance inflation factor (Chapter 4)
∇	difference operator: $\nabla x_t = x_t - x_{t-1}$ (Chapter 7)
∇_d	seasonal difference operator: $\nabla x_t = x_{t-d}$ (Chapter 7)

ω	frequency of a sine or cosine wave (Chapter 7)
W	weighted similarity coefficient (Chapter 5)
WSC	weighted similarity coefficient (Chapter 5)
w,x,y,z	values for numbers of joint positive and negative characters between two characters; $w = +/+$, $x = +/-$, $y = +/-$, $z = -/-$ (Chapter 6)
w	weights used in weighted regression (Chapter 3)
w_{iAB}	weight assigned to the comparison of character i for individuals A and B (Chapter 6)
X_i	total of data at ith level of a factor in ANOVA (Chapter 2)
X_{iA}	state of character i for individual A (Chapter 6)
x	observation, single data point in ANOVA (Chapters 1 and 2)
x	independent or predictor variable in regression or a value of it (Chapters 3 and 4)
x_{ij}	attribute value (Chapter 5)
x_t	tth value in a time series (Chapter 7)
$\bar{x}$	mean of all x values in regression (Chapter 3)
$\bar{x}$	mean of replicates in a group (Chapter 1)
$\bar{x}_{.j}$	individual mean (Chapter 5)
$\bar{x}_{i.}$	attribute mean (Chapter 5)
$\hat{x}$	predicted value of x (Chapter 3)
$\hat{x}_a$	predicted value of x_a made at the end of a series (Chapter 7)
y	dependent variable in regression or a value of it (Chapters 3 and 4)
y_t	tth value in a time series after differencing (Chapter 7)
$\bar{y}$	mean of all y values in regression (Chapter 3)
$\hat{y}$	predicted y value (Chapter 3)
z	standardized predictor variable (Chapter 4)

Symbols and abbreviations used in Part 2

α_{ij}	resource refuge (minimum concentration available (Chapter 9)
α_{jj}	minimum response density (lower response threshold) (Chapter 9)
β_1	competitive effect of x_1 on x_2 relative to self inhibition (Chapter 9)
β_2	competitive effect of x_2 on x_1 relative to self inhibition (Chapter 9)
β_k	effect of competition (Chapter 9)
B	biomass of a cohort of fish (Chapter 8)
B_t	biomass of a cohort of fish at age t (Chapter 8)
C	limiting nutrient concentration (Chapter 8)
C'	rate of change of limiting nutrient concentration (Chapter 8)
CINT	communication interval (*ISIM* reserved variable) (Chapter 8)
c	correction term (Chapter 9)
D	dilution rate of medium in chemostat (Chapter 8)
Δt	time step (Chapter 8)
ΔX	change in value of X (Chapter 8)
d	phytoplankton mortality coefficient (Chapter 8)
ε_{ij}	fraction of ingested matter/energy that is egested (Chapter 9)
F	fishing mortality coefficient (Chapter 8)
F_{ij}	flux of energy/matter from X_i to X_j (Chapter 9)
f	flow rate of medium through chemostat (Chapter 8)
$f(X_i)$	function of compartment i (Chapter 9)
$f(X_j)$	function of compartment j (Chapter 9)
γ_{ij}	resource satiation (maximum) concentration (satiation level) (Chapter 9)
γ_{jj}	maximum crowding concentration (carrying capacity) (Chapter 9)
g	phytoplankton growth coefficient (Chapter 8)
g_m	nutrient saturated growth coefficient (Chapter 8)
H	coefficient in von Bertalanffy equation (Chapter 8)
η_j	minimum specific rate of excretion (Chapter 9)
K_s	half saturation coefficient (Chapter 8)
k	coefficient in von Bertalanffy equation (Chapter 8)
kQ	minimum intra-cellular nutrient concentration (Chapter 8)

λ	summed minimal losses (Chapter 9)
λ_j	loss or mortality term (Chapter 9)
λ_j	summed specific rate of loss from compartment j (Chapter 9)
μ	growth coefficient of bacteria or phytoplankton (Chapter 8)
μ_j	minimum specific rate of mortality (Chapter 9)
μ_m	maximum or nutrient saturated growth coefficient (Chapter 8)
M	natural mortality coefficient of fish (Chapter 8)
N	population density of phytoplankton or fish (Chapter 8)
N'	rate of change of population density (Chapter 8)
N_0	population density of fish at time zero (Chapter 8)
N_t	population density of fish at time t (Chapter 8)
P	population density of phytoplankton (Chapter 8)
Q	intra-cellular nutrient concentration (Chapter 8)
Q'	rate of change of intra-cellular nutrient concentration (Chapter 8)
q	nutrient depletion factor (Chapter 8)
R	rate of replenishment or input of limiting nutrient (Chapter 8)
ρ_j	minimum specific rate of respiratory loss (Chapter 9)
r	instantaneous rate of population growth (Chapter 8)
r_m	maximum or intrinsic specific rate of increase (Chapter 9)
S	limiting nutrient concentration (Chapter 8)
S'	rate of change of concentration (Chapter 8)
S_R	limiting nutrient concentration in chemostat reservoir (Chapter 8)
τ_{ij}	maximum specific rate of ingestion of matter/energy (Chapter 9)
τ_r	actual realized rate of ingestion (Chapter 9)
T	time (*ISIM* reserved variable) (Chapter 8)
TFIN	final value of T (*ISIM* reserved variable) (Chapter 8)
t	time or age of fish (Chapter 8)
t_c	age of fish at first capture (Chapter 8)
V	rate of uptake of nutrient by phytoplankton (Chapter 8)
V_{max}	maximum rate of uptake of nutrient by phytoplankton (Chapter 8)
v	volume of medium in chemostat (Chapter 8)
W	biomass of individual fish (Chapter 8)
W'	rate of change of biomass of individual fish (Chapter 8)
W_t	biomass of individual fish at age t (Chapter 8)
X	state variable (Chapter 8)
X'	rate of change of state variable with respect to time (Chapter 8)
X_i	donor compartment (Chapter 9)
X_j	recipient compartment (Chapter 9)

X_k	passive abiotic compartment (Chapter 9)
X_t	value of state variable at time t (Chapter 8)
x	biomass of bacteria in chemostat (Chapter 8)
x'	rate of change of bacterial biomass with respect to time (Chapter 8)
Y	yield coefficient (Chapter 8)
Z	total fish mortality coefficient (Chapter 8)

PART 1

Statistics

1

One-way analysis of variance

JOHN C. FRY

1. Introduction

One-way analysis of variance (ANOVA) is an extremely useful statistical approach in all branches of biology. It can be used to test whether there are any significant differences between a set of means from an experiment or survey and to identify where these differences lie. This chapter will give a succinct, but comprehensive account of how to do a one-way ANOVA with computer based statistical packages. General tests that describe one-way ANOVA in more detail for non-mathematicians are those of Winer (1) and Sokal and Rohlf (2), whilst Miller (3) gives a more mathematical account. I have found all of these texts fairly easy to understand and so they should be useful for those who need amplification of the text written here.

1.1 Data structure

A typical data structure for one-way ANOVA is drawn diagrammatically in *Figure 1*. This is for a case when there are equal numbers (n) of replicate values (x) for each of a groups. I shall use groups here, but other terms are commonly used for the same thing; these include treatments and sets. It is perfectly permissible to have unequal numbers of replicates in the groups. In the case of one-way ANOVA there is only one factor, and this can be compared with crossed and hierarchical designs (see Chapter 2) where there is more than one factor.

	Factor					
	1	2	3	4	. . . .	a
replicates (*n* per group)	*x*	*x*	*x*	*x*	. . . .	*x*
	x	*x*	*x*	*x*	. . . .	*x*
	x	*x*	*x*	*x*	. . . .	*x*

Figure 1. Typical data structure for one-way analysis of variance with *a* groups in the factor being tested and *n* replicates per group. Each *x* represents an individual value; One group is indicated with a rounded box.

Table 1. Numbers of mayfly larvae (per $0.05\,m^2$ quadrats) in six sites from a river[a]

Site					
1	**2**	**3**	**4**	**5**	**6**
7	61	50	11	0	1
4	13	155	6	0	4
0	0	106	2	0	1
5	42	100	13	1	0

[a] Details of the river topography are described in text

Two data sets will be used illustratively throughout this chapter. The first (*Table 1*) has equal *n* and was obtained by counting the number of mayfly larvae in 0.05 m^2 quadrats from riffles in a local river. Sites 1–6 were sampled sequentially downstream. Site 1 was more rocky than the other sites and a tributary joined the river between sites 3 and 4. The second set of data (*Table 2*) has unequal *n* and are prolactin concentrations in the pituitary glands dissected from nine-spined sticklebacks. The fish were kept in either saltwater or freshwater prior to assay and were obtained from the same pond on three

Table 2. Prolactin concentrations (units g^{-1}) in the pituitary glands of nine-spined sticklebacks with different treatments[a]

Saltwater, cysts, day 1	Freshwater, no cysts, day 1	Freshwater, no cysts, day 2	Freshwater, cysts, day 3
14.5	52.7	36.0	31.0
11.1	44.4	28.0	69.0
15.0	125.0	97.0	115.0
14.3	66.0	26.0	53.0
25.7	23.3	38.0	52.0
		25.0	53.0
		70.0	66.0
		127.0	44.0
		264.0	31.0
		48.0	37.0
		88.0	
		101.0	
		16.0	
		46.0	
		52.0	

[a] Treatments are described in the text

different occasions. Cysts tend to develop in these fish when kept in saltwater and sometimes develop naturally in freshwater populations. The four different groups of fish were used in a preliminary experiment to examine the effects of cysts, whether induced by saltwater or normally present, on the prolactin production of the pituitary gland.

1.2 Assumptions and experimental design

The main statistical assumptions which underpin one-way ANOVA are as follows:

- randomness of replicates within a group
- independence of errors
- homogeneity (equality) of group variances
- normality of errors

When designing experiments for analysis by one-way ANOVA these assumptions must be carefully considered (4). Randomness and independence will be considered first. The replicates for the mayfly data were collected randomly at the sites. However, if they had been collected at fixed intervals across the river or only at spots which looked promising for mayfly larvae within the site area, the assumption of randomness might have been violated. With the prolactin data, independence could have been violated if, say, only the larger sticklebacks developed cysts or all males were chosen for some treatments and females for others. The remaining two assumptions are very important, but can only be tested once the data have been obtained, and so will be discussed later.

Some other points may also be considered when designing experiments for analysis by one-way ANOVA. If the assumptions are even slightly violated it becomes harder to rely on the results from the analysis, as sample sizes become more unequal (5). Thus one-way ANOVA and the associated tests are less robust for unequal n than for equal n. So every attempt should be made to ensure equal numbers of replicates per group, particularly if the data are prone to unequal variances. One-way ANOVA can be used to analyse virtually any type of biological data in which there is a large range of possible values. However, it should not be used to investigate categorical data where a response is divided into a finite number of values. Such results include presence/absence data and abundance categorized into, say, six possible values.

1.3 Computer packages

There is a very wide range of statistical computer packages available that will carry out the basic data handling and statistical computations necessary for one-way ANOVA. However, I have yet to find a package that has simple commands for all the tests described in this chapter. Readers should therefore use a package that will cope with most things and which works well for the other statistics they intend to carry out. Most good packages allow you to combine commands together in command files and so construct macros that will perform the other tests needed. I use mainly *Minitab* for my statistical requirements which is very easy to use and flexible. However, in this chapter I also explain how three other good packages, namely *SPSS/PC+*, *Systat*, and *Statgraphics*, can be used for one-way ANOVA. All statistical packages take considerable time and effort to learn how to use, so the novice computer statistician should be prepared for hard work. The effort required can be minimized considerably by attending a suitable course.

2. The basic ANOVA

The first step is to enter the data in the correct form. Most packages require all the data to be in a single column or variable. These data are then labelled with a set of integer numbers in another column or variable. The column containing these integer codes, which assign the data points to the factors, is called the subscript, labelling, level or category variable. The mayfly data arranged in this way are in *Appendix 1.1* and the prolactin data is in *Appendix 1.2*.

Once the data have been entered the analysis can start. The basic order in which one-way ANOVA is done is given in *Protocol 1*. Following this route through the analysis will ensure that mistakes are not made and that the results from the ANOVA and the subsequent comparisons of group means are reliable.

Protocol 1. Route through a one-way ANOVA[a]

1. Compute one-way ANOVA table.
2. Check assumptions of ANOVA.
   (a) Tests for homogeneity of variances
   - Bartlett's χ^2
   - Hartley's F_{max}
   - Cochran's C

   (b) Tests for normality of residuals
   - normal probability plots
   - Shapiro–Wilk test
   - boxplots
3. Transform data if assumptions do not hold (see *Protocol 2*) and repeat steps 1 and 2. (If assumptions do not hold after transformation, firstly check step 4, to see if outliers are responsible for some large variances, and secondly follow *Protocol 3*.)
4. Examine residuals of transformed data and test for outliers, consider removing outliers from groups if there is justification. Tests for outliers are

- Dixon's test ($n < 25$)
- Grubb's test ($n > 25$)

5. Comparisons of group means (see *Protocol 3* if assumptions do not hold).
   (a) *A priori* tests (could be planned before results obtained)
   - calculate LSD for pairs of means
   - orthogonal decomposition for more than two means; sometimes called contrasts

   (b) *A posteriori* tests (could not be planned before results obtained)
   - calculate MSD by Tukey–Kramer method for pairs of means
   - use SS-STP procedure for more than two means

[a] Abbreviations are: ANOVA, analysis of variance; LSD, least significant difference; MSD, minimum significant difference; SS-STP, sum of of squares simultaneous test procedure.

The next step is to compute the basic ANOVA table by using the appropriate command from the package being used. It is also useful to save the residuals at this stage for use later. The residuals are our best estimate of the error in the analysis and are calculated by

$$\text{residuals} = x - \bar{x},$$

where x are the data values and $\bar{x}$ are the group means.

The ANOVA table from the raw mayfly data (*Figure 2a*) shows important features which should be noted. The mean squares for between groups (MS_{group}) and within groups (MS_{error}) are calculated by dividing the appropriate sum of squares by the corresponding degrees of freedom. These mean squares

(a)

Analysis of variance

Source of variation	Sum of Squares	d.f.	Mean square	F-ratio	Sig. level
Between groups	31810.000	5	6362.0000	14.440	.0000
Within groups	7930.500	18	440.5833		
Total (corrected)	39740.500	23			

(b)

Analysis of variance

Source of variation	Sum of Squares	d.f.	Mean square	F-ratio	Sig. level
Between groups	9.2421696	5	1.8484339	10.490	.0001
Within groups	3.1718378	18	.1762132		
Total (corrected)	12.414007	23			

Figure 2. One-way ANOVA table for (a) the raw and (b) the $\log_{10}(x + 1)$ transformed mayfly data produced by *Statgraphics*.

are measures of the variation between sites (MS_{group}) and within the sites (MS_{error}). The latter is an average variance over all the groups in the ANOVA and is hence an estimate of the error variance, so it is designated MS_{error}; it is sometimes also called the residual mean square. The *F*-ratio is calculated as

$$F_{calc} = \frac{MS_{group}}{MS_{error}},$$

and is compared with the Table $F_{P(a-1,df_{error})}$ (*Appendix B.1*) to find the probability level at which F_{calc} is significant. This is normally given by the package but it is useful to know that F_{calc} should be large for the result to be significant. Thus for the raw mayfly data F_{calc} is significant at $P \ll 0.001$ as $F_{calc} > F_{P(a-1,df_{error})}$ because

$$F_{0.1(5,18)} = 2.20,$$
$$F_{0.05(5,18)} = 2.77,$$
$$F_{0.01(5,18)} = 4.25,$$

and

$$F_{0.001(5,18)} = 6.81.$$

This procedure is logical: a moment's thought will show that a high error variance results in a low *F*-ratio and a non-significant *F*-test.

A significant *F*-test means that there are significant differences somewhere between the group means, providing the variances are homogeneous and the errors are normally distributed (step 2, *Protocol 1*). It does not indicate which means are different from each other; this is examined by the tests for comparisons of means (step 5, *Protocol 1*).

3. Checking assumptions

The two important assumptions to confirm, before the results of the one-way ANOVA can be relied upon, are homogeneity of variance and normality of errors. The former can be tested directly and the latter by using the residuals, as they are our best estimates of the real errors.

3.1 Homogeneity of variances

This is the most important assumption for ANOVA and must always be tested. The three most useful tests for variance equality are Bartlett's χ^2, Hartley's F_{max} and Cochran's *C*. These are also the most commonly applied and available in many computer packages. All three tests are calculated in *SPSS/PC+* and *Statgraphics*, while *Systat* only calculates Bartlett's χ^2, but provides an alternative *F*-statistic for small sample sizes. *Minitab* does not have commands for any of these statistics. However, I provide a set of *Minitab* macros (BART.MTB, BART1–BART4.MTB; *Appendix 1.3*) that will calculate all three statistics and store group means and variances for subsequent use.

Bartlett's test is best calculated by computer (see (2), p. 404 for method). The two other tests can be calculated more easily from computer output if the group variances (s^2) or standard deviations (s) are provided (*Minitab, Systat*). Hartley's F_{max} and Cochran's C are calculated by

$$F_{max} = \frac{s^2_{max}}{s^2_{min}} \quad \text{and} \quad C = \frac{s^2_{max}}{\sum^{a} s^2_i},$$

where s^2_{max} is the largest group variance, s^2_{min} is the smallest group variance and s^2_i are all the group variances. For the mayfly data (*Table 1*) the group standard deviations are 2.94, 27.6, 42.9, 4.97, 0.500, and 1.73, so

$$F_{max} = \frac{(42.9)^2}{(0.50)^2} = \frac{1840}{0.25} = 7360$$

and

$$C = \frac{(42.9)^2}{(2.94)^2 + \ldots\ldots + (1.73)^2} = \frac{1840}{2639} = 0.697.$$

These values are compared with tabulated values at $P = 0.05$ (*Appendices B.2* and *B.3*). So with F_{max} at a and n-1 degrees of freedom the tabulated value for $F_{max(a,n\text{-}1)} = F_{max(6,3)} = 62.0$, and this is below the calculated F_{max} so the variances are heterogeneous. Similarly, the tabulated value for $C_{(a,n\text{-}1)} = C_{(6,3)} = 0.532$ is smaller than the calculated value, so the variances are also declared heterogeneous. In all three of these tests, calculated values smaller than the table values are required for the variances to be homogeneous and this assumption of ANOVA to be upheld. The result from Bartlett's χ^2 test on the raw mayfly data (*Table 3*) agrees with these two tests. Note the more accurate calculation of F_{max} in *Table 3* as there is no rounding error.

The F_{max} and C tables are designed for equal group sizes. If the data have unequal n then the tables can still be used to give an approximate result. The prolactin data have $n = 5$–15 with $F_{max} = 148.8$ and $C = 0.651$ (*Table 3*). The tabulated values for highest and lowest n are $F_{max(4,15)} = 4.01$, $F_{max(4,5)} = 13.7$, $C_{(4,16)} = 0.437$ (the nearest value in the table, *Appendix B.3*, to $C_{(4,15)}$), and $C_{(4,5)} = 0.590$. Thus the calculated values are larger than all possibilities from the tables and so it is clear that the variances are once again declared heterogeneous. If the calculated value for either of these tests was between the two tabulated values the result would be uncertain, but if either is less than the smallest tabulated value (that for the largest n) then the variances would be homogeneous. Examples of tests giving these results are seen for the prolactin data in *Table 3*. The calculated values for F_{max} and C are in the uncertain region for $\log_{10}$ transformed data and below the lowest table value for data transformed by the reciprocal root.

Table 3. Tabulated and calculated values for statistics[a] used to test homogeneity of variance before and after transformation of the data

	Calculated values using the following transformation								
	Cube	**Square**	**Raw data**	**Square root**	**$\log_{10}$**	**Reciprocal root**	**Reciprocal**	**Reciprocal square**	**Table values at $P = 0.05$[b]**
(i) Mayfly data									
Bartlett's χ^2	210.5	127.9	45.9	19.09	9.80	13.99	23.5	47.7	11.07
Hartley's F_{max}	$>10^6$	$>10^6$	7374	218.4	29.0	263.6	7065	$>10^6$	62.0
Cochran's C	0.9	0.964	0.697	0.587	0.620	0.482	0.309	0.309	0.532
(ii) Prolactin data									
Bartlett's χ^2	80.02	46.76	20.43	11.63	5.98	3.60	5.05	20.46	7.81
Hartley's F_{max}	700 747	8329	148.8	26.96	6.43	3.44	5.27	46.0	13.7/4.01
Cochran's C	0.962	0.860	0.651	0.549	0.470	0.397	0.395	0.762	0.59/0.437

[a] All statistics calculated with the BART series of *Minitab* macros in *Appendix 1.3*

[b] For the prolactin data the tabulated values given for F_{max} and C are for 4,5 and 4,15 or 4,16 degrees of freedom; see text for details; the Bartlett's χ^2 tabulated value is from *Minitab*[a]

(a)

```
Tests for Homogeneity of Variances

      Cochrans C = Max. Variance/Sum(Variances) =   .6974, P =  .002 (Approx.)
      Bartlett-Box F =                            10.192  , P =  .000
      Maximum Variance / Minimum Variance       7374.333
------------------------------------------------------------------------------
```

(b)

```
Tests for Homogeneity of Variances

      Cochrans C = Max. Variance/Sum(Variances) =   .6204, P =  .011 (Approx.)
      Bartlett-Box F =                             1.983  , P =  .080
      Maximum Variance / Minimum Variance         28.967
------------------------------------------------------------------------------
```

Figure 3. Sections of output from *SPSS-PC+* showing results of tests for homogeneity of variance on (a) the raw and (b) the $\log_{10}(x + 1)$ transformed mayfly data.

Care must be taken when interpreting the results of computer output with these tests. The probability values often given (*SPSS/PC+*, *Systat*, *Statgraphics; Figure 3*) should be greater than $P = 0.05$ for the variances to be significantly homogeneous. Notice that for these tests the desirable outcome is for the P value to be large and not small, as is the case for many other tests. We can then be confident about proceeding with the one-way ANOVA assuming equal variances.

3.2 Tests for normality of residuals

One-way ANOVA and the tests for comparisons of means carried out subsequently (*Protocol 1*; Section 6) are not as sensitive to lack of normality of errors as they are to heterogeneity of variances. However, all the tests for homogeneity of variances discussed here (Section 3.1) are susceptible to lack of normality and so can give misleading results if errors are badly non-normal. For this reason it is essential to carry out some sort of test for this condition.

Some of the best tests for normality are cumulative normal probability plots against the residuals (2,3). Most statistical packages allow such plots to be prepared easily (*Systat, Statgraphics*) with simple plotting commands. *Minitab* allows the calculation of normal scores with the NSCORE command: these are a set of expected points from a normal distribution with a mean of zero and one value for each of the residuals. Plotting the residuals against the normal scores gives the usual cumulative normal probability plot. These plots will be straight lines if the residuals are normally distributed and curved if not. The residuals from the raw mayfly data are clearly not on a straight line (*Figure 4a*) whilst those from the $\log_{10}$ transformed data lie on a much straighter line.

Although the linearity of the probability plot can be assessed by eye, a

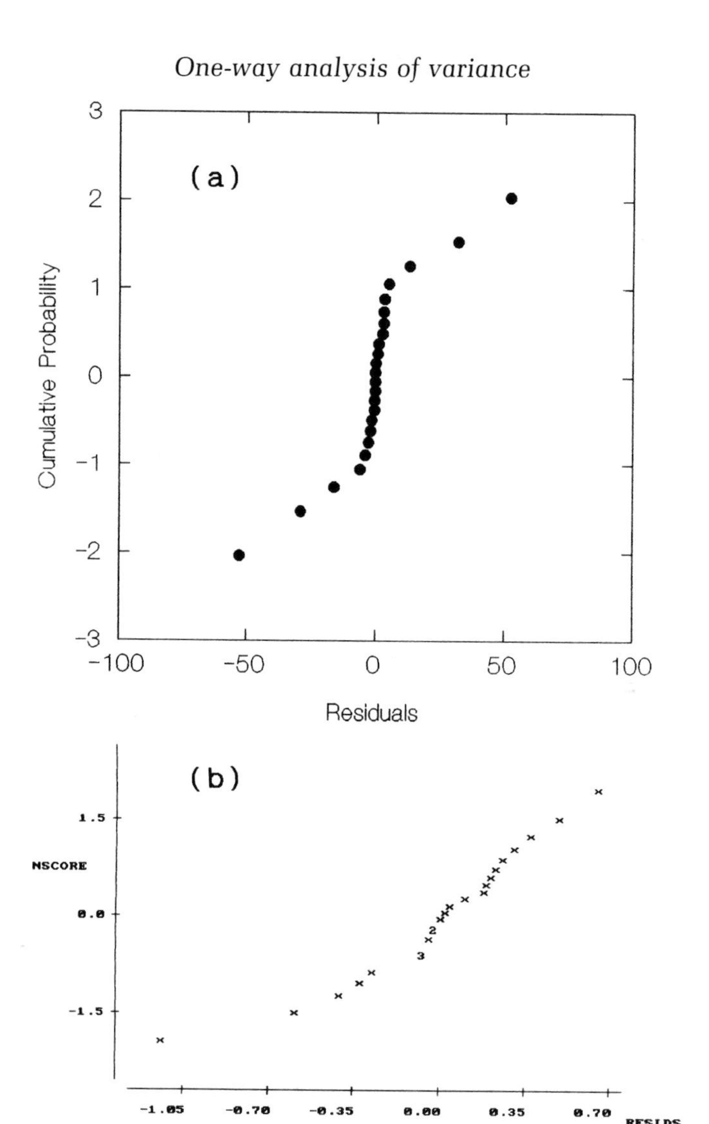

Figure 4. Cumulative normal probability plots of residuals from one-way ANOVA of (a) the raw mayfly data produced by *Systat* and (b) the $\log_{10}(x + 1)$ transformed data produced by *Minitab*.

specific test for linearity is useful. Correlation of the normal scores and residuals gives a coefficient which can be compared with table values (*Appendix B.4*) to see if the hypothesis of normality is acceptable. The correlation coefficients from the raw and $\log_{10}$ transformed mayfly data are 0.871 and 0.952 respectively. The table value for N (total number of data points in the one-way ANOVA = 24) degrees of freedom is 0.956 for 24 degrees of freedom. As a high calculated value indicates normality the raw data are very clearly non-normal, but the $\log_{10}$ data only just fail the test. Failure by such a narrow margin would lead to very few errors in the final stages of the analysis of variance and so would probably be an acceptable deviation from normality. This test is essentially the same as the powerful Shapiro–Wilk test for normality.

Another straightforward graphical way to examine residuals is by using the Box-and-Whiskers plot or boxplot. This is really a graphical representation of a letter value display (see Section 4.3 for more details). It shows (*Figure 5a*) the median (middle data point) and hinges (middle points between the median and maximum and minimum values), adjacent values (the ends of the whiskers), and the more extreme values outside these values (outside and far outside values). Thus residuals that are evenly distributed will show symmetrical boxplots and uneven residuals will give non-symmetrical boxplots. As the normal distribution is even, normally distributed residuals will give an even boxplot with a central median and slightly longer whiskers than the median–hinge distance. Thus the residuals from the raw prolactin data are clearly non-normal (*Figure 5b*; normal score correlation = 0.868), whilst those from the reciprocal root transformed data are acceptably normal (*Figure 5c*; normal score correlation = 0.990). Boxplots are part of a useful, wider group of statistical procedures called exploratory data analysis (6).

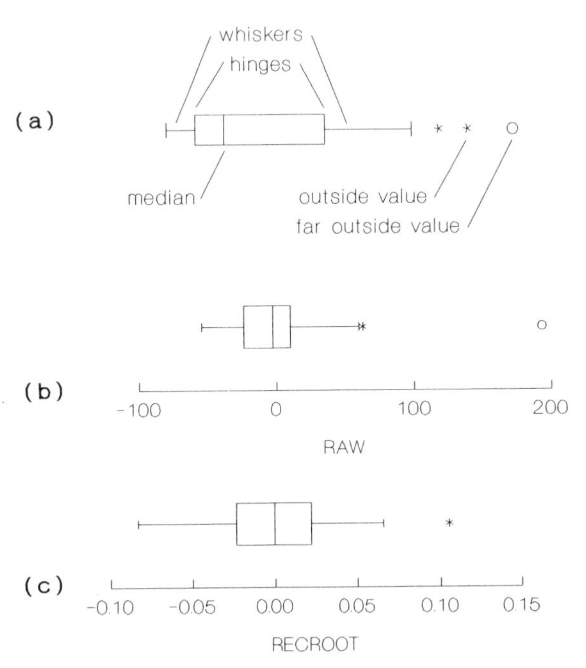

Figure 5. Boxplot of residuals. (a) Diagram of a typical boxplot and boxplots for the residuals from ANOVA on the prolactin data when (b) untransformed and (c) transformed by the reciprocal root. Plots (b) and (c) produced by *Systat*.

4. Transformations

If analysis of the raw data shows that the variances are not homogeneous and the residuals are not normally distributed then none of the results of the one-way ANOVA can be relied upon. The usual action is to search for a suitable transformation which will modify the scale upon which the data are expressed so that the two critical assumptions are valid. Biologists often think that transformation somehow corrupts the original data, but this is not so. It is a perfectly valid procedure and will often make understanding the data easier as well as enabling ANOVA to be carried out. Readers who need convincing should read the excellently argued case for using the logarithmic transformation for population data made by Wiliamson (7). *Protocol 2* gives a summary of how to select an appropriate transformation and is based on the discussion below. After transformation the critical assumptions must be examined again to check that the transformation has worked (*Protocol 1*; Section 3).

Protocol 2. Choosing an appropriate transformation

The approaches outlined in steps 2–5 below are given in order of ease of computation with most computer packages.

1. Select an appropriate method according to the data structure and ease of computation:
- any data: steps 2 and 5
- several groups with small numbers of replicates: steps 2 and 3
- at least one large group: step 4

2. Choose a transformation based on theory; some examples follow:
- population data: $\log_{10} x$ or $\log_{10} (x + 1)$
- low counts in quadrats: $\sqrt{x}$ or $\sqrt{x + 1}$
- percentages or proportions: the arcsine transformation: $\sin^{-1} \sqrt{x/100}$ or $\sin^{-1} \sqrt{x}$

3. Taylor's power law
(a) calculate group means ($\bar{x}$) and variances (s^2) for raw data
(b) plot $\log_{10} s^2$ against $\log_{10}\bar{x}$ for raw data
(c) calculate slope (b) of the regression line from the above plot where

$$\log_{10}s^2 = a + b \log_{10}\bar{x}$$

(d) calculate appropriate power (p) for transformation where

$$p = 1 - \frac{b}{2}$$

(e) use power directly to transform by x^p or choose nearest power transformation from the ladder of powers (*Table 4*)

4. Letter value display method
  (a) transform data according to ladder of powers (*Table 4*)
  (b) compute midsummaries for all transformations
  (c) calculate σ_e from spreads/normal spreads for all transformations
  (d) the best transformation has the most even range of midsummaries and σ_e values

5. Minimization of homogeneity of variance statistics
  (a) transform all data according to ladder of powers (*Table 4*)
  (b) calculate Hartley's F_{max}, Cochran's C, and Bartlett's χ^2 statistics for all transformations
  (c) use transformation giving the minimum value for most statistics

Table 4. The ladder of powers[a]

Power	Transformation: Name	Transformation: Formula	Addition of small number needed for zero values
3	cube	x^3	no
2	square	x^2	no
1	raw data	x	no
0.5	square root	$\sqrt{x}$	no[b]
0	logarithm	$\log_{10}x$	yes
−0.5	reciprocal root	$1/\sqrt{x}$	yes
−1	reciprocal	$1/x$	yes
−2	reciprocal square	$1/x^2$	yes

[a] The table can be extended beyond the extremes by logical extension: based on a table in Velleman and Hoaglin (6)
[b] Not needed, but $\sqrt{x+1}$ or $\sqrt{x+1/2}$ is often used

It is also possible that the critical assumptions might not be valid because of severe outliers within the data. Hence this possibility should be considered whilst the data are being examined (*Protocol 1*; Section 5).

4.1 Choices based on theory or experience

This topic has been carefully considered by Underwood (4) and Elliott (8), and will be briefly covered here. Biologists who regularly analyse their data with correctly applied statistical procedures will soon find the best transformations for the different types of data they generate. Thus the more time-consuming methods of searching for a good transformation will rarely need to be routinely applied.

4.1.1 Logarithmic transformations

As mentioned above, a $\log_{10}$ transformation is often suitable for population data. If the data contain zero values then a small constant number should be added to all data points. This constant should represent the smallest number that could sensibly be found, that is the limit of detection. Thus for the mayfly data a $\log_{10}(x + 1)$ transformation might well be appropriate. Other population-related variables can also be sensibly transformed by logarithms. Enzyme activities of bacteria, primary production in seawater, and grazing rates of zooplankton are all examples of this. Data collected from survival experiments often naturally follow a logarithmic decline and hence can be $\log_{10}$ transformed. In all the above examples I used $\log_{10}$ because this base of logarithms is easy to understand as the number of orders of magnitude: 1 million insects is 10^6, or 6.0 when transformed. However, logarithms to any base can be used and some may prefer $\log_e$. These two forms can be easily interconverted in statistical packages without one or the other transformations as $\log_{10}x$ is equal to $\log_e x$ divided by $\log_e 10$.

4.1.2 Square root transformations

Data collected in quadrats are distributed according to the Poisson distribution. Haemocytometer counts of blood cells, counts of bacteria in petri dishes, and plants in quadrats are examples of this type of data collection. When the counts are low (< 20) the distributions are very skewed and are best transformed by the square root of x or $x + 1$. When counts are high (> 20) the Poisson and normal distributions are so similar that transformation might not be necessary.

4.1.3 The arcsine transformation

This is a special transformation which is used for proportions or percentages and can be applied almost automatically to data of this type. The transformation for proportions is

$$\text{arcsine } x = \sin^{-1}\sqrt{x},$$

and has been designed to make the variances homogeneous. With percentages the values should be converted to proportions by division by 100. It can be looked up in tables (9) but is most conveniently calculated in degrees by computer. Below I give the *Minitab* command for this conversion which assumes the raw data are percentages in column 2 (C2) and the transformed data are to be stored in column 3 (C3).

```
LET C3 = (ASIN(SQRT(C2/100))) * 57.296
```

Other packages make use of similar commands.

4.2 Taylor's power law

This provides a very convenient method for finding the best transformation for a set of data. It works best when there are several groups (≥ 6) and is effective even when the group size is small. The method (*Protocol 2*, step 3) works by calculating the slope (b) of the regression line of the $\log_{10}$ of the group variances upon $\log_{10}$ group means. The power (p) for the tansformation (x^p) is then calculated by $p = 1 - b/2$. For the resulting power transformation to be effective the plot of $\log_{10}s^2$ versus $\log_{10}\bar{x}$ should be linear, that is, all the points should lie close to a straight line. The slope from this regression of the mayfly data is 1.56; hence the power suggested is $1 - 1.56/2 = 0.22$, and this would seem reliable as the points on the corresponding graph are close to a straight line (*Figure 6a*). Thus the transformation suggested is $x^{0.22}$. A similar plot from the prolactin data (*Figure 6b*; $p = -0.54$) shows the problem with too few groups because the slope of the regression line will be too reliant on the group with the lowest variance and mean.

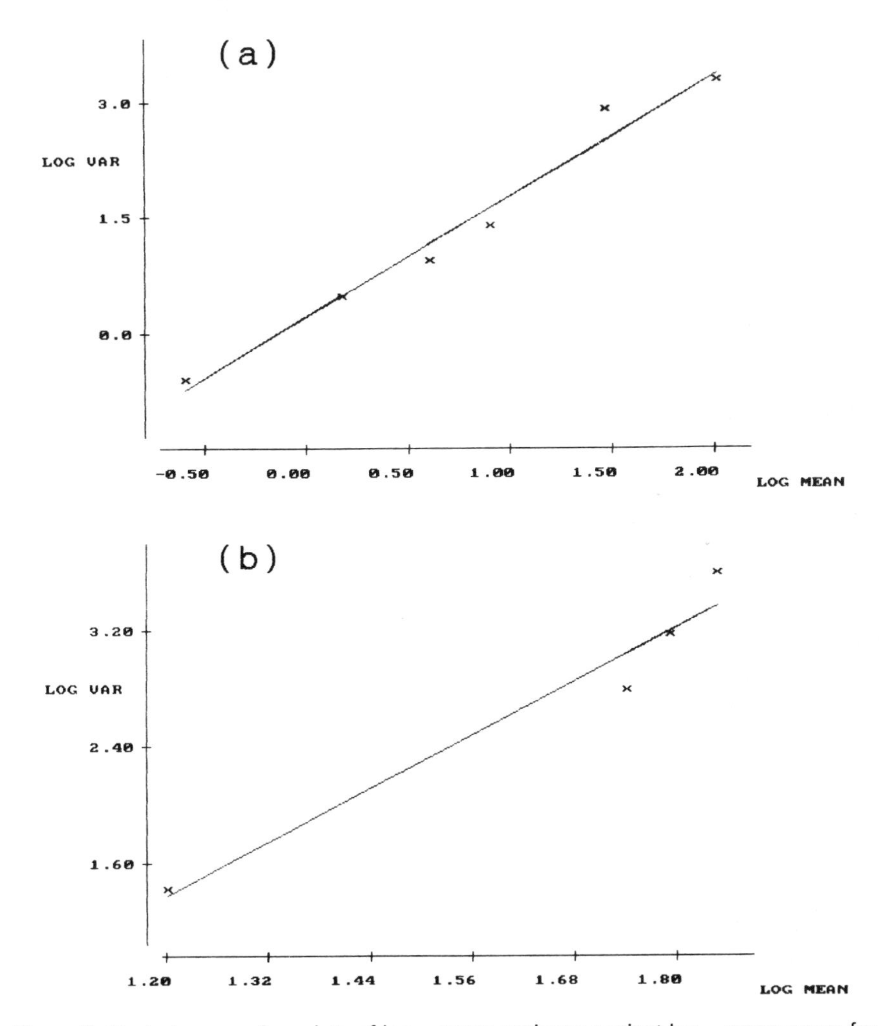

Figure 6. Taylor's power law plots of $\log_{10}$ group variance against $\log_{10}$ group mean for (a) the mayfly and (b) prolactin data; plots produced by *Minitab*.

The power transformations indicated by the Taylor's power law method will be slightly different for each new set of data collected, and so do not provide continuity of statistical analysis within a research programme. It would be better to use the calculated power as an indication of the best transformation to use. The ladder of powers (6) provides a logical way of doing this. It puts the raw data and a range of equivalent transformations into a logical sequence (*Table 4*) from which a suitable transformation can be selected from the power suggested from Taylor's power law. Thus, with $x^{-0.54}$ from the prolactin data a reciprocal root transformation is indicated. The power from the mayfly data was 0.22, which is midway between the $\log_{10}$ and the square root transformation. This uncertainty is perhaps to be expected, because the mayfly counts are essentially population data collected from quadrats with many low counts (see Section 4.1).

4.3 Letter value displays

This is another technique of exploratory data analysis, which is fully described by Velleman and Hoaglin (6), and *Minitab* allows calculation of the associated statistics. *Figure 7* gives a diagrammatic representation of how the letter

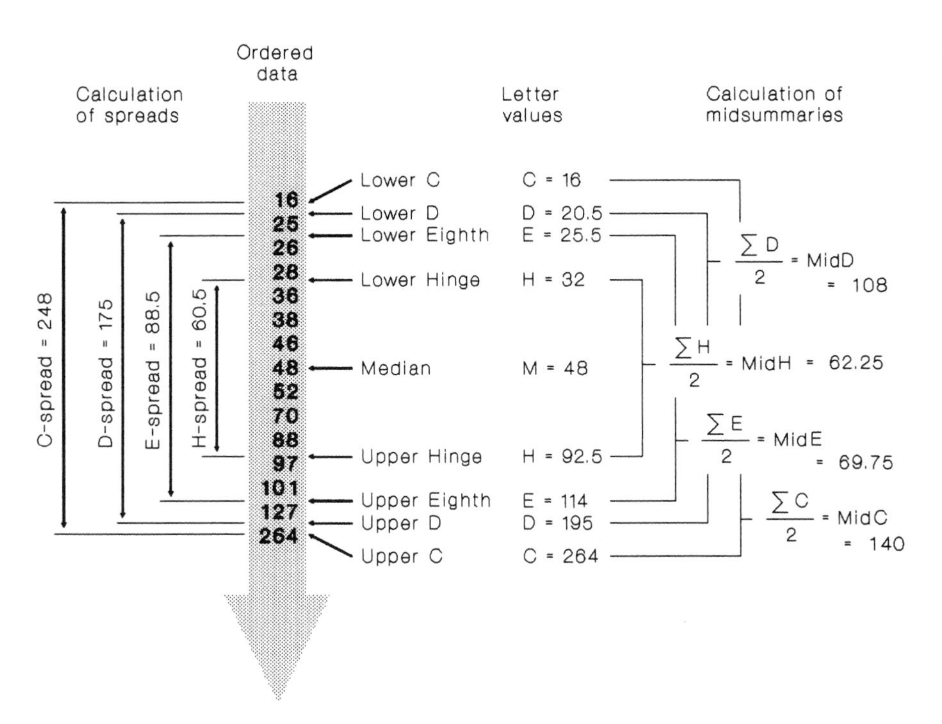

Figure 7. Diagram illustrating how letter values are assigned and how midsummaries and spreads are calculated. The data used is the largest group ($n = 15$) from the prolactin data set.

values are assigned and the midsummaries and spreads calculated. Briefly, the calculations are done as follows. When the data are ordered, the median is the middle data point and is assigned the letter value M. The two middle data points between the median and the lowest and highest values are called hinges and assigned H. This principle continues through eighths (E) and letter values D,C,B,A,Z, etc. which do not have names. When there is not a single central value the central two data points are averaged to calculate the number required (see *Figure 7*). The midsummaries are then calculated from averages of the pairs of letter values; hence, for example, mid H = (upper H + lower H)/2. For a perfectly symmetrical distribution these midsummaries will all be equal, but for a distribution skewed to the left they will increase and will decrease for one skewed right. Spreads are calculated as the differences between the letter values and so are the magnitudes of ranges between the letter values. Hence for a normal distribution they will be entirely predictable. The values of the spreads from a standard normal distribution (mean = 0, standard deviation = 1) are called normal spreads and are given in *Table 5*. Thus the relationship between a normal distribution and the data being analysed can be examined from the ratios of the calculated spreads and the normal spreads. This ratio is an estimate of the standard deviation of the data (σ_e), so

$$\sigma_e = \frac{\text{spread}}{\text{normal spread}},$$

and will be constant if the distribution of the data is close to normal. As with the midsummaries, the normal spreads will increase or decrease for skewed distributions.

These ideas have been used to make a test to select the best transformation for a set of data (6). This test should be done on data from a single group in the one-way ANOVA and only works well for data sets with at least one large

Table 5. Spreads for letter values from a standard normal distribution[a]

Letter value	Normal spread
H	1.349
E	2.301
D	3.068
C	3.726
B	4.308
A	4.836
Z	5.320

[a] Reproduced with permission from (6)

group (> *c.* 12). The test is done by transforming the data from the largest group by all the transformations in the ladder of powers (*Table 4*), taking care to add an appropriate constant (perhaps 1 or 0.5) to all the values if zeros are present. The midsummaries and σ_e values are then calculated and the best transformation is the one in which these values remain constant and do not increase or decrease in a regular manner. I provide a *Minitab* macro (LADDER.MTB; *Appendix 1.4*) to calculate the midsummaries and σ_e values and part of the output from this macro for the largest group in the prolactin data (n = 15) is in *Figure 8*. This shows that the midsummaries for the cube through to square root transformations clearly increase, whilst those

```
(2) RESULTS FOR CHOOSING BEST TRANSFORMATION

*************LADDER OF POWERS*************************************
TRANS. = CUBE  SQUARE  RAW  ROOT  LOG  REC.ROOT  RECIP  REC.SQ
POWER  =  +3      +2    +1   +.5   0      -.5      -1      -2


************MIDSUMMARIES OF TRANSFORMATIONS***********************
---------LOOK FOR MOST EVEN VALUES DOWN COLUMNS FOR MOST
                SYMETRICAL TRANSFORMATION-------------------------

 ROW     CUBE..  SQUARE..     RAW..     ROOT..       LOG..    REC.RT..       RECIP..     REC.SQ..

   1     110592    2304.0     48.00     6.9282   1.68124   -0.144338   -0.0208333   -0.0004340
   2     415688    4808.3     62.25     7.6303   1.73368   -0.140946   -0.0212912   -0.0005706
   3     777971    6907.7     69.75     7.8546   1.73026   -0.146089   -0.0240591   -0.0008098
   4    5116962   21676.5    108.00     9.1294   1.78187   -0.150070   -0.0285405   -0.0013956
   5    9201920   34976.0    140.00    10.1240   1.81286   -0.155773   -0.0331439   -0.0019603


***********SIGMAS FOR TRANSFORMATIONS*****************************
--------LOOK FOR THE MOST EVEN VALUES FOR THE TRANSFORMATION
            THAT MOST CLOSELY FITS THE NORMAL DISTRIBUTION---------

 ROW     CUBE..  SQUARE..      RAW..     ROOT..       LOG..     REC.RT..      RECIP..     REC.SQ..

   1     565433    5586.7    44.8480    2.94225    0.343882    0.0546753    0.0155001    0.0006715
   2     661774    5438.7    38.4615    2.43813    0.281445    0.0451710    0.0131870    0.0006343
   3    3329271   13843.5    57.0404    3.01785    0.313453    0.0488459    0.0148041    0.0008849
   4    4937103   18636.6    66.5593    3.28719    0.326754    0.0505782    0.0157574    0.0010445
```

Figure 8. Part of the output from the *Minitab* macro LADDER.MTB (*Appendix 1.4*) which calculates midsummaries and σ_e values for transformed and raw data used to select an optimal transformation from a single large group. The largest group (n = 15) from the prolactin data was used as input for the macro.

for the reciprocal and reciprocal square decrease. All but one of the midsummaries from the $\log_{10}$ transformed data increase slightly and those for the reciprocal root are almost constant. Thus the reciprocal root is indicated as the best transformation. The σ_e values follow a similar trend, but give a less precise indication of the best transformation.

Although this approach to selecting a transformation might not appear very precise, it works remarkably well. Readers will note that the power transformation suggested here, $x^{-0.5}$ (*Table 4*), is very close to that calculated from Taylor's power law of $x^{-0.54}$ (Section 4.2).

4.4 Minimization of homogeneity of variance statistics

The three statistics used to check data for homogeneity of variance (Bartlett's χ^2, F_{max}, C) can also in principle be used to select a good transformation. This can be done by calculating these statistics for data transformed according to the ladder of powers. This has been done for the mayfly and prolactin data (*Table 3*). By comparing the critical values from tables at $P = 0.05$ with the calculated values for the different transformations a suitable transformation can be chosen. For the mayfly data Bartlett's χ^2 and F_{max} both reach acceptable minima at the logarithmic transformation, but C is below the critical value for all three types of reciprocal transformation. With the prolactin data the reciprocal root is fully acceptable for all the test statistics. Additionally Bartlett's χ^2 indicates that $\log_{10}x$ and $1/x$ are acceptable and C suggests $1/x$ is satisfactory. Clearly, with different data sets these tests are likely to have different discriminatory powers. Once again the overall conclusion is that $\log_{10}x$ works best for the mayfly data and $1/\sqrt{x}$ is optimal for the prolactin results.

4.5 Conclusions about selecting transformations

Although the best transformation could not have been selected for the prolactin data before the analysis, all the methods of choosing a good transformation for both sets of data used here support each other. There is no need to use all the methods suggested here to choose a transformation for unfamiliar data sets. It is best to select one of these methods and to base the choice on the arrangement of the data and the ease with which the computations can be done with the computer package being used. A guide for selection is given in step 1 of *Protocol 2*.

5. Tests for outliers

Sometimes data sets might contain one or more very extreme values that may not really be part of the same data. Such values are outliers and can occur for a variety of reasons, such as transcription or experimental errors. Outliers can sometimes be seen when residuals are being tested for normality (3). For example, the probability plot of the $\log_{10}$ mayfly residuals (*Figure 4b*) shows one value with the lowest residual that might be an outlier. Inspection of a table of residuals shows that the suspect point from the mayfly data is the zero value at site 2. This is the seventh point (*Appendix 1.1*), and can also be detected easily by plotting the residuals against the order of the data. *Minitab* has a time series plot for this purpose and this confirms (*Figure 9*) that the seventh point is suspect. Similarly, the boxplot of the reciprocal root prolactin residuals (*Figure 5c*) also throws suspicion on the point with the highest residual. In this case the 23rd point is the one of interest, which is the value of 16 in the third and largest group (*Appendix 1.2*).

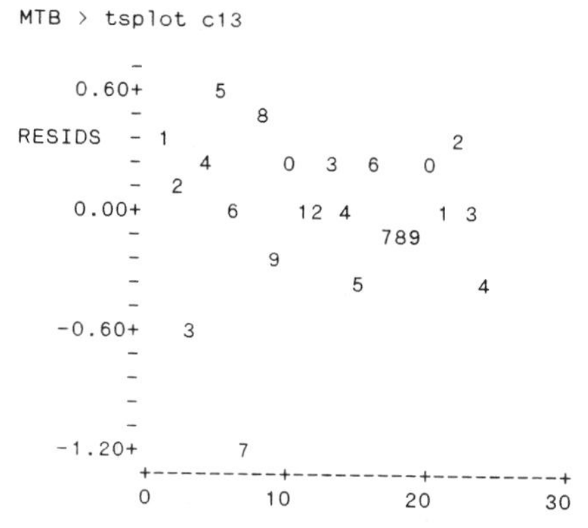

Figure 9. Time series plot of the residuals from a one-way ANOVA of the $\log_{10}(x + 1)$ transformed mayfly data; plot produced by *Minitab*.

The most useful test for the significance of outliers is Dixon's test, which is designed for small group sizes ($n < 25$) and will be described here. However, Grubb's test (see (2), p. 413) is available for data sets with large group sizes ($n > 25$). To test the possible outlier in the mayfly data from site 2 the $\log_{10}(x+1)$ transformed values must be used because Dixon's test only works with normally distributed data. *Appendix B.5* must be consulted to find the correct formula for a group size of $n = 4$ which is

$$r_{10} = \frac{x_2 - x_1}{x_n - x_1}.$$

The data in the group with the suspect point are then ordered and values corresponding to x_1, x_2, and x_n determined. The outlier of interest is assigned x_1, whether it is the smallest or largest value, and the rest of the order maintained accordingly. Hence, for these data

x	$x + 1$	$\log_{10}(x + 1)$	
0	1	0.00	x_1
13	14	1.15	x_2
42	43	1.63	x_3
61	62	1.79	x_4

so

$$r_{10} = \frac{x_2 - x_1}{x_4 - x_1} = \frac{1.15 - 0}{1.79 - 0} = 0.642.$$

Consulting the table of critical values (*Appendix B.5*) at $n = 4$ shows that r_{10} is smaller than the table values at all three probabilities quoted, so the outlier is not significantly ($P > 0.1$) lower than the other values in the group. Similar calculations on the suspect point in the largest group ($n = 15$) of the reciprocal root transformed prolactin data show $r_{22} = 0.358$ (see *Appendix B.5* for formula), which again is not significant ($P > 0.1$). Thus neither of these values should be considered for exclusion from the analysis. If an outlier is significant it should not automatically be excluded from the data set. Firstly, field and/or laboratory notebooks should be consulted to see whether the data point is correct or whether there is a good scientific reason for exclusion.

6. Comparisons of means

The result of the basic one-way ANOVA only says whether or not there are any significant differences between the means of the groups in the data set. It does not tell which means are different from each other, and a highly significant ANOVA might contain only a few large differences. Thus we need tests to compare means after the basic analysis is complete. Note that all these tests must be carried out on the data transformed in the most appropriate way to ensure that the assumptions are upheld. There are a great number of such tests described in the literature and particularly good explanations will be found in the books by Winer (1) and Sokal and Rohlf (2). This is an area of active mathematical research and it is hard to decide which tests are the best to use. The excellent review of Day and Quinn (5) has carried out comparisons between the efficacy of these tests and it is basically their recommendations I follow.

These tests are divided into two types:

- *a priori* tests or planned comparisons
- *a posteriori* tests or unplanned comparisons.

Both types of test can be divided into two further divisions:

- tests for comparing pairs of means
- tests for comparing groups of means

The latter division includes tests for comparing single means or groups of means with one or more other groups of means or single means. The *a priori* versions of these tests are sometimes called contrasts. This division also includes tests for similarity between means as opposed to differences between means. Readers requiring tests of similarity or between complex groups of means should consult other books (2). I will provide one example of each type of test which should provide an effective suite of tests for most purposes. For pairwise comparisons I use the version of the tests that work for both equal and unequal sample sizes.

These tests are very patchily represented in computer packages. *Minitab* does not have any commands for these tests in release 7.1. *SPSS/PC+*, *Systat*, and *Statgraphics* have several tests of this type. All three of these packages currently allow computation of the pairwise comparisons I describe and *SPSS/PC+* and *Systat* allow *a priori* contrasts to be performed as well.

6.1 *A priori* tests

These tests can only be done for groups which could sensibly have been tested before the experiment was done. Thus for the mayfly data set the researcher could sensibly have planned to compare the sites immediately above and below the tributary sites 3 and 4; (see *Table 6* and Section 1.1. for site details)

Table 6. Group means and sums for the $\log_{10}(x + 1)$ transformed mayfly data ($n = 4$) with notes on site details given in Section 1.1

Site	Group mean	Group sum	Site details
1	0.595	2.380	← most rocky site
2	1.143	4.571	
3	1.983	7.933	
4	0.887	3.547	← tributary enters
5	0.075	0.301	
6	0.325	1.301	

and so these are candidates for an *a priori* pairwise comparison. Similarly, the rocky above tributary station (site 1) could be compared *a priori* with the other two less rocky sites above the tributary (sites 2 and 3). These tests are more powerful at detecting differences than the *a posteriori* tests, and so stringent rules must be followed. These rules are

- tests can be applied regardless of significance of basic ANOVA
- the maximum number of comparisons allowed is $a - 1$ (where a = total number of groups in the ANOVA)

Because these tests are so powerful they should be used in preference to *a posteriori* tests wherever validly possible.

6.1.1 Least significant difference (LSD)

This pairwise comparison is valid only as an *a priori* test, despite being linked with *a posteriori* tests in the *SPSS/PC+* command structure. The LSD is the smallest difference between two means that is significant; one value is calculated for all the comparisons to be made. Calculation of LSD is straightforward:

$$\text{LSD} = t_{P(\text{df}_{\text{error}})} \sqrt{\left[\frac{1}{n_i} + \frac{1}{n_j}\right] \text{MS}_{\text{error}}},$$

where the two-tailed t-statistic (t; *Appendix B.6*) is quoted at a probability P and for within groups degrees of freedom (df_{error}) from the one-way ANOVA table (see *Figure 2* for the mayfly data); n_i and n_j are the number of replicates in the largest and smallest groups. So for the mayfly data at $P = 0.05$:

$$LSD = 2.101 \sqrt{\left[\frac{1}{4} + \frac{1}{4}\right] 0.176} = 0.623,$$

where 0.176 is the MS_{error} from the $\log_{10}(x + 1)$ transformed data (*Figure 2b*). As the difference between the group means (*Table 6*) at the sites above and below the tributary is 1.096 there is a significant difference between them.

6.1.2 Orthogonal decomposition

These tests are to allow comparisons among groups of group means. The method essentially performs a new one-way ANOVA on a restructured set of data. A test sum of squares (SS_{test}) is calculated according to the following type of formula;

$$SS_{test} = \left[\underset{\text{term 1}}{\frac{(g_1 + g_2 + \ldots)^2}{n_1 + n_2 + \ldots}} + \underset{\text{term 2}}{\frac{(g_3 + g_4 + \ldots)^2}{n_3 + n_4 \ldots}}\right] - \frac{(g_1 + g_2 + g_3 + g_4 + \ldots)^2}{n_1 + n_2 + n_3 + n_4 + \ldots},$$

where g_1 to g_4 are the sums of the values in the four groups used in this test and n_1 to n_4 are all the numbers of replicates in the corresponding groups. This formula can be extended (indicated by dots) or contracted to test more or fewer group means in each of the terms, or by adding more terms. A test mean square (MS_{test}) and F (F_{test}) are then calculated:

$$MS_{test} = \frac{SS_{test}}{df_{test}} \qquad F_{test} = \frac{MS_{test}}{MS_{error}},$$

where df_{test} is one less than the number of terms used to calculate SS_{test}. F_{test} is then compared with a table value ($F_{P(df_{test},\, df_{error})}$; *Appendix B.1*) and if $F_{test} > F_{table}$ the result is significant.

Thus to compare the mayfly data at site 1 with those at sites 2 and 3 (group sums, g, in *Table 6*; MS_{error} in *Figure 2b*) the calculations are

$$SS_{test} = \frac{(2.380)^2}{4} + \frac{(4.571 + 7.933)^2}{4 + 4} - \frac{(2.380 + 4.571 + 7.933)^2}{4 + 4 + 4}$$

$$= \frac{(2.380)^2}{4} + \frac{(12.504)^2}{8} - \frac{(14.884)^2}{12}$$

$$= 2.499,$$

$$MS_{test} = \frac{2.499}{1} = 2.499,$$

and

$$F_{test} = \frac{2.499}{0.176} = 14.197.$$

From the table in *Appendix B.1*, $F_{P(1,18)}$ is

4.41 for $P = 0.05$,
8.28 for $P = 0.01$, and
15.4 for $P = 0.001$.

Hence there is a significant difference in mayfly numbers due to rockiness above the tributary at the $P = 0.01$ level but not at the $P = 0.001$ level.

Particularly with larger data sets, these calculations can be tedious and can easily be done by computer by re-labelling the groups appropriately. *Table 7* shows how this is done for the above example (column 'rocky') and for a comparison of all the three sites below the tributary (column 'below'). Performing a one-way ANOVA using either of these new sets of subscripts will show the SS_{test} in the normal SS_{groups} position. The F_{test}, however, must be calculated with the MS_{error} from the entire original one-way ANOVA table. By this method the SS_{test} below the tributaries is 1.382 and so $MS_{test} = 1.382/2 = 0.691$ and hence $F_{test} = 0.691/0.176 = 3.926$. In this test df_{test} is 2 because there were three terms compared and can be found as df_{groups} in the modified ANOVA table used to calculate SS_{test}. As $F_{0.05(2,18)}$ is 3.55 there is just a significant difference between these means.

We have now done four means comparisons by *a priori* tests (above and below tributary = 1; 'rocky' = 1; 'below' = 2; total = 4) and we are very close to the upper limit of 5 $(a - 1)$, so it would be unwise to search artificially for a fifth *a priori* comparison.

6.2 *A posteriori* tests

These tests are less stringent than the *a priori* tests, but allow us to look for means and groups of means which appear to be different in the data after they have been collected. This feature makes them very powerful and they can be used extensively. The basic rules for most *a posteriori* tests are as follows:

- the initial ANOVA on all the data must be significant before these tests are attempted
- large numbers of comparisons are allowed, always more than $\{a(a - 1)\}/2$

The limit set above is a lower limit and essentially allows all possible pairs to be compared. As we are rarely interested in absolutely all pairwise comparisons, there are essentially comparisons available for some groups of means to be compared also.

6.2.1 Tukey–Kramer method

The best *a posteriori* pairwise comparison is the Kramer modification of the

Table 7. The method of labelling groups[a] for calculating sums of squares by computer for *a priori* orthogonal decomposition and the *a posteriori* SS-STP test used to compare multiple groups of means. The $\log_{10}(x + 1)$ transformed mayfly data are used

log10	Sites	Rocky	Below	Lowest
0.903	1	1	*	*
0.699	1	1	*	*
0.000	1	1	*	*
0.778	1	1	*	*
1.792	2	2	*	*
1.146	2	2	*	*
0.000	2	2	*	*
1.633	2	2	*	*
1.707	3	2	*	*
2.193	3	2	*	*
2.029	3	2	*	*
2.003	3	2	*	*
1.079	4	*	1	1
0.845	4	*	1	1
0.477	4	*	1	1
1.146	4	*	1	1
0.000	5	*	2	2
0.000	5	*	2	2
0.000	5	*	2	2
0.301	5	*	2	2
0.301	6	*	3	1
0.699	6	*	3	1
0.301	6	*	3	1
0.000	6	*	3	1

[a]The labels in the column headed 'rocky' compare means at site 1 with those at sites 2 and 3. Those in column headed 'below' compare the means at sites 4, 5, and 6. Those in the column headed 'lowest' compare site 5 with sites 4 and 6. The data are in the column headed 'log10' and the labels used for the entire one-way ANOVA are in the column headed 'sites'. Missing values are labelled with an asterisk

Tukey method (5). With this test, a minimum significant difference (MSD) is calculated which is analogous to the LSD described previously.

$$\text{MSD} = Q_{P(a,\text{df}_{\text{error}})} \sqrt{\frac{\text{MS}_{\text{error}}\{(1/n_i) + (1/n_j)\}}{2}},$$

where Q is the studentized range statistic (*Appendix B.7*) and so for the mayfly data $Q_{0.05(6,18)}$ is 4.495. Hence

$$\text{MSD} = 4.495\sqrt{\frac{0.176\{(1/4) + (1/4)\}}{2}} = 0.943,$$

and so none of the group means (*Table 6*) below the tributary are different from each other. We can also use this statistic to investigate the mayfly numbers above the tributary in more detail. It is clear that site 1 is the only individual significantly different from site 3 and not from site 2. This does not invalidate our previous *a priori* conclusion because it is perfectly possible for *a priori* and *a posteriori* tests to give conflicting results, because they have markedly different powers.

6.2.2 Sum of squares, simultaneous test procedure (SS-STP)

This is a very powerful *a posteriori* test (2) for comparing groups of means. An SS_{test} is calculated longhand or by computer in an identical manner to that previously described for orthogonal decomposition (Section 6.1.2). The SS_{test} is then compared with a critical value (SS_{crit}) calculated as follows:

$$SS_{crit} = (a - 1) \times MS_{error} \times F_{P(a-1, df_{error})}.$$

If $SS_{test} > SS_{crit}$ then the comparison being made is significant. Thus for the mayfly data at $P = 0.05$:

$$SS_{crit} = 5 \times 0.176 \times 2.77 = 2.438.$$

This statistic can be used to investigate groups of means further in the mayfly data. For example the SS_{test} calculated from the column headed 'lowest' in *Table 7* would compare the group with the lowest group mean (site 5) below the tributary with the other two below tributary sites (4 and 6). In this case SS_{test} is 0.751 and so the difference is not significant. However, using the same principles a test between sites 1–4 and sites 5 and 6 is significant ($SS_{test} = 4.831$).

6.3 Computer output for pairwise comparisons

Several statistical computer packages give tables as part of the output for one-way ANOVA which indicate results for pairwise means comparisons. This output can take several forms. *Systat* gives two matrices to indicate differences: one contains absolute mean differences and the other probabilities for the differences being significant and both are organized in an $a \times a$ triangular matrix (*Figure 10*). *SPSS/PC+* gives either a similar type of matrix, but with significant differences, marked with an asterisk and/or a table of homogeneous subsets, which is a list of groups which do not have mean values that are significantly different. *Statgraphics* indicates homogeneous subjects by labelling the groups in a list with a system of asterisks.

7. What to do if the assumptions do not hold true

In almost all cases the above procedures will find a transformation, if one is required, that ensures that the assumptions of ANOVA are upheld. However, occasionally data will be collected that cannot be made to fit the assumptions

```
MATRIX OF PAIRWISE ABSOLUTE MEAN DIFFERENCES

              1         2         3         4         5         6

    1       0.000
    2       0.548     0.000
    3       1.388     0.840     0.000
    4       0.292     0.256     1.097     0.000
    5       0.520     1.068     1.908     0.811     0.000
    6       0.270     0.818     1.658     0.562     0.250     0.000


TUKEY HSD MULTIPLE COMPARISONS
MATRIX OF PAIRWISE COMPARISON PROBABILITIES

              1         2         3         4         5         6

    1       1.000
    2       0.464     1.000
    3       0.002     0.097     1.000
    4       0.918     0.951     0.018     1.000
    5       0.519     0.022     0.000     0.117     1.000
    6       0.939     0.112     0.000     0.438     0.955     1.000
-------------------------------------------------------------------------------
```

Figure 10. Part of the *Systat* computer output from a one-way ANOVA of the $\log_{10}(x + 1)$ mayfly data giving results of pairwise group comparisons for sites 1–6 by the Tukey–Kramer method.

by transformation. A summary of what to do under these circumstances is provided in *Protocol 3* which has been referred to earlier (*Protocol 1*).

Protocol 3. What to do if ANOVA assumptions do not hold

1. If ANOVA shows no significant differences with the best transformation, accept the result.
2. If ANOVA shows large differences ($P < 0.001$) and assumptions are only slightly violated, continue with ANOVA but use a more stringent probability level to detect differences (e.g. $P \leqslant 0.01$). Check results with non-parametric tests (see steps 3 and 4).
3. Use a non-parametric test that is equivalent to one-way ANOVA to detect a significant overall ANOVA:
   - Kruskal–Wallis
   - Mood median
4. Use non-parametric tests to compare pairs of means:
   - notched boxplots of grouped data
   - multiple Mann–Whitney tests
5. Consider using parametric tests to compare pairs of means when variances are unequal:
   - Games and Howell procedure
   - T3 method

7.1 Robustness of one-way ANOVA

One-way ANOVA is a fairly robust procedure and so small deviations from homogeneity of variances (which is the most important assumption) rarely give large errors. This is particularly true if the basic ANOVA is highly significant and the group sizes are equal. However, it is wise to confirm the results obtained with the best transformation which can be obtained with the results obtained by the non-parametric procedures described below.

7.2 Non-parametric tests equivalent to one-way ANOVA

There are two tests which are widely available, and both determine whether the group medians are significantly different. Both tests work best with fairly large numbers of observations in each group ($n \geqslant 6$), but the major statistical packages normally give results for smaller n and print warnings. Both tests perform calculations on the ranks of the numbers in the data and so depend on the order of the data not the value. For this reason transformation is normally not needed. Data are usually submitted as a data column and a labelling column, as described for one-way ANOVA.

The Kruskal–Wallis test is the most commonly used procedure of this type. The result for the mayfly data is $P = 0.009$ and so is similar to the parametric one-way ANOVA. The Mood median test is at present only available in *Minitab* and gives a more conservative result for the mayfly data ($P = 0.016$). However, this test also allows calculation of confidence intervals which can be used to make an initial assessment of the differences between means. These intervals are value sensitive and so should be done on the best data transformation. Some example output from these two tests is provided in *Figure 11*.

7.3 Comparisons of means

7.3.1 Non-parametric tests

I have found the most useful non-parametric test of this type to be the notched boxplot (6), which is yet another exploratory data analysis technique. The 'notches' are confidence intervals provided as extra information to a standard boxplot of all the groups placed side by side. If the notches of two groups do not overlap then the group medians are significantly different. This test is value-sensitive and so the best transformation should be used. Notched boxplots are produced by *Minitab*, *Statgraphics*, and *Systat*. The former two packages print the notches in the boxplots as brackets whilst *Systat* uses spikes to indicate the notches when they lie outside the hinges (*Figure 12*). Comparison of the results from the notched boxplot in *Figure 12* with the matrix of *a posteriori* comparisons (*Figure 10*) for the $\log_{10}$ mayfly data show that the results are very similar.

(a)

Kruskal-Wallis analysis of raw by sites

Level	Sample Size	Average Rank
1	4	10.7500
2	4	15.2500
3	4	22.2500
4	4	14.3750
5	4	4.62500
6	4	7.75000

Test statistic = 15.7839 Significance level = 7.48902E-3

(b)

```
MTB > mood c4 c2

Mood median test of LOG10

Chisquare = 14.00    df = 5    p = 0.016

                                          Individual 95.0% CI's
 SITES   N<=    N>   Median     Q3-Q1  +---------+---------+---------+------
     1     2     2     0.74      0.70  (-----------+--)
     2     1     3     1.39      1.47  (----------------------+------)
     3     0     4     2.02      0.37                            (-----+--)
     4     1     3     0.96      0.56         (-------+--)
     5     4     0     0.00      0.23  +----)
     6     4     0     0.30      0.52  (----+------)
                                       +---------+---------+---------+------
                                     0.00      0.60      1.20      1.80
Overall median = 0.74
* NOTE * Levels with < 6 obs. have confidence < 95.0%
```

Figure 11. Computer output giving the results of the (a) Kruskal–Wallis (raw data; *Statgraphics*) and (b) Mood median test ($\log_{10}(x + 1)$ data; *Minitab*) on the mayfly results.

7.3.2 Parametric tests

Some authorities have recommended (2,5) that specially designed parametric tests should be used when variances are not homogeneous. Two of the best tests of this type are the Games and Howell procedure and the T3-test. However, computation is in both cases difficult as a separate estimate of the variance and the degrees of freedom must be calculated for each comparison made. For this reason computers are almost essential for these tests. Unfortunately they are not provided as standard features in the major statistical packages I have used. There is a suite of programs (*BIOM*) written in Fortran to accompany the book by Sokal and Rohlf (2) which is available free from W. H. Freeman. This contains a program which performs the Games and Howell procedure (*MCHETV*). Although using this program is probably the best approach for those wishing to undertake the best possible test on data with heterogeneous variances, the notched boxplot will probably be more cost effective in time.

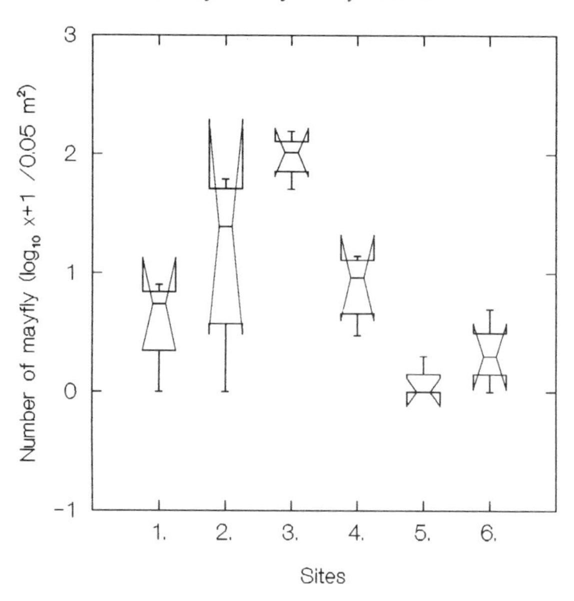

Figure 12. Notched boxplot of the $\log_{10}(x + 1)$ mayfly data produced by *Systat*. The notches are either at the hinges or are the spikes which extend beyond the hinges either side of the 'waisted' median.

References

1. Winer, B. J. (1971). *Statistical principles in experimental design*. McGraw-Hill, New York.
2. Sokal, R. R. and Rohlf, F. J. (1981). *Biometry*. W. H. Freeman, San Francisco.
3. Miller, R. G. (1986). *Beyond ANOVA: basics of applied statistics*. John Wiley, New York.
4. Underwood, A. J. (1981). *Oceanogr. Mar. Biol. Annu. Rev.*, **19**, 513.
5. Day, R. W. and Quinn, G. P. (1989). *Ecol. Monogr.*, **59**, 433.
6. Velleman, P. F. and Hoaglin, D. C. (1981). *Applications, basics, and computing of exploratory data analysis*. Duxberry Press, Boston.
7. Williamson, M. (1972). *The analysis of biological populations*. Edward Arnold, London.
8. Elliott, J. M. (1977). *Some methods for the statistical analysis of samples of benthic invertebrates*. Freshwater Biological Association, Ambleside.
9. Rohlf, F. J. and Sokal, R. R. (1981). *Statistical tables*. W. H. Freeman, New York.

Appendix 1.1. Contents of file MAYFLY.DAT[a]

RAW	SITES
7	1
4	1
0	1
5	1
61	2
13	2
0	2
42	2
50	3
155	3
106	3
100	3
11	4
6	4
2	4
13	4
0	5
0	5
0	5
1	5
1	6
4	6
1	6
0	6

[a] The file is organized as 25 rows, the top row contains variable labels for the data (RAW: number of mayfly 0.05 m^{-2}) and a labelling variable SITES: 1–6) for the six sites sampled. The top row may have to be removed before the file can be read into some packages. Data provided by Dr. M. A. Learner

Appendix 1.2. Contents of file PROLACT.DAT[a]

Prolact	Expt
14.5	1
11.1	1
15.0	1
14.3	1
24.7	1
52.7	2
44.4	2
125.0	2
66.0	2
23.3	2
36.0	3
28.0	3
97.0	3
26.0	3
38.0	3
25.0	3
70.0	3
127.0	3
264.0	3
48.0	3
88.0	3
101.0	3
16.0	3
46.0	3
52.0	3
31.0	4
69.0	4
115.0	4
53.0	4
52.0	4
53.0	4
66.0	4
44.0	4
31.0	4
37.0	4

[a] The file is organized as 36 rows, the top row contains variable labels for the data (Prolact: prolactin concentration, units g^{-1}) and a labelling variable (Expt: labelled as four groups, 1–4). The top row may have to be removed before the data can be read into some packages. Data provided by Dr. T. Wigham

Appendix 1.3. Listings of a set of *Minitab* macros (BART.MTB, BART1.MTB, BART2.MTB, BART3.MTB, BART4.MTB) for calculating Bartlett's χ^2, Hartley's F_{max}, and Cochran's C tests for homogeneity of variance

To run these macros only BART.MTB needs to be called. All the files must be present in the directory being used by *Minitab*. The raw data must be in C91 and the group labels in C92. The macro stores values for n, df, $\bar{x}$, s, s^2, $\log_e s^2$ for each group in C93–C98, in numerical order according to the magnitude of the group labels. Constants K90–K100 are also used by the macro. The macros have been constructed for *Minitab* release 7.1 and might need modification for other releases.

```
# BART.MTB (needs BART1.MTB, BART2.MTB,
                                BART3.MTB and BART4.MTB)
# Set of Minitab macros (for version 7.1) to test for
# homogeneity of variances by Bartlett's, Hartley's, and
# Cochran's tests. Written by J.M. Getliff 1990 and
# modified by J.C. Fry 1991
#
# Data in C91 groups in C92
# *******************************************************************
# *                                                                 *
# *   DO NOT USE ANY GROUPS WITH ONLY ONE DATA POINT                *
# *                                                                 *
# *******************************************************************
# c91-c98 and k90-k100 are used
# c95 stores Group means
# c96 stores Group std. deviations
# c97 stores Group variances
# c94 stores Group sizes
#
noecho
oh=0
sort c92 c91 c92 c91
copy c91 c92 c91 c92;
omit c91 '*'.
count c92 k90
let k90=k90-1
let k91=1
let k92=2
let k93=1
exec 'bart1' k90
erase k91-k92
erase k94-k96
print k93
let k91=c92(1)
let k92=1
let k94=0
exec 'bart2' k93
erase k90-k97
exec 'bart4.mtb'
```

Appendix 1.3. *(contd.)*

```
# BART1.MTB
# compares adjacent subscripts
# to determine the number of groups
let k94=c92 (k91)
let k95=c92 (k92)
let k96=(k94 ne k95)
let k91=k91+1
let k92=k92+1
let k93=k93+k96
```

```
# BART2.MTB
copy c91 c93;
use c92 (k91).
count c93 k95
mean c93 k96
stdev c93 k97
let k98 = (k94 < (k93 - 1))
exec 'bart3' k98
let k94=k94+1
let c94 (k94)=k95
let c95 (k94)=k96
let c96 (k94)=k97
```

```
# BART3.MTB
let k92=k92+k95
let k91=c92(k92)
end
```

```
# BART4.MTB
name c91 'data' c92 'groups' c93 'Df'
name C94 'N' c95 'means' c96 'stdev'
name c97 'variance' c98 'ln_Var'

let 'df'='N'-1
let 'variance'='stdev' * 'stdev'
let 'ln_var'=logE('variance')
sum 'df' k90
let k91=(sum('df'*'variance'))/k90
let k92=loge(k91)
let k93=sum('df'*logE('variance'))
let k94=(k90*k92)-k93
let k95=N('variance')-1
let k96=1/(3*k95)
let k96=1+k96*((sum(1/'df'))-(1/sum('df'))))
let k97=k94/k96
print c94 c93 c95-c98
max 'variance' k98
min 'variance' k99
let k100=k98/k99
echo
# --------------------------------------------------------------------------------
```

Appendix 1.3. (*contd.*)

```
# Bartlett's calculated Chi squared
# compare with table chi square for k95 degrees of freedom
# if table Chi Sq. > calc Chi Sq. variances are homogeneous
#
# the table Chi Sq. value at P=0.05 is
noecho
invcdf 0.95;
chisquare k95.
echo
# the calculated Chi Sq. value is
noecho
print k97
echo
# -------------------------------------------------------------------------------
# The value for Hartley's Fmax is
noecho
print k100
echo
# -------------------------------------------------------------------------------
# The value for Cochran's C is
noecho
let K100=(max(c97))/(sum(c97))
print k100
echo
```

Appendix 1.4. Listing of a *Minitab* macro (LADDER.MTB) for calculating midsummaries and σ_e values for transformed and raw data; used to select the best transformation for the data.

To run this macro the file must be present in the directory being used by *Minitab*. The raw data from the largest group must be put in C75; all columns above this are used by the macro, as are K1 and K2. The macro puts the useful output in EDALET.LIS and puts the other output not required but produced by *Minitab* in RUBBISH.LIS. The macro was constructed for *Minitab* release 7.1 and might need modification for other releases.

```
NOTE LADDER.MTB
NOTE EDA:LETTER VALUE DISPLAY ANALYSIS
NOTE COMPUTING NOW
NOTE EDA:LETTER VALUE DISPLAY ANALYSIS
NOTE DATA IN COLUMN C75
NOTE DON'T USE ANY COLUMNS ABOVE THIS NUMBER OR K98
NOTE WRITTEN BY J.C. FRY 1990 FOR MINITAB VERSION 7.1
```

Appendix 1.4. *(contd.)*

```
NOTE          ------------------------------------------------------------------
NOTE          *******     OUTPUT IN EDALET.LIS     **********
NOTE          ------------------------------------------------------------------
NOTE          *******     WASTE IN RUBBISH.LIS     **********
NOTE          ------------------------------------------------------------------
NOECHO
NOTE A. TRANSFORMATIONS
LET C76=C75*C75*C75
LET C77=C75*C75
LET C78=C75
LET C79=SQRT(C75)
LET C80=LOGTEN(C75)
LET C81=-1/C79
LET C82=-1/C75
LET C83=-1/C77
NAME C76 'CUBE..' C77 'SQUARE..' C78 'RAW..' C79 'ROOT'..' C80
'LOG..'
NAME C81 'REC.RT..' C82 'RECIP..' C83 'REC.SQ..'
OUTFILE 'EDALET';
OW 132;
NOTERM.
NOTE ******   MACRO FOR CHOOSING THE BEST TRANSFORMATION    ******
NOTE ******           FROM A SINGLE LARGE GROUP             ******
NOTE ******            BY LETTER VALUE DISPLAYS             ******
NOTE
NOTE (1) RAW DATA & TRANSFORMATIONS
NOTE
PRINT C76-C83
NOTE
NOOUTFILE
NOTE B. LETTER VALUES FOR ALL TRANSFORMATIONS
NOTE   MIDSUMMARIES AND SPREADS STORED
OUTFILE 'RUBBISH';
NOTERM.
LVALS CUBE C76 C75 C84 C92
LVALS SQUARE C77 C75 C85 C93
LVALS RAW C78 C75 C86 C94
LVALS ROOT C79 C75 C87 C95
LVALS LOG C80 C75 C88 C96
LVALS REC.ROOT C81 C75 C89 C97
LVALS RECIP C82 C75 C90 C98
LVALS REC.SQ C83 C75 C91 C99
NOOUTFILE
NOTE C. CALCULATE SIGMAS FROM SPREADS
ERASE C75
SET C75
1.349 2.301 3.068 3.726 4.308 4.836 5.320
END
COPY C92-C99 C92-C99;
```

Appendix 1.4. *(contd.)*

```
OMIT C92=0.0.
LET K98=COUNT(C92)
COPY C75 C75;
USE 1:K98.
LET C92=C92/C75
LET C93=C93/C75
LET C94=C94/C75
LET C95=C95/C75
LET C96=C96/C75
LET C97=C97/C75
LET C98=C98/C75
LET C99=C99/C75
NOTE D. OUTPUT MAIN RESULTS
OUTFILE 'EDALET';
OW 132;
NOTERM.
NOTE (2) RESULTS FOR CHOOSING BEST TRANSFORMATION
NOTE
NOTE
NOTE *************LADDER OF POWERS*********************************************
NOTE TRANS. = CUBE  SQUARE  RAW  ROOT  LOG  REC.ROOT  RECIP  REC.SQ
NOTE POWER =  +3      +2      +1    +.5    0        -.5        -1       -2
COPY C84-C91 C76-C83
NOTE
NOTE
NOTE
NOTE ************MIDSUMMARIES OF TRANSFORMATIONS**********************
NOTE ---------LOOK FOR MOST EVEN VALUES DOWN COLUMNS FOR MOST
NOTE                  SYMMETRICAL TRANSFORMATION---------------------------------
PRINT C76-C83
NOTE
NOTE
NOTE
COPY C92-C99 C76-C83
NOTE ***********SIGMAS FOR TRANSFORMATIONS*******************************
NOTE --------LOOK FOR THE MOST EVEN VALUES FOR THE TRANSFORMATION
NOTE             THAT MOST CLOSELY FITS THE NORMAL DISTRIBUTION--------
PRINT C76-C83
ERASE C75-C99 K1 K2
NOOUTFILE
ECHO
NOTE COMPUTING COMPLETED
NOTE        MORE DATA IN C75
```

2

Crossed and hierarchical analysis of variance

TERENCE C. ILES

1. Introduction

This chapter describes the analysis of experiments where measurements are made of the response to several factors, extending the one-way ANOVA where just one factor is investigated. Experiments where the response is measured at all combinations of levels of several factors are called factorial experiments. The value of such experiments is in the opportunity of assessing the interrelationships or interactions between factors; it is possible that the response to one factor may differ according to the levels of a second factor. Also, a single well-designed factorial experiment is usually more efficient than a series of single-factor experiments. Texts that describe details of the analysis of variance of factorial experiments for non-mathematicians are Winer (1) and Sokal and Rohlf (2). Further information, though in a more mathematical style, can be found in Miller (3) and Milliken and Johnson (4).

An important prerequisite of any factorial experiment is a consideration of the experimental design so that the experiment satisfies the objectives of the investigation, and also that the experiment is efficient in its use of information. It is convenient to defer the discussion of experimental design until Section 7, but it must be stressed that to make the best possible use of experimental resources the design should be considered before data are collected and analysis attempted.

1.1 Data structure

Figures 1 and *2* are schematic diagrams for the two forms of factorial experiment with two factors, the crossed layout and the hierarchical or nested layout respectively. Each observation is represented by a cross (X) and here there are two replicated data for each combination of levels of the two factors. One combination of levels, called a cell, is indicated with a rounded box. Each X in these diagrams represents an independent measurement of the response at the indicated levels of the two factors. Each measurement needs an amount of experimental material, often called a plot or experimental unit.

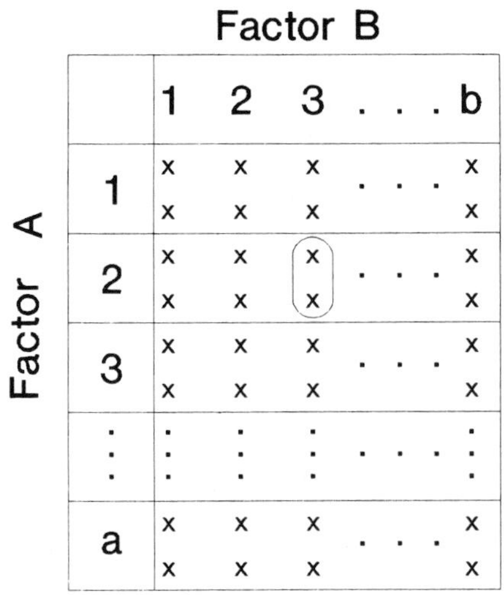

Factor A \ Factor B	1	2	3	. . .	b
1	x x	x x	x x	. . .	x x
2	x x	x x	(x x)	. . .	x x
3	x x	x x	x x	. . .	x x
⋮	⋮	⋮	⋮	. . .	⋮
a	x x	x x	x x	. . .	x x

Figure 1. Typical data structure for a two-factor crossed analysis of variance with *a* levels of factor *A* crossed with *b* levels of factor *B*. There are two replicate data in each cell.

Factor A	1	2	3	. . .	a
Factor B	1 2 ... b	1 2 ... b	1 2 ... b	. . .	1 2 ... b
	x x ... x x x ... x	x x ... x x x ... x	x (x) ... x x (x) ... x	. . . . . .	x x ... x x x ... x

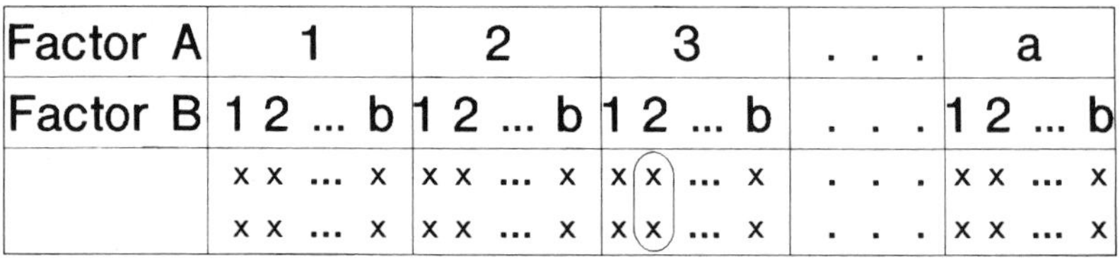

Figure 2. Typical data structure for a two-factor hierarchical or nested analysis of variance with *b* levels of factor *B* nested hierarchically within *a* levels of factor *A*. There are two replicate data in each cell.

Two replicate data in a cell require two independent plots to be made available for each cell. A genuine replicate cannot be obtained by simply duplicating the measurement made on a single plot. In some factorial experiments it may be expedient to have more than two replicates in each cell.

The distinction between a crossed layout and a hierarchical layout is most easily clarified by an example. *Table 1* gives the yields of four varieties of wheat. So as to obtain enough replicate data to enable comparisons to be made, three farms were used in the experiment. At each farm eight similar plots of land were selected and each variety was sown on two replicate plots. This experiment is described as crossed because each variety is grown at each farm. All the data in the first row have in common that they are measurements from farm number 1. The average, across the four varieties, represents an average for that farm. The three farm averages are compared to determine

Table 1. Yields (tonnes per hectare) of four varieties of wheat at three farms

	Variety 1		**Variety 2**		**Variety 3**		**Variety 4**	
Farm 1	0.327	0.280	0.500	0.510	0.442	0.360	0.471	0.460
Farm 2	0.532	0.526	0.599	0.637	0.516	0.499	0.638	0.455
Farm 3	0.269	0.277	0.308	0.286	0.241	0.328	0.305	0.314

if there are differences between farms. Similarly the data in the first two columns have in common that they are measurements of variety number 1. The average, across the three farms, represents an average for that variety. The four variety averages are compared to determine if there are differences between varieties.

Suppose the experiment had been conducted differently, although still comparing four varieties by measuring the yields from 24 plots of land. If the farms used for variety 1 differ from those for variety 2 and those for varieties 3 and 4 then the experiment is described as hierarchical or nested, with differences between farms nested within varieties. The comparison of the four variety means is still made, averaging each variety across farms. However, there is no meaning in a comparison of the three row averages since the farms differ from variety to variety. Instead, the farm averages (of two data) are compared within varieties. This experiment might be difficult to interpret. If differences between farms are found to exist then such differences could well affect the comparison of varieties. In this context the crossed experiment is preferred. However, in other contexts hierarchical experiments give useful information.

Notice that although it is a convention to arrange the data for a crossed experiment in a table resembling *Figure 1* and those for a hierarchical experiment in a table like *Figure 2*, the layout of the data is not enough to allow the correct relationship between the factors to be established. *Figure 1* can readily be rearranged into the form of *Figure 2* and vice versa. It is the interrelationships of the factors themselves that determine whether they are crossed or hierarchical.

In factorial experiments with two or more factors it is an advantage to have a balanced experiment. In such experiments the number of levels of one factor for which measurements are made is the same at every level of all other factors, and the number of replicate data is the same for all cells. There are three advantages of balanced experiments in preference to unbalanced ones:

- they are easier to analyse
- they are usually much easier to interpret
- they are more robust to departures from statistical assumptions used to justify the analysis.

Table 2. Numbers of seedlings produced by fixed numbers of loblolly pine seeds

	Number of seedlings[a]			
Sowing date in March	**Burnt ground**		**Conventionally cleared ground**	
2	900*	810	880	1100
	760	1040	960*	1040
6	880*	1170	1050*	1240
	1060	910*	1110	1120
10	1530	1160	1140*	1270
	1390*	1540	1320	1080
14	1970*	1890	1360*	1510
	1820	2140*	1490*	1270
18	1960	1670	1270	1380
	1310	1480*	1500	1450
22	830	420	150	380*
	570	760	420	270

[a] Observations marked with an asterisk (*) are assumed to be missing in some examples

Three sets of data are used for illustration of ANOVA techniques in this chapter. The experiment whose data are given in *Table 1* has already been described. The data in *Table 2* are the numbers of seedlings produced from loblolly pine seeds. A fixed number of seeds were sown randomly on six dates in spring into four replicate plots on land cleared by burning and, on the same dates, in another four plots cleared by conventional means. The data for the third experiment, in *Table 3* were obtained by students in Cardiff. Twelve students were involved, six postgraduates (PG) and six undergaduates (UG). Each student made three replicate determinations of the number of viable

Table 3. Estimated numbers ($\times 10^3\ ml^{-1}$) of viable heterotrophs in waters from three sources

Water type	**Student**	**Postgraduates**			**Undergraduates**		
Sewage	1	2700	2800	1700	4900	3600	1300
	2	2600	3000	3200	3500	4100	2500
Polluted river	1	52	49	61	60	140	75
	2	68	75	83	40	60	80
Clean stream	1	5.9	7.6	16.0	6.4	4.2	4.1
	2	5.6	5.9	6.3	8.3	3.1	5.2

heterotrophic bacteria present in water samples (by a plate count determination). Four students, two undergraduates and two postgraduates, worked on water from sewage, four worked on water from a polluted river and four on water from a clean stream. Notice that in *Table 3* the students have been labelled 1 or 2 in pairs for each water source/PG–UG combination. This convention for labelling is the one used in texts on ANOVA, and also for data entry in statistical computer packages.

Two points should be made about these data. In all three experiments the data are an independent series of measurements made on a set of plots. The analysis of variance is not suitable for the analysis of categorical data where a population is categorized, possibly by several classifications simultaneously, and the numbers in a sample from the population are counted in each category. A χ^2 contingency table may be suitable for the analysis of such data. Neither should the analysis of variance be used for experiments where measurements of a number of variables are made on a sample from a population. Such data may be analysed by a method of multivariate analysis.

1.2 The assumptions of the analysis of variance

The key to the correct analysis of a factorial experiment and the correct interpretation of the ANOVA is an understanding of the mathematical assumptions underlying the analysis. Even if the calculations are done by a standard computer package, this understanding is necessary for the correct analysis to be selected. For that reason the mathematical models of factorial experiments are described in some detail in subsequent sections, and details are given here of the linear model of the one-way ANOVA described in Chapter 1.

Underpinning the analysis of the one-way experiment is an additive or linear model in which each observation is supposed to consist of three components added together. The first is an overall mean, common to all of the data, the second is an adjustment that is specific to the group to which the observation belongs, and the third is an error term unique to the particular observation. In mathematical terms the model is:

$$x_{ij} = \mu + \gamma_i + \varepsilon_{ij}.$$

Here i is an index for the groups, (ranging between 1 and a) and j is an index for the replicates within the groups, and thus ranges between 1 and n_i (or n if the number of replicates is the same for all groups). Thus x_{ij} denotes the jth observation in group i, μ is the overall mean, and γ_i the adjustment for the ith group. The error terms ε_{ij} are assumed to be independent random variables and to be normally distributed with a mean of 0 and variance of σ^2. (The errors are thus assumed all to have the same variance.)

There are two sorts of experiment that are analysed by the one-way ANOVA: fixed and random effects models. In the fixed effects model the group adjustments γ_i are assumed to be a set of fixed but unknown parameters. The usual criterion for estimation is to find μ and γ_i that minimize the sum of squares of the errors $\Sigma(x_{ij} - \mu - \gamma_i)^2$. If a set of values of the $a + 1$ parameters that minimize this expression are found, then a solution with the same minimum sum of squares of errors is obtained by adding a constant to the estimate of μ and subtracting the same constant from each of the γ_i. The parameters in the model are not uniquely identifiable. The usual convention is to impose a restriction on the parameters γ_i representing them as the average discrepancy from the overall mean. Mathematically this restriction is $\Sigma n_i\gamma_i = 0$. Fixed effects models are appropriate for the analysis of experiments where the groups represent specific levels of a factor, determined in advance by the experimenter. The detection of significant differences in the means for the levels (groups) and, if identified, the isolation of those levels whose means differ significantly from the others is the appropriate approach for analysis.

In a random effects model the γ_i in the model are assumed to be an independent set of random variables, independent from the errors ε_{ij}, and also normally distributed with mean zero. The variances of the γ_i are assumed all to be equal, but this variance σ_G^2 is not necessarily equal to the error variance σ^2. Such models are appropriate for experiments in which the levels of the factor represent different individuals in some population, either finite or infinite, which are sampled by a random selection. The means for the particular levels observed would not be of any interest; if the experiment were repeated different levels would be observed. (In the fixed effects case the same levels would be observed in any repetition of the experiment.) It is the variance σ_G^2 of the γ_i that is estimated in random effects models. This, together with the error variance σ^2, enables the components of variability in the model to be identified. It is my view that random effects models are often wrongly used. They should be reserved for those experiments in which the identification of the levels of a factor involves random sampling from some population. Deciding the levels of measurement of a factor, or those treatments to use as levels of a factor in an experiment, does not represent random sampling and such factors should be regarded as fixed effects. Statements of the variability in average measurements at different levels of fixed effects can be made by quoting ranges of means for the levels observed in the experiment.

Linear models for factorial experiments with two or more factors are similar to those for the one-way ANOVA, but contain more terms. On the left-hand side is an x with a set of indices. There is one index for each factor in the model and an additional index for the replicates. The right-hand side consists of several terms separated by + signs, indicating the assumption of a model in which the various adjustments are additive. The first term is always an overall mean μ, and this is always assumed to be fixed. The last term is always assumed to be an error ε, followed by all the indices, and these are assumed to be independent normally distributed random variables with mean zero and variance σ^2. These assumptions should always be confirmed by diagnostic checking (see Section 2).

The terms on the right-hand side of the linear model between μ and ε are assumed to be fixed constants, with restrictions imposed for unique estimates to be defined, or random variables depending on the assumptions made about the factors as fixed or random effects. *Protocol 4*, following the detailed descriptions of factorial experiments (Section 4) describes how to write down the correct linear model.

1.3 The general principles of ANOVA

The idea of ANOVA is that the overall variability of the data, measured by a sum of squares (of deviations of the data from the overall mean), can be partitioned into several components. The size of these depends on the absolute magnitude of the terms corresponding to an effect or interaction in the linear model. Thus, if one of the components is small then a corresponding term in the linear model can be ignored. Conversely, if a component is large then the corresponding term is judged to be significant, and further explanation of the effects corresponding to that term is needed. The calculations of these components or sums of squares is easy in a balanced experiment (see *Appendix 2.1* for details, or consult Winer (1) or Sokal and Rohlf (2)). Associated with each sum of squares is a number called the degrees of freedom, df. These too are simply calculated in a balanced experiment. A sum of squares is divided by its degrees of freedom to give a mean square, and it is these that are tested against each other to determine the significance of effects. The mean squares also enable variances to be estimated for random effects. So as to determine the appropriate testing procedure, the theoretical average values of the mean squares in terms of variances (for random effects) and constants (for fixed effects) is worked out. Rules for the evaluation of these expected mean squares, or E[MS], for balanced experiments, are given in *Appendix 2.2*. For balanced experiments both *Minitab* (release 7) and *SAS* (version 6) allow the E[MS] column to be printed. For unbalanced experiments, however, the calculation of sums of squares, degrees of freedom, and mean squares is computationally more difficult. Statistical packages such as *Minitab, SPSS/PC+*, and *SAS* enable these calculations to be done, but they can be time-consuming. Only *SAS* of these three packages evaluates the E[MS] column for unbalanced data.

In experiments where all factors are fixed (except the error term) all mean squares are tested against the error mean square by an F-ratio. If a random effect is present, the testing is usually more complicated. To test for the significance of an effect, two mean squares are identified whose E[MS] differ just by a single term reflecting on the effect to be tested. The ratio of the MS including the extra term to that without it thus tests the significance of an effect in the model. In more complicated experiments, such pairs of E[MS] cannot be identified and the ratio of one MS to a combination of other MSs has to be calculated. The difficulty there is in the calculation of the degrees of freedom, and such models will not be considered in this chapter. Further details of the use of such combinations of MSs, using an approximation to the df due to Satterthwaite, are given by Winer (1), p. 377.

Once the significance of effects is established, the nature and magnitude of the effects is described. For fixed effects, the identification of significantly different means is done by multiple range tests, such as those described in Section 6 of Chapter 1. Graphs of means for different levels of a factor or interaction are especially valuable for the presentation of information. In the case of random effects, variance components are identified, using the *E*[MS] expressions.

1.4 Organizing data for computer solutions of factorial ANOVA

The form in which data have to be entered for statistical packages is not usually that of a table as presented in *Tables 1–3*. In *Minitab, SPSS/PC+*, and *SAS* all the data are entered in one column. A further column is needed for each factor in the model giving the levels of the factors. These columns are called indicator variables. *Tables 4–6* are the data and indicator variable

Table 4. Format for entering data of *Table 1* into statistical packages and contents of file FARM.DAT[a]

ROW	Yield	Farm	Variety
1	0.327	1	1
2	0.280	1	1
3	0.500	1	2
4	0.510	1	2
5	0.442	1	3
6	0.360	1	3
7	0.471	1	4
8	0.460	1	4
9	0.532	2	1
10	0.526	2	1
11	0.599	2	2
12	0.637	2	2
13	0.516	2	3
14	0.499	2	3
15	0.638	2	4
16	0.455	2	4
17	0.269	3	1
18	0.277	3	1
19	0.308	3	2
20	0.286	3	2
21	0.241	3	3
22	0.328	3	3
23	0.305	3	4
24	0.314	3	4

[a] The file actually contains the data only for Yield, Farm, and Variety in three columns; the row number is not included

Table 5. Format for entering data of *Table 2* into statistical packages and contents of file LOBLOLLY.DAT[a]

ROW	Seedling	Date	Burning
1	900	1	1
2	880	2	1
3	1530	3	1
4	1970	4	1
5	1960	5	1
6	830	6	1
7	880	1	2
8	1050	2	2
9	1140	3	2
10	1360	4	2
11	1270	5	2
12	150	6	2
13	810	1	1
14	1170	2	1
15	1160	3	1
16	1890	4	1
17	1670	5	1
18	420	6	1
19	1100	1	2
20	1240	2	2
21	1270	3	2
22	1510	4	2
23	1380	5	2
24	380	6	2
25	760	1	1
26	1060	2	1
27	1390	3	1
28	1820	4	1
29	1310	5	1
30	570	6	1
31	960	1	2
32	1110	2	2
33	1320	3	2
34	1490	4	2
35	1500	5	2
36	420	6	2
37	1040	1	1
38	910	2	1
39	1540	3	1
40	2140	4	1
41	1480	5	1
42	760	6	1
43	1040	1	2
44	1120	2	2
45	1080	3	2
46	1270	4	2
47	1450	5	2
48	270	6	2

[a] File format as *Table 4*

Table 6. Format for entering data of *Table 3* into statistical packages and contents of file HETERO.DAT[a]

ROW	Count	Waters	Students	PG–UG
1	2700.0	1	1	1
2	2800.0	1	1	1
3	1700.0	1	1	1
4	4900.0	1	1	2
5	3600.0	1	1	2
6	1300.0	1	1	2
7	2600.0	1	2	1
8	3000.0	1	2	1
9	3200.0	1	2	1
10	3500.0	1	2	2
11	4100.0	1	2	2
12	2500.0	1	2	2
13	52.0	2	1	1
14	49.0	2	1	1
15	61.0	2	1	1
16	60.0	2	1	2
17	140.0	2	1	2
18	75.0	2	1	2
19	68.0	2	2	1
20	75.0	2	2	1
21	83.0	2	2	1
22	40.0	2	2	2
23	60.0	2	2	2
24	80.0	2	2	2
25	5.9	3	1	1
26	7.6	3	1	1
27	16.0	3	1	1
28	6.4	3	1	2
29	4.2	3	1	2
30	4.1	3	1	2
31	5.6	3	2	1
32	5.9	3	2	1
33	6.3	3	2	1
34	8.3	3	2	2
35	3.1	3	2	2
36	5.2	3	2	2

[a] File contents as *Table 4*

columns for the data of *Tables 1–3* respectively. Notice the convention for the numbering of the nested students factor in *Table 6*. Although in the experiment there were 12 students, the numbering for entry into the computer is the students within water types, hence 1 and 2 are repeated six times.

2. Diagnostic checking

The diagnostic checks to justify the assumptions of the ANOVA model in multi-factorial experiments are similar to those used in the one-way ANOVA and described in detail in Chapter 1, Section 3. Diagnostic checking is an important part of the ANOVA procedure, and genuine differences may not be detected if the assumptions of the model do not hold. Often a simple transformation of the data is all that is needed to enable a standard ANOVA to be done. The main distinction between the multi-factorial and one-way cases is in the tests for homogeneity of variance. These tests are done on variances calculated from the cell means, and these are not normally calculated as part of a multi-factorial ANOVA table, though the within group variances (or standard deviations) are often presented in a standard one-way analysis. The tests on residuals, however, are done on the residuals calculated from the full model. *Protocol 1* describes the procedure for diagnostic checking in a multi-factorial experiment.

Protocol 1. Diagnostic checking for a multi-factorial ANOVA

1. Compute the cell variances (or standard deviations). This can be done in *Minitab* by a one-way ANOVA with cells as groups, or by the TABLE command.
2. Check for homogeneity of variance (see Chapter 1, Section 3.1):
   - Bartlett's χ^2
   - Hartley's $F_{\max}$
   - Cochran's C
3. Compute the residuals from the full ANOVA.
4. Check the residuals for normality (see Chapter 1, Section 3.2):
   - normal probability plots
   - Shapiro–Wilk test
   - boxplots
5. Check for outliers (see Chapter 1, Section 5) and for patterns in the residuals:
   - Dixon's test ($n < 25$)
   - Grubb's test ($n > 25$)

   Look for patterns in the residuals, for example in time of data measurement.
6. If these tests indicate that the assumptions do not hold, transform the data (see *Protocol 2* of Chapter 1) and repeat the checks.

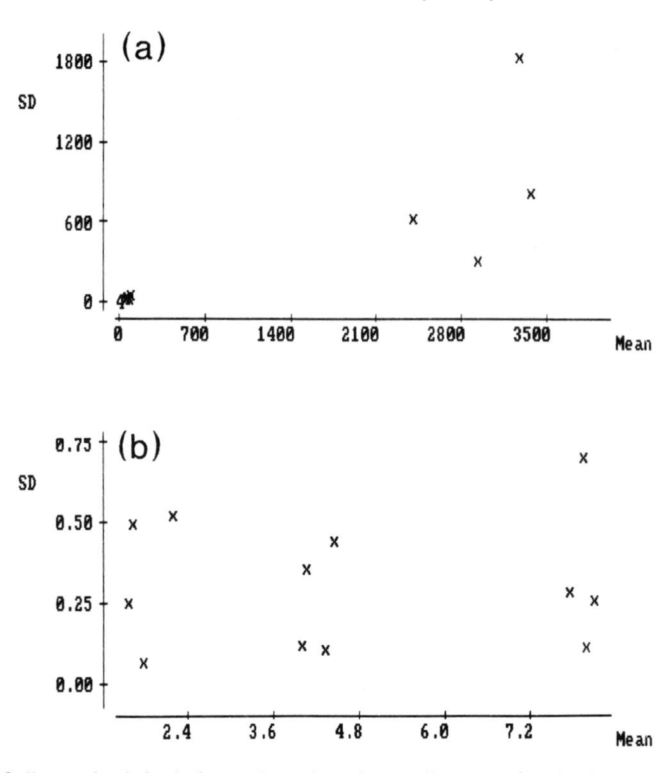

Figure 3. Cell standard deviations plotted against cell means for the heterotroph count data in *Table 3*; (a) raw data, (b) logged data.

The diagnostic checking procedure is illustrated by the heterotroph count data of *Table 3*. *Figure 3* indicates the heterogeneity of variance of the raw data. The cell means of each set of three counts made by a student are plotted against the cell standard deviations. It is plain from *Figure 3a* that there is a strong tendency for larger standard deviations (hence variances) to be associated with higher estimated counts of bacteria. No such trend is apparent in the graph of cell standard deviation against cell mean for the logged data in *Figure 3b*. The heterogeneity of variance in the untransformed data is confirmed by the three tests described in Section 3.1 of Chapter 1. The *Minitab* macros BART.MTB, BART1–BART4.MTB in *Appendix 1.3* were used to calculate Bartlett's χ^2, Hartley's F_{max} and Cochran's C. The values obtained were respectively 129.215, 26 945 926 and 0.748 104. The critical values for these tests are 19.68, the upper 95th percentile of χ^2 with $P = 0.05$ and 11 df (*Appendix B.8*), 704 (from *Appendix B.2*), and a value between 0.335 and 0.445 (from *Appendix B.3*). All three statistics considerably exceed their critical values, so heterogeneity of variance is strongly indicated. The same data when transformd by taking the logarithm have homogeneous cell

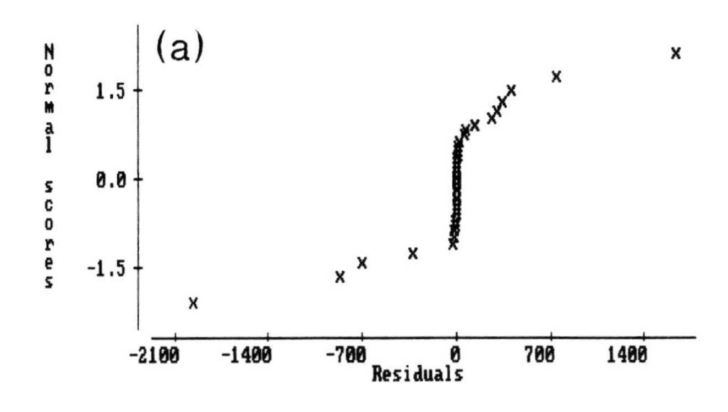

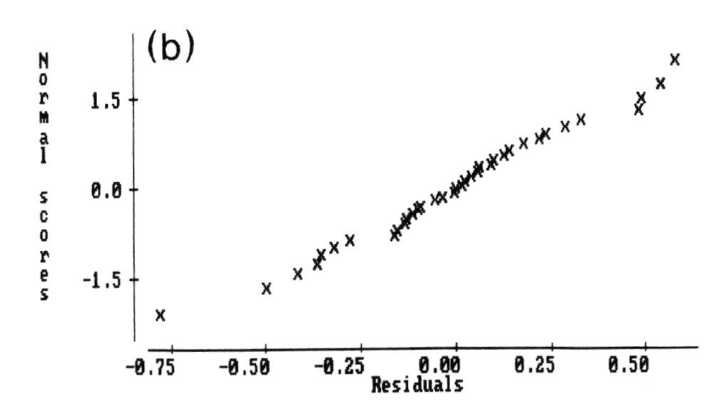

Figure 4. Normal scores plotted against residuals from an ANOVA for the heterotroph count data in *Table 3*; (a) raw data, (b) logged data.

variances, however. The three statistics are 16.671 for Bartlett's χ^2, 138.43 for Hartley's F_{max} and 0.3112 for Cochran's C.

The assumption of normality in the raw data is also doubtful, as indicated by *Figure 4*. A full ANOVA model was fitted (described in Section 4) and the residuals computed. *Minitab* was used to do this, the RESIDUALS sub-command of the ANOVA command makes it easy. The NSCORE command was then used to calculate normal scores corresponding to these residuals. *Figure 4* is a plot of the normal scores against the residuals for the raw data and logged data respectively. The curvature of the plot for the raw data is evident. The correlation coefficients are 0.798 for the raw data and 0.989 for the logged data. Comparison with the table for critical values for the correlation coefficient in *Appendix B.4* shows that the former is not significant, but the latter is significant, indicating normality for the residuals of the logged data. (The critical value is for N = 24 and equals 0.956.)

3. Balanced experiments with two factors

3.1 Two crossed factors, no replicates

The factorial experiment with two crossed factors and no replicates is the simplest multi-factorial experiment, and for that reason will be described first. In the absence of replications it is not possible to assess whether the effect of factor B is consistent from one level of factor A to another. Such an inconsistency is called an interaction between the factors A and B, and the assessment of interactions in two-factor experiments is described in Section 3.2. Two factor experiments with no replicates are limited, therefore, and in general I advise replicate measurements to be made wherever this is possible.

The linear model to describe such an unreplicated experiment is

$$x_{ij} = \mu + \alpha_i + \beta_j + \varepsilon_{ij}.$$

Here i denotes the levels of factor A and j the levels of factor B. The model is an extension of the one-way model, but with main effects terms for both factors. In this model the replicates for factor A are considered to be the b levels of factor B, and those for B the a levels of factor A. There is an implicit assumption that the effects are additive, that the effect of factor A does not change with levels of factor B; that is, that there is no interaction between A and B. (A test that validates this assumption is Tukey's non-additivity test, for details of which see Winer (1) or Sokal and Rohlf (2).) The absence of replicate data for any cells also precludes the calculation of cell variances, so that diagnostic checking for homogeneity of variance can only be done crudely by an examination of the residuals. If these increase markedly with the levels of one or other of the factors, then the homogeneity of variance assumption may be called into question.

A particular case of the two-factor crossed experiment with no replicates is the randomized block experiment. Here a treatments (or levels of a factor A) are compared and b replicates per level are required. This requires ab observations to be made. The randomized block experiment is used where the experimental material or plots on which measurements are made can be naturally divided into b sets called blocks, each block containing a plots. The purpose in designing the experiment in this way is that differences between blocks can be allowed for in assessing the effect of factor A. In each block one plot is used for each level of factor A. The efficiency of the design depends on the plots within the blocks being roughly similar.

There is a non-parametric equivalent, called Friedman's test, of the randomized block ANOVA based on the ranks of the data within the blocks. This test is useful if the errors in the data are so markedly different from normally distributed that no simple transformation enables a standard ANOVA to be done. The test is described in detail by Winer (1) and Sokal and Rohlf (2), and is readily available on statistical packages, for example *Minitab* and

Table 7. Expected mean squares for the two-factor crossed ANOVA with no replicates

	***E*[MS]**		
Source	**Fixed effects model**	**Random effects model**	**Mixed model, factor *B* random**
Factor *A*	$\sigma^2 + b\,\Sigma\alpha_i^2/(a-1)$	$\sigma^2 + b\sigma_A^2$	$\sigma^2 + b\,\Sigma\alpha_i^2/(a-1)$
Factor *B*	$\sigma^2 + a\,\Sigma\beta_j^2/(b-1)$	$\sigma^2 + a\sigma_B^2$	$\sigma^2 + a\sigma_B^2$
Error	σ^2	σ^2	σ^2

SPSS/PC+. For more complicated factorial experiments, non-parametric methods are still being developed. Hoaglin *et al.* ((5), Chapter 6; (6), Chapters 3 and 4) give further details on approaches to these methods.

Table 7 gives the column of expected mean squares (E[MS]) for the three possible cases, where both effects are fixed, where both are random, and the mixed model where one effect is fixed and the other random. In this table σ^2 represents the error variance, σ_A^2 the variance for factor A and σ_B^2 the variance for factor B. This table shows that the appropriate tests for the significance of factors A and B are to take the ratios of the MS for A and B respectively to the error MS. If a factor is significant then the variance for that factor is estimated. If B is a random effect the error variance σ_B^2 is estimated by subtracting MS_{error} from MS_B and dividing the difference by a. A similar rule enables σ_A^2 to be estimated.

As an illustration of the two-factor ANOVA with no replicates the wheat yield data in *Table 1* will be used. Assume that only the first of each pair of data in each cell is available. The two factors are here crossed, all the data in the first row are from one farm, all those in the second row from a second farm, etc. Similarly the columns correspond to varieties of wheat. The factor representing varieties is regarded as fixed but the interpretation of the farms factor is open to question. If these are the only farms from which data are of any interest, such as would probably be the case for the farmers, then a fixed effects model is appropriate; the mean yields for the particular farms are of interest. If on the other hand the three farms were chosen at random from a population of farms, so as to obtain sufficient replicate data, then the farms factor would be regarded as random. This latter assumption will be made here. The farms factor could have been included as blocks, and the experiment is then a randomized block.

Figure 5 gives the two-way ANOVA table from *Minitab* using the ANOVA command, together with the sub-commands used to obtain the output. In SAS use the VARCOMP procedure to give similar results, with the METHOD = TYPE1 option and specifying only the class variable for farms as random on the MODEL line. The F-ratio for varieties is 4.75 (with 3 and 6 df) and this is just significant, as indicated by the P value of 0.050. Thus a

```
MTB > anova c1=c2 c3;
SUBC> random c2;
SUBC> ems.

Factor      Type Levels Values
Farm      random      3      1      2      3
Variety    fixed      4      1      2      3      4

Analysis of Variance for Yield

Source        DF         SS          MS        F       P
Farm           2   0.168996    0.084498    56.86   0.000
Variety        3   0.021185    0.007062     4.75   0.050
Error          6   0.008917    0.001486
Total         11   0.199098

Source        Variance Error Expected Mean Square
             component  term (using unrestricted model)
 1 Farm        0.02075     3    (3) + 4(1)
 2 Variety                 3    (3) + Q[2]
 3 Error       0.00149          (3)

MTB >
```

Figure 5. Two-way ANOVA table from *Minitab* for the first replicate of each cell of the wheat yield data in *Table 1*.

marginally significant difference in the varieties has been indicated by these data. The F-ratio for farms is 56.86 (with 2 and 6 df) and this is highly significant, with a P value of < 0.001. The Expected Mean Square column uses (3) as the symbol for the error variance σ^2, (1) as the symbol for the farms variance σ_F^2 and Q[2] for the quadratic expression in the adjustments for the fixed varieties effects. The use of the unrestricted model refers to assumptions made about a mixed model with replicate data and can be ignored here. The two components of variance are 0.020 75 for farms and 0.001 49 for error. (Notice that no variance component is attributed to varieties. The varieties are a fixed effect and they are assessed by comparing their means). Since a linear model is assumed, the variance of any observation is the sum of the variance components. Thus, in this case the variability in farms represents an estimated proportion of $0.020\,75/(0.020\,75 + 0.001\,49) = 0.933$ of the total variance of any observation (for any particular variety). This division of variability into proportions attributable to the random components of the model is more easily understood than a simple reporting of the variances.

Friedman's test is designed specifically for randomized block experiments, not for general two-factor experiments with no replications. So that a comparison can be made with the parametric method, the same data will be used for illustration. This supposes that the experiment is viewed in a slightly different light. The varieties are regarded as the factor under investigation and the farms will be treated as blocks. Each variety is measured on three plots, but these plots are on different farms. All four varieties are measured

```
MTB > friedman c1 c3 c2

Friedman test of Yield by Variety blocked by Farm

S = 7.40  d.f. = 3  p = 0.061

                       Est.    Sum of
 Variety        N    Median     RANKS
       1        3   0.40825       5.0
       2        3   0.48175      11.0
       3        3   0.41075       4.0
       4        3   0.48925      10.0

Grand median   =    0.44750

MTB >
```

Figure 6. Friedman's non-parametric analysis of variance for the first replicate of each cell of the wheat yield data in Table 1. Output from *Minitab.*

on each farm. Differences between varieties are to be investigated, making allowance for differences between the farms. Differences between the farms are allowed for but not themselves assessed by Friedman's test.

Figure 6 is the output from *Minitab*'s FRIEDMAN command for the same data. The P value of 0.061 associated with the χ^2 test of the hypothesis that the median yield is the same for each variety confirms the ANOVA result: that there is only marginally significant difference in the yields for the four varieties. The similarity of the median yields is evident from the column of medians. For these data the conclusions drawn from Friedman's test are similar to those of the parametric analysis of variance.

3.2 Two crossed factors with replicates

The linear model is

$$x_{ijk} = \mu + \alpha_i + \beta_j + \alpha\beta_{ij} + \varepsilon_{ijk}.$$

There are two differences between this model and that used to describe the model for experiments with no replicates. There is an additional index k, for the replicates, and an additional term $\alpha\beta_{ij}$ on the right-hand side as well as the main effects α_i and β_j for factors A and B respectively. $\alpha\beta_{ij}$ is called the interaction and represents the possibility that the response to the levels of factor A differs from one level of B to another—that the response to factors A and B is non-additive. Either or both of the factors can be regarded as random and if one is random then both the main effect for that factor and the interaction are regarded as independent random variables with associated variances.

Table 8 gives the E[MS] and restrictions for four assumptions made about the random or fixed nature of the effects in the model. In this table n is the number of replicates per cell and σ^2_{AB} is the variance of the interaction term

Table 8. Expected mean squares and restrictions on fixed effects for the two-factor crossed ANOVA with n replicates per cell

Source	**Fixed effects model**	**Random effects model**	**Mixed model, *B* random (unrestricted)**	**Mixed model, *B* random (restricted)**
Factor A	$\sigma^2 + nb\ \Sigma\alpha_i^2/(a-1)$	$\sigma^2 + n\sigma_{AB}^2 + nb\sigma_A^2$	$\sigma^2 + n\sigma_{AB}^2 + nb\ \Sigma\alpha_i^2/(a-1)$	$\sigma^2 + n\sigma_{AB}^2 + nb\ \Sigma\alpha_i^2/(a-1)$
Factor B	$\sigma^2 + na\ \Sigma\beta_j^2/(b-1)$	$\sigma^2 + n\sigma_{AB}^2 + na\sigma_B^2$	$\sigma^2 + n\sigma_{AB}^2 + na\sigma_B^2$	$\sigma^2 + na\sigma_B^2$
Interaction $A \times B$	$\sigma^2 + n\ \Sigma\Sigma\alpha\beta_{ij}^2/(a-1)(b-1)$	$\sigma^2 + n\sigma_{AB}^2$	$\sigma^2 + n\sigma_{AB}^2$	$\sigma^2 + n\sigma_{AB}^2$
Error	σ^2	σ^2	σ^2	σ^2
Restrictions	$\Sigma\alpha_i = 0$ $\Sigma\beta_j = 0$ $\Sigma_i\alpha\beta_{ij} = 0$ $\Sigma_j\alpha\beta_{ij} = 0$	N/A	$\Sigma\alpha_i = 0$	$\Sigma\alpha_i = 0$ $\Sigma_i\alpha\beta_{ij} = 0$

$\alpha\beta_{ij}$. Notice that two alternatives are presented for the mixed model, where the one effect is fixed and the other random. In the restricted model, as well as assuming that the fixed effects α_i sum to zero, we assume that the interaction effects sum to zero over the levels of the fixed effect. This assumption is not made in the unrestricted model. Both models give sensible statistical estimates of the parameters of the model, and it is an unresolved question of which is to be preferred. Many texts assume the restricted model and Miller (3), p. 144, quotes studies that suggest that the restricted model is usually the more appropriate. The issue is also discussed by Searle (7), pp. 400–4. He does not clearly recommend one of the models in preference to the other, but points out that the unrestricted model is the one usually assumed for unbalanced data. *SAS* assumes the unrestricted model, but *Minitab* enables a choice to be made. Fortunately, this unresolved problem in statistics does not cause any difficulties of interpretation for the practician. The difference between the models will be clarified after the example immediately following *Protocol 2*. The main difference is that in the unrestricted model both effects are tested against the interaction. In a restricted model the random effect is tested against the error.

With the model determined, *Table 8* enables the correct tests and estimation procedure to be adopted. These are summarized in *Protocol 2*. The overall principle, as in the no replicate case, is to identify pairs of MSs whose E[MS] differs just by a single term. The F-ratio of these MSs then tests the significance of a single effect or interaction.

Protocol 2. Testing and estimation procedures for a two-factor crossed ANOVA with replications

1. Decide whether the factors are fixed or random and, in the mixed model, choose between the restricted and unrestricted models.

2. If both effects are fixed, the three F-tests for significance of effects are as follows:

- factor A: $F_A = \dfrac{\text{MS}_A}{\text{MS}_{\text{error}}}$
- factor B: $F_B = \dfrac{\text{MS}_B}{\text{MS}_{\text{error}}}$
- interaction: $F_{\text{interaction}} = \dfrac{\text{MS}_{\text{interaction}}}{\text{MS}_{\text{error}}}$

Significant effects are further investigated using multiple comparison tests (see Section 5 and Chapter 1, Section 6). There is only one variance component in this model, the error variance σ^2. This is estimated by MS_{error}

Protocol 2. *Continued*

3. If both effects are random, the three tests are:

- factor A: $F_A = \dfrac{MS_A}{MS_{interaction}}$
- factor B: $F_B = \dfrac{MS_B}{MS_{interaction}}$
- interaction: $F_{interaction} = \dfrac{MS_{interaction}}{MS_{error}}$

There are four variance components. The formulas for estimating these from the MSs are:

- error variance: MS_{error}
- interaction variance: $(MS_{interaction} - MS_{error})/n$
- factor A variance: $(MS_A - MS_{interaction})/bn$
- factor B variance: $(MS_B - MS_{interaction})/an$

4. In a mixed model with no restrictions on the interaction term in the model, proceed exactly as step 3, but no estimate is made of a variance for the fixed effect; there are three variance components.

5. In a mixed model with restrictions, the formulas for the F-test statistics are as follows (assuming factor A to be the fixed effect and factor B random):

- factor A: $F_A = \dfrac{MS_A}{MS_{interaction}}$
- factor B: $F_B = \dfrac{MS_B}{MS_{error}}$
- interaction: $F_{interaction} = \dfrac{MS_{interaction}}{MS_{error}}$

Notice that the fixed effect is tested against the interaction and the random effect against the error. This is the opposite of what might be expected from the purely fixed and purely random models.

There are three variance components. The formulas for estimating these are:

- error variance: MS_{error}
- factor B: $(MS_B - MS_{error})/an$
- interaction: $(MS_{interaction} - MS_{error})/n$

Some statisticians recommend a modification to this suggested procedure called pooling. The procedure is modified if any term fails to be significant. Start by testing the interaction, then, if it is not significant, calculate a new estimate of the error variance by adding the sums of squares for interaction and error and dividing by the total of their df. Then set σ^2_{AB} or $\alpha\beta_{ij}$ to zero in other expressions for E[MS] and thus test the factor B MS against this new MS. I do not recommend this procedure since it can distort the interpretation of results, and it is not done by any of *Minitab, SPSS/PC+*, or *SAS*.

Figure 7 is the output from MINITAB analysing the complete set of data in *Table 1* on wheat yields, together with the commands to obtain the output. So that a comparison can be made between the restricted and unrestricted models in the mixed model case, and also to make a comparison with *SAS* output, *Figure 8* gives the output for the same data (stored on drive A of my PC as A:FARM.DAT) from the *SAS* package using the VARCOMP procedure. The *SAS* statements to execute the analysis are included in *Figure 8*. There are slight differences in the statistics calculated, but the main distinction is the difference in the E[MS] column, *SAS* assuming an unrestricted model. The VARCOMP procedure does not calculate the F-ratios, though it does calculate the rest of the analysis of variance table. The ANOVA command in *SAS* allows random factors and this command calculates the F-ratios.

The output is interpreted by first checking for significant effects. Neither the interaction F-ratio nor the variety F-ratio is significant ($P = 0.190$ and 0.098 respectively). This indicates that the varieties do not differ significantly from farm to farm (the non-significant interaction) and that there is little evidence of overall significant differences between varieties. There is,

```
MTB > anova c1=c2 c3 c2*c3;
SUBC> random c2;
SUBC> restricted;
SUBC> ems.


Factor      Type Levels Values
Farm      random      3      1      2      3
Variety    fixed      4      1      2      3      4

Analysis of Variance for Yield

Source           DF         SS          MS        F       P
Farm              2   0.268861    0.134430    61.33   0.000
Variety           3   0.038494    0.012831     3.32   0.098
Farm*Variety      6   0.023206    0.003868     1.76   0.190
Error            12   0.026305    0.002192
Total            23   0.356866

Source             Variance Error  Expected Mean Square
                  component  term  (using restricted model)
 1 Farm             0.01653   4    (4) + 8(1)
 2 Variety                    3    (4) + 2(3) + 6Q[2]
 3 Farm*Variety     0.00084   4    (4) + 2(3)
 4 Error            0.00219        (4)
```

Figure 7. Two-way ANOVA table from *Minitab* for the wheat yield data in *Table 1*. Mixed model with restrictions assumed.

```
data farm;
infile 'a:farm.dat';
input yield farm variety;
proc varcomp method=type1;
     class farm variety;
     model yield = variety farm variety*farm/fixed=1;
run;
```

```
                   Variance Components Estimation Procedure

Dependent Variable: YIELD

Source                   DF         Type I SS          Type I MS

VARIETY                   3        0.03849433         0.01283144

FARM                      2        0.26886100         0.13443050

FARM*VARIETY              6        0.02320567         0.00386761

Error                    12        0.02630500         0.00219208

Corrected Total          23        0.35686600


Source                   Expected Mean Square

VARIETY                  Var(Error) + 2 Var(FARM*VARIETY) + Q(VARIETY)

FARM                     Var(Error) + 2 Var(FARM*VARIETY) + 8 Var(FARM)

FARM*VARIETY             Var(Error) + 2 Var(FARM*VARIETY)

Error                    Var(Error)


Variance Component                   Estimate

Var(FARM)                          0.01632036

Var(FARM*VARIETY)                  0.00083776

Var(Error)                         0.00219208
```

Figure 8. Two-way ANOVA table from *SAS* for the wheat yield data in *Table 1*. Mixed model with no restrictions assumed.

however, a significant difference within the farms ($P < 0.0005$). Farms is assumed here to be a random effect and associated with it is a variance. Wherever a model contains a random component, the variance of the observations is a sum of variances, including the error variance, variance of the random effect and the variance of the interaction including the random effect. The easiest way of expressing the elements of this variance is to calculate the proportions attributable to the different components. In this example the proportion of variation accounted for by differences in farms is estimated as $0.016\,53/(0.016\,53 + 0.000\,84 + 0.002\,19) = 0.845$. Since the interaction is judged not significant in the F-test, it may be preferable to conclude that the interaction variance is zero, in which case the proportion of variation due to farms is $0.016\,53/(0.016\,53 + 0.00219) = 0.883$. These results are more or less in agreement with those of the analysis of the first replicate alone. This new analysis is of value in confirming the lack of a significant interaction. We can here be confident in reporting the significance of the main effect of farms, secure in the knowledge that this difference does not change from one variety to another. This confirms the value of genuine replicates in interpreting factorial experiments.

The difference between the interpretation of the *Minitab* output (with restricted model selected) and *SAS* output (with unrestricted model assumed) lies in the interpretation of the farms effect. From the *SAS* expected mean square column it can be seen that MS_{farms} should be compared with $MS_{interaction}$. The *F*-ratio is 0.134 430 50/0.003 867 61 = 34.76, with 2 and 6 df. From the *F* table in *Appendix B.1* it is apparent that this ratio is highly significant ($P < 0.001$) so the conclusion is the same as that reached from the restricted model. In this example the interaction is not significant and no conflict of interpretation arises. Such a conflict could arise if the interaction effect is significant and therefore $MS_{interaction}$ is larger than MS_{error}. Assuming a restricted model, the random effect is compared with the error. In the unrestricted model it is compared with the interaction. Thus in the restricted model the overall random effect may be judged significant whereas in the unrestricted model it may be judged non-significant. However, even if overall it is deemed not to be a significant effect the presence of the significant interaction indicates that the effect of the random effect differs according to the level of the fixed effect, so some differences in the random effect are indicated.

The loblolly pine data are also analysed by a two-factor crossed ANOVA, but here both factors (date of sowing and method of ground clearing) are fixed effects. This second example is included to illustrate the interpretation of a fixed effects model, and the identification of interaction effects. *Figure 9* is the *Minitab* output for these data using the ANOVA command. (The data were stored in column C2 of the worksheet and the dates and burning

```
MTB > anova c2=c3¦c4

Factor      Type Levels Values
date       fixed      6      1      2      3      4      5      6
burning    fixed      2      1      2

Analysis of Variance for seedling

Source            DF          SS          MS        F        P
date               5     7500086     1500017    68.88    0.000
burning            1      369252      369252    16.96    0.000
date*burning       5      686385      137277     6.30    0.000
Error             36      783925       21776
Total             47     9339648

MTB >
```

Figure 9. Two-way ANOVA table from *Minitab* for the loblolly pine data in *Table 2*. Fixed effects model assumed.

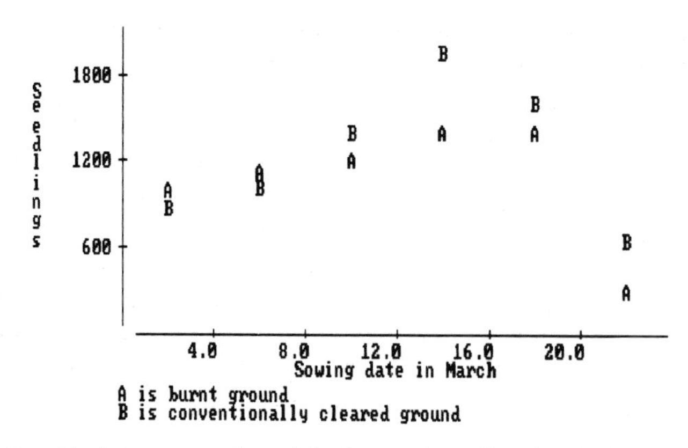

Figure 10. Graphical demonstration of the interaction effect for the loblolly pine data in *Table 2*.

classifications were in columns C3 and C4. Notice the abbreviated form of the model on the command line compared with *Figure 7*; a similar convention is used in *SAS*. Both abbreviated and full forms of the command have the same meaning. The *F*-ratios for both main effects, date, and burning, and for the interaction, are all significant with *P*-values less than 0.001. The conclusions are that there are overall differences in the mean number of seedlings germinated at different dates, and overall differences depending on whether the ground was cleared by burning or not. The significant interaction confuses this interpretation somewhat and is most easily sorted out by a graph. *Figure 10* is a plot of the cell means against date of sowing, with the different methods of ground clearing identified. It is clear from this figure that seedlings do better on burnt ground if sown early in March, but otherwise do worse. Also seedlings on conventionally cleared ground do much better than on burnt ground if sown in the middle of the month; the differences are not so great at other times. I strongly recommend the use of graphs to present information following an ANOVA. The ANOVA confirms that the differences presented are statistically significant, but the picture is worth the proverbial thousand words, and rather more than the raw statistics. *Figure 10* also suggests the possibility of using a parabola to predict the number of seedlings. This is investigated further in Chapter 4.

3.3 Two factors with one hierarchically nested within the other

It is vital to have replicates with hierarchically nested designs since, in the absence of replicate data, it is not possible to differentiate between the effect of the nested factor and the error. The linear model to describe the two-factor hierarchical design with factor B nested within A is

$$x_{ijk} = \mu + \alpha_i + \beta(\alpha)_{j(i)} + \varepsilon_{ijk}.$$

The third term on the right-hand side represents the effect of the jth level of factor B within the ith level of factor A. This replaces the two terms $\beta_j + \alpha\beta_{ij}$ in the two-factor crossed model, and in a balanced experiment with equal numbers of replicates per cell the sum of squares for the B within A effect can be derived by treating both factors as crossed and adding the factor B and interaction sums of squares. *Table 9* gives the E[MS] and restrictions for the various combinations of fixed and random effects. Notice that there is only one type of mixed model possible. If factor A is assumed random the effect $\beta(\alpha)_{j(i)}$ is assumed to be random whether the nested factor were assumed to be fixed or random. The mixed model with factor B assumed random does not impose any restrictions on the terms $\beta(\alpha)_{j(i)}$. The protocol for a two-factor hierarchical analysis of variance is as follows.

Table 9. Expected mean squares and restrictions on fixed effects for the two-factor hierarchical ANOVA with n replicates per cell

Source	**Fixed effects model**	**Random effects model**	**Mixed model, *B* random (unrestricted)**
Factor A	$\sigma^2 + nb\,\Sigma\alpha_i^2/(a-1)$	$\sigma^2 + n\sigma^2_{B(A)} + nb\sigma^2_A$	$\sigma^2 + n\sigma^2_{B(A)} + nb\,\Sigma\alpha_i^2/(a-1)$
B within A	$\sigma^2 + n\,\Sigma\beta(\alpha)^2_{j(i)}/a(b-1)$	$\sigma^2 + n\sigma^2_{B(A)}$	$\sigma^2 + n\sigma^2_{B(A)}$
Error	σ^2	σ^2	σ^2
Restrictions	$\Sigma\alpha_i = 0$ $\Sigma_j\alpha\beta_{j(i)} = 0$	N/A	$\Sigma\alpha_i = 0$

Protocol 3. Testing and estimation procedure for a two-factor hierarchical ANOVA

1. Decide whether the effects are fixed or random.
2. If both effects are fixed the F-tests for significance of effects are:
   - factor A: $F_A = \mathrm{MS}_A/\mathrm{MS}_{\mathrm{error}}$
   - factor B within factor A: $F_{\mathrm{B\ within\ }A} = \mathrm{MS}_{\mathrm{B\ within\ }A}/\mathrm{MS}_{\mathrm{error}}$

   Investigate significant effects further using multiple comparisons tests.
3. If both effects are random the F-tests are:
   - factor A: $F_A = \mathrm{MS}_A/\mathrm{MS}_{B\ \mathrm{within}\ A}$
   - factor B within factor A: $F_{B\ \mathrm{within}\ A} = \mathrm{MS}_{B\ \mathrm{within}\ A}/\mathrm{MS}_{\mathrm{error}}$

   There are three variance components. The formulas for estimating these from the MSs are:
   - error variance: $\mathrm{MS}_{\mathrm{error}}$
   - B within A: $(\mathrm{MS}_{B\ \mathrm{within}\ A} - \mathrm{MS}_{\mathrm{error}})/n$
   - factor A variance: $(\mathrm{MS}_A - \mathrm{MS}_{B\ \mathrm{within}\ A})/bn$

Protocol 3. *Continued*

4. If factor A is fixed and factor B random (a mixed model), the tests are exactly as in step 3, and the formulas for the error variance and B within A variance are also the same. No variance is calculated for the fixed factor A.

The two-factor hierarchical analysis of variance is illustrated by using just the data relating to postgraduate students from *Table 3*. Here the students are a hierarchical factor within water types because there are six students, two for each water type, and the students numbered 1 do not have anything in common with each other, no distinctive feature. Before the data are analysed, it is necessary to make a transformation to justify the assumptions of the ANOVA. A suitable transformation is $\log_e$. The necessity for this transformation was demonstrated in the example in Section 2. *Figure 11* is the *Minitab* output from the ANOVA for these logged data. The logged data were stored in column C2, the water type in C3 and the student number in C4. Note the specification of C4 as nested within C3 as C4(C3) in the model specification. The same convention is used in *SAS*. The F-ratio for students is 2.58 with 3 and 12 df, and this is not significant ($P = 0.102$), so no significant differences are identified between students. The F-ratio for waters is 321.42, with 2 and 12 df. This is highly significant ($P < 0.001$), so there are big differences between the mean numbers of heterotrophs from the three water types. (This probably would not surprise a microbiologist.) In view of the non-significant students' effects, the extraction of a variance component for students is

```
MTB > anova c2=c3 c4(c3);
SUBC> random c4;
SUBC> ems.

Factor              Type Levels Values
Waters             fixed      3      1      2      3
Students(Waters) random      2      1      2

Analysis of Variance for log N

Source              DF         SS         MS        F      P
Waters               2    106.269     53.135   321.42  0.000
Students(Waters)     3      0.496      0.165     2.58  0.102
Error               12      0.768      0.064
Total               17    107.533

Source              Variance Error  Expected Mean Square
                   component  term  (using unrestricted model)
 1 Waters                        2  (3) + 3(2) + Q[1]
 2 Students(Waters)  0.03378     3  (3) + 3(2)
 3 Error             0.06398        (3)

MTB >
```

Figure 11. Hierarchical ANOVA table from *Minitab* for the postgraduate data from *Table 3*. Mixed model assumed with students random and waters fixed.

unlikely to be of any practical importance, but for the purposes of illustration the calculation will be outlined. The variance for students is estimated as 0.033 78 and that for error as 0.063 98. Thus variation between students accounts
for 0.033 78/(0.033 78 + 0.063 98) = 0.346 of the total variance.

4. Balanced experiments with more than two factors

The general rules for writing down the linear model of a factorial experiment are now presented as *Protocol 4*.

Protocol 4. Rules for writing down the linear model for a factorial experiment

1. On the left-hand side write x followed by a list of subscripts, one for each factor and an additional one for the replicates.
2. On the right-hand side write a series of terms separated by + signs. The first term is μ (overall mean) and the last is ε (error).
3. Decide whether the factors are crossed or hierarchical.
4. Where there are two crossed factors, include both main effects and the two-factor interaction. If there is a third crossed factor, include the three-factor interaction as well as the additional main effect and two-factor interactions. With four factors there is a four-factor interaction, etc.
5. If one factor is hierarchically nested within another main factor, include only the main effect for the main factor and a single effect for the nested factor within the main factor. If a factor is nested within several other factors, all terms in the model relating to the nested factor include the factors within which it is nested.
6. Decide whether the factors are fixed or random. (If factors are fixed, restrictions are imposed but these are not of practical importance in balanced experiments.)
7. If any factor is assumed to be random then any term in the model including that factor is assumed to be a random variable. Ascribe a variance to each of these terms. The error is always assumed random and the mean is always fixed.

Protocol 5 describes the general procedure for the analysis of a balanced factorial experiment. A similar procedure is adopted in unbalanced experiments, but there are complications in the calculation of sums of squares and E[MS] (see Section 6).

Protocol 5. Procedure for the analysis of a balanced factorial experiment

1. Write down the linear model to describe the experiment, using *Protocol 4*.
2. Perform diagnostic checks using *Protocol 1* and transform the data if necessary.
3. Compute the ANOVA table with the correct model specified.
4. If all the effects are fixed, all MSs are compared with MS_{error}. If there are random effects work out the E[MS]. (*Minitab* or *SAS* can be used for this.)
5. Test for the significance of effects by finding MSs whose E[MS] differ by just one term.
6. Test the highest order interaction [a] first. If this is significant, investigate the interaction by graphs of means for the combinations of levels of factors in the interaction. If it is not significant test the next higher order interactions.
7. Test the next highest order interactions, and use graphical procedures to identify effect of significant interactions.
8. If no interactions are significant test the main effects. If interactions are significant the main effects are more complicated. The effect of a factor depends on the levels of other factors.
9. For significant fixed effects use multiple range tests (see Section 5) to identify those levels of the factor differing from others.
10. For random effects extract components of variance using the E[MS].

[a] The highest order interaction is that containing the most terms. Thus in a three-factor fully-crossed design the highest order interaction is the $A \times B \times C$ interaction.

The data on numbers of heterotrophs counted by Cardiff students and presented in *Table 3* will be used to illustrate these procedures. There are three factors: waters, PG–UG (whether a student is post or undergraduate), and students. Waters and PG–UG are crossed fixed factors. Students is hierarchically nested within waters and PG–UG, and could be regarded as fixed or random, depending on the desired interpretation. Here it is regarded as random. The linear model is

$$x_{ijkl} = \mu + \omega_i + \gamma_j + \omega\gamma_{ij} + \kappa(\omega\gamma)_{k(ij)} + \varepsilon_{ijkl}.$$

Here, i represents waters and ω_i their effects; j and γ_j are for PG–UG, and $\omega\gamma_{ij}$ is the interaction between these factors. The term $\kappa(\omega\gamma)_{k(ij)}$ is the effect for the kth student within the ith water jth PG–UG combination and are

```
MTB > anova c2=c3¦c5 c4(c3 c5);
SUBC> random c4;
SUBC> ems.


Factor                      Type Levels Values
Waters                     fixed      3      1      2      3
PG-UG                      fixed      2      1      2
Students(Waters PG-UG) random      2      1      2

Analysis of Variance for log N

Source                    DF         SS          MS        F       P
Waters                     2    230.897     115.449   898.56   0.000
PG-UG                      1      0.016       0.016     0.13   0.734
Waters*PG-UG               2      0.535       0.268     2.08   0.206
Students(Waters PG-UG)     6      0.771       0.128     1.00   0.451
Error                     24      3.099       0.129
Total                     35    235.318

Source                    Variance Error  Expected Mean Square
                         component  term  (using unrestricted model)
 1 Waters                              4  (5) + 3(4) + Q[1,3]
 2 PG-UG                               4  (5) + 3(4) + Q[2,3]
 3 Waters*PG-UG                        4  (5) + 3(4) + Q[3]
 4 Students(Waters PG-UG)  -0.00021    5  (5) + 3(4)
 5 Error                    0.12912       (5)

MTB >
```

Figure 12. ANOVA table from *Minitab* for the heterotroph data in *Table 3*. The model is discussed in the text.

assumed to have variance $\sigma^2_{K(WG)}$. The errors ε_{ijkl} are assumed to have variance σ^2.

In Section 2 the necessity of a transformation of these data was demonstrated to justify the assumptions of ANOVA. *Figure 12* is the *Minitab* output for the ANOVA of the logged data. The conclusion is straightforward: only the waters effect has a significant *F*-ratio, and that is hugely significant ($P < 0.001$). Notice the negative variance estimate for students within waters and PG–UG in the *E*[MS] table. Negative variances are impossible, and all that is indicated here is that, since there is no significant students' effect, the students and error mean squares are estimates of the same thing, the error variance σ^2. The sensible estimate of $\sigma^2_{K(NG)}$ is 0.

It was tempting for this example to invent more interesting data that showed significant differences in students that would have to be interpreted. However, experience with successive groups of students in Cardiff has shown that the main sources of variation in this plate-count method of estimation of bacterial counts are in different sample bottles and between plates from the same bottle and not between students. In the analysis just described, all 36 data have been treated as replicate plots, tacitly assuming that 12 equal samples of water were randomly selected from each water source and randomly divided up amongst postgraduates and undergraduates for counts to be estimated.

If the experiment were conducted differently and two sample bottles of each water type used, one each for postgraduates and undergraduates and the replicate counts were merely sub-samples from each bottle, then the interpretation would have been different. There are then two different kinds of plot. The first, called the main plot, is of sample bottles. The factors waters and PG–UG apply to these main plots. The second, called the sub-plot, is the sub-sample taken from each bottle and plated out. The factor students applies to these sub-plots. Such an experiment is called a split-plot, and requires a different model with two error terms, one for main plots and one for sub-plots. There is insufficient space here for further description of split-plots, Winer (1) gives further details. They are often performed unwittingly, and incorrect interpretation may follow. If the heterotroph counting experiment had been done this way then there would be no replicate for the waters × PG–UG combinations, and the only way of proceeding with an analysis would use the waters × PG–UG interaction as the main plot error.

5. Tests on means of main effects

A posteriori or *a priori* tests on means of main effects are done in multi-factorial experiments in the same way as described in Section 6 of Chapter 1. The method of orthogonal decomposition of sums of squares described in Section 6.1.2 of Chapter 1 is sometimes useful in identifying particular levels of a factor that differ from others. In principle the sum of squares due to a main effect in an ANOVA can be partitioned into components each of one df and each representing the amount of variability explained by a linear combination of effects in the model. It is not possible so to partition the sums of squares for every linear combination of effects. Some linear combinations of effects are said not to be estimable, that is, no combination of the observations exists whose expected value is the required linear combination. In a balanced experiment a linear contrast, that is, a linear combination of effects whose coefficients sum to zero, is always an estimable function. Moreover, two linear contrasts that are orthogonal (that is the sum of products of the corresponding coefficients is zero) have sums of squares that are independent of the order of inclusion of the contrasts in the model, and so may be independently assessed for significance. For further information on estimable functions, see Winer (1) and Milliken and Johnson (4). The decomposition of interactions by contrasts is described by Winer (1) and Sokal and Rohlf (2).

A linear contrast of effects α_i in a balanced experiment is a linear combination $\Sigma c_i\alpha_i$ such that $\Sigma c_i = 0$. Such a contrast is estimated by the linear combination $\Sigma c_i\bar{x}_i$ of the means $\bar{x}_i$ for the levels of the factor. Two contrasts $\Sigma c_i\alpha_i$ and $\Sigma d_i\alpha_i$ are orthogonal if $\Sigma c_i d_i = 0$. The formula for the sum of squares due to a linear contrast is $n' [\Sigma c_i\bar{x}_i]^2/\Sigma c_i^2$, where n' is the number of observations at each level of the factor. This formula gives the same answer as that given in Chapter 1. A sum of squares with a-1 df can be decomposed into

a-1 components, each with 1 df, representing orthogonal linear contrasts, and the sums of squares for these contrasts adds to the sum of squares for the effect.

To illustrate the calculations, and the ideas of linear contrasts, the wheat yield data of *Table 1* will be further analysed. In this analysis the farms will be regarded as fixed effects and the reason for the significance of the farms effect is identified. The mean yields for the three farms are respectively 0.418 75, 0.550 25, and 0.291 00. Each mean is calculted from 8 observations, so $n' = 8$. If the three farm effects are represented as ϕ_1, ϕ_2, and ϕ_3, the linear combination $\phi_1 - 0.5\phi_2 - 0.5\phi_3$ effects a comparison between farm 1 and the average of the other two. The estimate of the contrast is $0.418\,75 - 0.275\,13 - 0.145\,50 = 0.001\,88$ and the sum of squares is $8 \times (0.001\,88)^2/\{1^2 + (-0.5)^2 + (-0.5)^2\} = 1.885 \times 10^{-5}$. Once the first contrast has been chosen, the choice of a second is restricted by the requirement for orthogonality $\Sigma c_i d_i = 0$, and with only 2 df there is only one remaining orthogonal contrast. This is $\phi_2 - \phi_3$, and this contrast compares farms 2 and 3. The value of this contrast is $0.550\,25 - 0.291\,00 = 0.259\,25$ and the sum of squares is $8 \times (0.259\,25)^2/(1^2 + (-1)^2 = 0.268\,842$. These two components add to the sum of squares for farms with 2 df in the analysis of these data in Section 3.2 (the difference in the fifth place of decimals is due to rounding error in the calculations just presented). Sums of squares due to contrasts are available within the GLM procedure of *SAS*, and are specified by the CONTRAST statement. *Figure 13* gives part of the *SAS* output for these data with the two contrasts selected as above. It can be verified that the sums of squares for the contrasts add to the farms sum of squares. It is clear that the contrast

```
data farm;
infile 'a:farm.dat';
input yield farm variety;
proc glm;
     class farm variety;
     model yield=farm|variety;
     contrast 'farm 1 v others' farm 1 -.5 -.5;
     contrast 'farm 2 v farm 3' farm 0 1 -1;
run;
```

Source	DF	Type I SS	Mean Square	F Value	Pr > F
FARM	2	0.26886100	0.13443050	61.33	0.0001
VARIETY	3	0.03849433	0.01283144	5.85	0.0106
FARM*VARIETY	6	0.02320567	0.00386761	1.76	0.1895

Source	DF	Type III SS	Mean Square	F Value	Pr > F
FARM	2	0.26886100	0.13443050	61.33	0.0001
VARIETY	3	0.03849433	0.01283144	5.85	0.0106
FARM*VARIETY	6	0.02320567	0.00386761	1.76	0.1895

Contrast	DF	Contrast SS	Mean Square	F Value	Pr > F
farm 1 v others	1	0.00001875	0.00001875	0.01	0.9278
farm 2 v farm 3	1	0.26884225	0.26884225	122.64	0.0001

Figure 13. Part of *SAS* output for ANOVA on wheat yield data in *Table 1*, illustrating the specification of contrasts in the GLM procedure.

comparing farms 2 and 3 is the major component of the difference between farms, caused by the low yields obtained on farm 3.

In a model with all terms fixed the LSD or Tukey–Kramer procedures described respectively in Sections 6.1.1 and 6.2.1 of Chapter 1 are easily adapted to multi-factorial models. The n_i and n_j are the number of data from which the means to be compared are calculated and a is the total number of means amongst which the comparisons are made. Thus for a comparison of the farm means $n_i = n_j = 8$ and $a = 3$ (the total number of farms). $MS_{error} = 0.002\,192$ (from *Figure 7*; the error is calculated in the same way regardless of the factors being fixed or random). $Q_{0.05(3,12)} = 3.773$ (from *Appendix B.7*). Thus

$$\text{MSD} = 3.773\sqrt{\frac{0.002\,192(1/8 + 1/8)}{2}} = 0.062\,45.$$

The difference in mean yields for farms 2 and 3 is greater than this (0.2593), so these farms are significantly different. Farms 1 and 3 and farms 1 and 2 also differ significantly. The differences in means are 0.1278 and 0.1315 respectively and both differences are more than 0.062 45.

6. Unbalanced experiments

In principle it is possible to work out the sums of squares corresponding to the effects in a linear model for unbalanced data, though the formulas given in *Appendix 2.1* do not apply. The calculations needed for unbalanced data are lengthy, and computer packages therefore have to be used, but there are also difficulties of interpretation. In a balanced experiment the sum of squares due to the main effect of a factor A plus the sum of squares due to a factor B with which A is crossed is the same as the sum of squares for both main effects together. The effects are said to be orthogonal. In an unbalanced experiment the effects are not orthogonal and the change in the sum of squares when the effect corresponding to factor A is introduced into the model depends on the other factors included. Several ways have been suggested for interpreting unbalanced experiments. Four such ways, called Types I to IV, are identified by Milliken and Johnson (4), and these are calculated in the *SAS* GLM procedure. *Minitab* (release 7) and *SPSS/PC+* also allow the calculation of ANOVA tables for unbalanced data. It is particularly difficult to analyse data sets for factorial experiments where some cells have no data. In general, care has to be exercised in the use of packages since it is easy to misunderstand the manuals and wrongly interpret the output.

Further difficulties arise in the calculation of the E[MS] tables for unbalanced data where there are random effects in the model. There are several ways of obtaining estimates of variance components. *SAS* gives a choice of methods in the VARCOMP and GLM procedures. Neither *Minitab* nor *SPSS/PC+* have commands for these calculations.

6.1 Missing data

Where observations are missing in an otherwise balanced experiment an approximate procedure is to fill in the missing observations with values derived from the remaining data and analyse the experiment as if it were balanced, but reducing the total and error df by the number of missing observations. In an experiment with replicates the cell mean is often used as the surrogate for the missing observation. In the two-factor crossed experiment with no replicates a single missing observation, i in the (i,j)th cell, is replaced by the value calculated from the formula:

$$\hat{x}_{ij} = (a\, X_i + b\, X_j - G)/(a - 1)(b - 1),$$

where X_i is the total of the $b - 1$ observations actually obtained at the ith level of factor A, X_j is the total of the $a - 1$ observations obtained at the jth level of factor B, G is the overall total of all the data obtained, and a and b are the number of levels of factors A and B respectively.

Suppose the first replicate only of the wheat yield data in *Table 1* is analysed and that the observation of 0.500 for variety 2 in farm 1 is missing. The total X_1 of the three observations available from farm 1 is 1.24 and the total X_2 of the two observations for variety 2 is 0.907. The overall total of the 11 data is 4.648. The formula for the missing value then gives $(3 \times 1.24 + 4 \times 0.907 - 4.648)/2 \times 3 = 0.45$. This value replaces the missing observation and the data analysed as if it were a genuine observation, but the error df are now 5 and the total df are 10. Since the error df is calculated automatically, assuming no missing data, in *Minitab, SPSS/PC+*, or *SAS*, MS_{error} has to be calculated by hand. Thus all F-ratios must also be recalculated.

6.2 The method of unweighted means

If the discrepancies in numbers of data n_{ij} in the cells of a factorial experiment are not large, an approximate procedure known as the method of unweighted means can be used. The method is described below for the two-factor crossed ANOVA. Calculate the harmonic mean $\tilde{n}$ of the n_{ij}s (by taking the arithmetic mean of the reciprocals of the n_{ij}s and taking the reciprocal of this mean). The formula for the harmonic mean of the n_{ij}s is

$$\tilde{n} = \left(\frac{\Sigma_i \Sigma_j (1/n_{ij})}{ab}\right)^{-1}.$$

Then perform a two-factor crossed ANOVA (with no replicates) on the arithmetic means of the data in each cell. The factor A and factor B sums of squares are multiplied by $\tilde{n}$ to give approximations to the correct main effects sums of squares. The error sum of squares is multiplied by $\tilde{n}$ to give an approximation to the interaction. The approximate table is completed by working out the pooled within cell sum of squares. The easiest way to do this is to do a one-way ANOVA with the cells as the groups.

(a)

ROWS: date COLUMNS: burning

	1	2	ALL
1	870.0	1006.7	938.3
2	1115.0	1156.7	1140.0
3	1410.0	1223.3	1316.7
4	1855.0	1390.0	1622.5
5	1646.7	1400.0	1505.7
6	645.0	280.0	488.6
ALL	1194.1	1076.7	1133.7

CELL CONTENTS --
seedling:MEAN

(b)

Analysis of Variance for meanseed

Source	DF	SS	MS	F	P
date	5	1812865	362573	13.46	0.006
burning	1	98102	98102	3.64	0.115
Error	5	134674	26935		
Total	11	2045641			

(c)

ANALYSIS OF VARIANCE ON seedling

SOURCE	DF	SS	MS	F	p
Cells	11	5899150	536286	19.70	0.000
ERROR	23	626267	27229		
TOTAL	34	6525417			

(d)

Source	DF	SS	MS	F
date	5	5020240	1004048	36.87
burning	1	271667	271667	9.98
date*burning	5	372943	74589	2.74
ERROR	23	626267	27229	
TOTAL	34	6525417		

Figure 14. Steps in the unweighted means ANOVA for the loblolly pine data in *Table 2* with observations marked * assumed missing: (a) table of cell means; (b) two-way ANOVA on cell means; (c) one-way ANOVA with cells as groups; (d) complete unweighted means ANOVA table.

The method is illustrated by an analysis of the data set obtained when those observations marked by an asterisk in *Table 2* are assumed to be missing. The harmonic mean of the n_{ij}s of this depleted data set is 2.769 23. *Figure 14* contains output from three steps in *Minitab* by which the unweighted means analysis can be done. *Figure 14a* is the table of cell means and in *Figure 14b* is the two-way crossed ANOVA for these cell means. *Figure 14c* is the one-way ANOVA for the depleted data with cells as groups. Finally, *Figure 14d* is the complete ANOVA table. This has to be calculated by hand. The last two lines for error and total are copied directly from the one-way ANOVA with cells as groups. The df for date, burning and the date × burning interaction are the same as those of the date burning and error respectively from the two-way ANOVA on cell means. The sums of squares for these three sources of variation are each multiplied by the harmonic mean $\tilde{n}$, in this case 2.769 23. Thus for the dates, the sum of squares is 2.769 23 × 1 812 865 = 5 02040. The MSs are calculated by hand by dividing the SS by the df. Finally the *F*-ratios are calculated according to the rules given in *Protocol 2*. In this case, with both effects assumed fixed, the denominator for all three ratios is MS_{error}.

6.3 An introduction to methods for unbalanced ANOVA

The calculation of the sums of squares will be illustrated by analyses of the depleted loblolly pine data using the *Minitab* GLM command (*Figure 15*) and the *SAS* GLM procedure (*Figure 16*). Notice first that the Source and df columns are the same for all analyses. Also the Total and Error sums of squares are the same as the one-way ANOVA with cells as groups (see *Figure 14c*). This will be the case whichever method of calculation is used: it is the decomposition of the sum of squares for the model which differs. In the sequential SS column of the *Minitab* output, the terms are included in the model in the order specified in the command line. Thus the SS due to date on its own is 5 267 869, and the extra SS accounted for by burning with date included is 274 345. The SS due to the interaction after both main effects are included is 356 938. The Type I SS given by *SAS* is the same as this sequential SS. The adjusted SS of *Minitab* gives the sums of squares for each term when that term is included last in the model. It is these sums of squares that *Minitab* uses for calculation of MS, *F*, and *P* columns. The Type III SS given by *SAS* is the same as this adjusted SS and if the tests of the hypotheses that the effects are zero are of interest, then it is these Type III (or adjusted) SS that should be interpreted. However, the Type III sums of squares do not, in an unbalanced experiment, add up to the total explained by the model, and if the building of a model is of interest, then the Type I (or Type II) sums of squares should be used. The Type II sums of squares are the extra explained when that term is included with all other terms of the same order. Thus the SS for dates when burning (but not the interaction) is included is 5 421 608. For data sets with no empty cells the Type III and Type IV SS are the same. For information on the distinction between these types see Milliken and Johnson (4). There is little difficulty in interpreting these data, though the interaction is only marginally significant. Compare this with the conclusion reached from the analysis of the complete data set in Section 3, where the interaction was highly significant. The assumed loss of the 13 observations has reduced the sensitivity of the statistical tests.

```
MTB > glm c2=c3¦c4

Factor    Levels Values
date           6      1      2      3      4      5      6
burning        2      1      2

Analysis of Variance for seedling

Source         DF      Seq SS      Adj SS      Adj MS        F       P
date            5     5267869     5515767     1103153    40.51   0.000
burning         1      274345      271667      271667     9.98   0.004
date*burning    5      356938      356938       71388     2.62   0.051
Error          23      626267      626267       27229
Total          34     6525417

Unusual Observations for seedling

Obs. seedling         Fit Stdev.Fit  Residual     St.Resid
  2   1960.00     1646.67      95.27     313.33        2.33R
 21   1310.00     1646.67      95.27    -336.67       -2.50R

R denotes an obs. with a large st. resid.

MTB >
MTB >
```

Figure 15. *Minitab* output of ANOVA for the loblolly pine data in *Table 2* with the observations marked * assumed missing.

Finally, the *Minitab* GLM output warns that two of the data should be considered as possible outliers, with large standardized residuals. These are not too far outside the criterion of ± 2.0 however, and have been included in the analysis.

7. Designing experiments

The design of experiments is often overlooked until the data are analysed, by which time inadequacies of the original design cannot be rectified. Winer (1) gives some guidance on the design of factorial experiments and most texts on experimental design discuss the conduct of the experiment. I recommend the first two chapters of Cochran and Cox (8) as particularly helpful. Cox (9) wrote a complete book on the subject of planning experiments. A most useful checklist was published some years ago by the Institute of Terrestrial Ecology (10), but this may not be easily available in libraries. The following list gives some guidance on the considerations of experimental design:

- state the objectives of the experiment and make sure that the experiment will answer the objectives
- consider all available relevant information, using a pilot experiment where necessary
- choose the response variable (the observation) so that it genuinely provides useful information

```
data pine;
infile 'a:pinedel.dat';
input seedling date burning;
proc glm;
     class date burning;
     model seedling=date|burning/ss1 ss2 ss3 ss4;
run;
```

```
                        General Linear Models Procedure

Dependent Variable: SEEDLING
                                      Sum of            Mean
Source                  DF           Squares          Square    F Value      Pr > F

Model                   11       5899150.476      536286.407      19.70      0.0001

Error                   23        626266.667       27228.986

Corrected Total         34       6525417.143

                  R-Square              C.V.        Root MSE          SEEDLING Mean

                  0.904027          14.55500        165.0121             1133.71429

Source                  DF       Type I SS     Mean Square    F Value      Pr > F

DATE                     5     5267868.333     1053573.667      38.69      0.0001
BURNING                  1      274344.607      274344.607      10.08      0.0042
DATE*BURNING             5      356937.535       71387.507       2.62      0.0512

Source                  DF      Type II SS     Mean Square    F Value      Pr > F

DATE                     5     5421607.563     1084321.513      39.82      0.0001
BURNING                  1      274344.607      274344.607      10.08      0.0042
DATE*BURNING             5      356937.535       71387.507       2.62      0.0512

Source                  DF     Type III SS     Mean Square    F Value      Pr > F

DATE                     5     5515766.343     1103153.269      40.51      0.0001
BURNING                  1      271667.308      271667.308       9.98      0.0044
DATE*BURNING             5      356937.535       71387.507       2.62      0.0512

Source                  DF      Type IV SS     Mean Square    F Value      Pr > F

DATE                     5     5515766.343     1103153.269      40.51      0.0001
BURNING                  1      271667.308      271667.308       9.98      0.0044
DATE*BURNING             5      356937.535       71387.507       2.62      0.0512
```

Figure 16. *SAS* output of ANOVA for the loblolly pine data in *Table 2* with the observations marked * assumed missing.

- choose the factors to investigate so that the experiment is representative and informative, paying particular attention to the control of the levels of the factors
- consider the nature of the experimental units or plots carefully, ensuring these are representative; watch out for split plots
- ensure that the plots are homogeneous and, if necessary, divide them into blocks and include blocks as a factor in the analysis
- make certain that sufficient replicates are used to assess all effects and interactions, using prior information on variability

- allocate combinations of factors to plots at random, within the constraints of the design, so as to eliminate bias
- monitor the conduct of the experiment and keep a detailed accurate record of all relevant facts
- use statistical analysis to show objectively those differences between factors that are genuinely significant and those that are merely random fluctuations.

References

1. Winer, B. J. (1971). *Statistical principles in experimental design*. McGraw-Hill, New York.
2. Sokal, R. R. and Rohlf, F. J. (1981). *Biometry*. W. H. Freeman, San Francisco.
3. Miller, R. G. (1986). *Beyond ANOVA: basics of applied statistics*. John Wiley, New York.
4. Milliken, G. A. and Johnson, D. E. (1984). *Analysis of messy data. Volume 1: Designed experiments*. Van Nostrand Reinhold, New York.
5. Hoaglin, D. C., Mosteller, F., and Tukey, J. W. (1983). *Understanding robust and exploratory data analysis*. John Wiley, New York.
6. Hoaglin, D. C., Mosteller, F., and Tukey, J. W. (1985). *Exploring data tables, trends and shapes*. John Wiley, New York.
7. Searle, S. R. (1971). *Linear models*. John Wiley, New York.
8. Cochran, W. G. and Cox, G. M. (1957). *Experimental designs*. John Wiley, New York.
9. Cox, D. R. (1958). *Planning of experiments*. John Wiley, New York.
10. Jeffers, J. N. R. *Statistical checklist 1. Design of experiments*. Institute of Terrestrial Ecology (Natural Environmental Research Council), Cambridge.

Appendix 2.1. Calculations for the analysis of variance of balanced factorial experiments

1. One-way ANOVA

Calculate the totals g_i for the data at each of the a levels of the factor, and also the overall total G of all the data. The correction factor, abbreviated to CF, is G^2/N, where N is the total number of data. A term denoted by SS_G is calculated from the group totals as $\Sigma g_i^2/n_i$, where n_i is the number of data in the ith group. Finally calculate the sum of squares Σx^2 of all the data. Then the ANOVA table is:

Source of variation	df	SS	MS	F
Groups	$a - 1$	$SS_G - CF$	*	*
Error	$N - a$	$\Sigma x^2 - SS_G$	*	
Total	$N - 1$	$\Sigma x^2 - CF$		

The two mean squares are calculated as the respective ratios of sum of squares to degrees of freedom. The F-ratio is the ratio of the two mean squares.

2. Two-way crossed ANOVA

Suppose the two factors are A and B with a and b levels respectively and that there are n replicate data in each cell. The sums of squares for the main effects of A and B are calculated in a manner analogous to that of the one-way layout as $SS_A - CF$ with $(a - 1)$ df and $SS_B - CF$ with $(b - 1)$ df respectively. To calculate the interaction sum of squares calculate the totals for each cell (each combination of levels of the two factors A and B). SS_{AB} is calculated from these totals by squaring the totals, dividing by n and adding. The interaction sum of squares is then $(SS_{AB} - SS_A - SS_B + CF)$ with $(a - 1)(b - 1)$ df. The layout of the ANOVA table is:

Source of variation	df	SS	MS	F
Factor A	$a - 1$	$SS_A - CF$	*	*
Factor B	$b - 1$	$SS_B - CF$	*	*
Interaction $A \times B$	$(a - 1)(b - 1)$	$(SS_{AB} - SS_A - SS_B + CF)$	*	*
Error	$ab(n - 1)$	$\Sigma x^2 - SS_{AB}$	*	
Total	$abn - 1$	$\Sigma x^2 - CF$		

Each mean square is the ratio of sum of squares to degrees of freedom. The F ratios calculated depend on whether the factors are fixed or random effects (see *Protocol 2*).

3. Hierarchical ANOVA (two factors)

Suppose factor B is nested within factor A. The ANOVA table, using the same notation as for the crossed ANOVA, is:

Source of variation	df	SS	MS	F
Factor A	$a - 1$	$SS_A - CF$	*	*
Factor B within A	$a(b - 1)$	$SS_{AB} - SS_A$	*	*
Error	$ab(n - 1)$	$\Sigma x^2 - SS_{AB}$	*	
Total	$abn - 1$	$\Sigma x^2 - CF$		

The mean squares are ratios of sums of squares to degrees of freedom, and the F ratios depend on whether the factors are fixed or random effects (see *Protocol 3*).

Appendix 2.1. *(contd.)*

4. More than two factors
The formula for the sum of squares of the $A \times B \times C$ interaction in an experiment where all three factors are crossed is

$$SS_{ABC} - SS_{AB} - SS_{AC} - SS_{BC} + SS_A + SS_B + SS_C - CF$$

with $(a-1)(b-1)(c-1)$ df.

If C is nested within B, and B is nested within A, the C within B within A sum of squares is $SS_{ABC} - SS_{AB}$ with $ab(c-1)$ df. If C is crossed with B and both are hierarchical within A, the $B \times C$ within A sum of squares is $SS_{ABC} - SS_{AB} - SS_{AC} + SS_A$ with $a(b-1)(c-1)$ df.

These examples identify the pattern in the calculation of sums of squares and degrees of freedom for any balanced factorial experiment.

Appendix 2.2. Expressions for the E[MS] in factorial experiments

The error term is assumed to have variance σ^2 and the variances associated with random effects are σ^2_X where X is a string of letters, for example σ^2_{AB} for $\alpha\beta_{ij}$ with A and B crossed or $\sigma^2_{B(A)}$ for $\beta(\alpha)_{j(i)}$ with B nested within A. Start off with variances for fixed effects as well, but at the end of the procedure these are changed to sums of squared effects divided by degrees of freedom, so σ^2_{AB} would be changed to $\Sigma\alpha\beta^2_{ij}/(a-1)(b-1)$. The rules for the E[MS] are:

1. The error MS has expectation σ^2. All other terms include a linear combination of other σ^2_X.
2. Each term in the E[MS], except σ^2, is multiplied by n (the number of replicates per cell) and possibly other factors.
3. The E[MS] for any effect or interaction includes terms for all σ^2_X where X includes all the letters in the effect. For example, in a three-factor crossed experiment the E[MS] for the $A \times B$ interaction includes σ^2_{ABC} and σ^2_{AB} (as well as σ^2). If an effect is nested the expected value of its MS includes σ^2_X where X includes the nested effect.
4. Multiply each σ^2_X by the product of numbers of levels of factors in the experiment, but not in the list X. For example, in a three-factor crossed experiment multiply the σ^2_{AB} term by c (as well as n).
5. Multiply each σ^2_X by a factor for each letter in X but which is not in the source of variation. Thus, in the E[MS] for $A \times B$ in a three-factor crossed experiment a factor is needed for factor C in the σ^2_{ABC} term. The factor is 1 for all bracketed factors (for factors in hierarchical experiments in which other factors are nested) or for random effects where an infinite population is assumed. It is $(1-f)$ for random effects where a finite population is assumed and the fraction of the population sampled is f. It is zero for fixed effects.

3

Bivariate regression

JOHN C. FRY

1. Introduction

All biologists will use regression analysis between two variables at one time or another and all statistical packages have commands for performing bivariate or simple linear regression. Whole books have been written about regression analysis, but many are mathematically complex and impenetrable for most biologists. The easiest text I have found is by Chatterjee and Price (1). For more detail Sokal and Rohlf (2) and Rawlings (3) are also useful. These texts should be consulted by readers requiring longer or different explanations. As in Chapter 1, I will use examples analysed with four statistical packages *Minitab, SPSS/PC+*, *Systat,* and *Statgraphics*. However, in this chapter almost all my sample output will be from *Minitab*. I will only provide sample output from the other packages when *Minitab* does not provide the necessary procedures. All four packages and many more besides provide excellent facilities for bivariate regression analysis.

1.1 Data structure

Any data set which has two variables in which the two sets of numbers are paired is a candidate for regression. This is the type of data which you would normally plot on a simple two-dimensional graph to examine the relationship between the two variables. One variable, y, would normally be plotted on the vertical axis and is called the dependent variable. The other variable x is plotted horizontally and is the independent or predictor variable. Each point on the graph is represented by a yx data pair and there are n points. Regression calculates a line of best fit through the data and aims to minimize in some way the distance between the data points and the line. These distances are called residuals (e) and are calculated from the difference between the y value of the data point, y_i, and the value of y at the corresponding value of x_i that lies on the line of best fit, called $\hat{y}$ or the predicted y value. The basic equation for the linear regression of y upon x is

$$y = \beta_o + \beta x + \varepsilon, \tag{1}$$

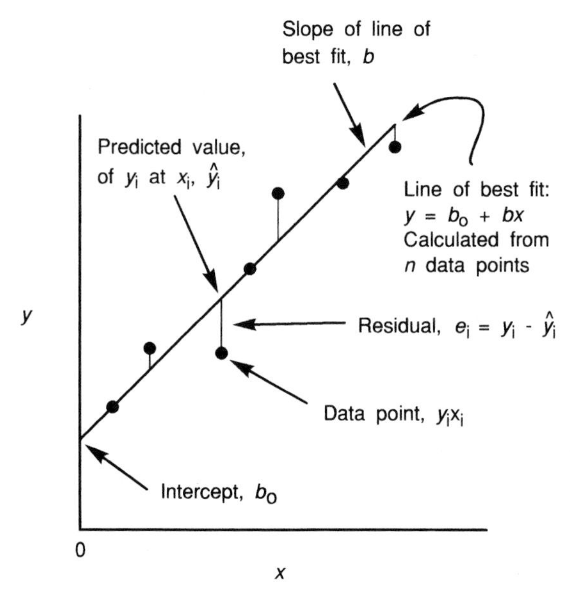

Figure 1. Diagrammatic representation of the key features of linear bivariate regression.

where β_o is the $\hat{y}$ value when $x = 0$, or the intercept of the line of best fit on the y axis, and β is the slope of the line. β_o and β are constants which are normally estimated as the regression coefficients b_o and b respectively, our best estimate of the error term ε comes from the residuals ($e_1 \ldots e_n$). This is represented diagrammatically in *Figure 1*.

1.2 Uses of regression

There are two main uses of bivariate regression:

- to provide a prediction equation for y based on x
- to understand the relationship between y and x

Prediction equations are useful for many diverse purposes, for example for calibration curves or for predicting simple relationships like the rate of an enzymic reaction given a certain concentration of substrate. Such equations use all the data and so provide summary statistics. Regression analysis is straightforward with most statistical packages and will provide much better estimates than those obtained from lines fitted by eye. Regression will also help biologists understand whether variables are linearly related or not, or whether the relationship is linear only after transformation of x or y by, say, $\log_{10}$, square root, or reciprocal. There are also techniques for fitting data which show non-linear or curved relationships.

1.3 Data sets used here

Four data sets are used in this chapter (*Appendix 3.1*). The optical density (OD) data are an example of a calibration curve in which the dry weight of bacteria in a culture could be estimated from the true optical density of the suspension. This was measured after dilution to less than OD = 0.6 and then back-calculated to allow for the dilution used; this should theoretically ensure a linear relationship between the two variables. The child data consist of children's heights over a narrow range of ages (4). The enzyme data are from an experiment to investigate the effect of puromycin treatment on the relationship between substrate concentration and reaction velocity for a simple enzymic reaction (5). The child and OD data have one value of y for each x value and the enzyme data have two values of y for all but one x value. This latter type of data structure is included because biologists often perform replicate estimations. The rotenone data are typical of the dose–response experiments often used in pharmacology, toxicology, and other branches of biology. These data (6) are derived from an experiment to test the effect of the pesticide rotenone on the chrysanthemum aphis, in batches of 50 insects for each of the pesticide concentrations used.

1.4 Simple plots of the data

The basic route through a bivariate regression problem is given in *Protocol 1*. Once it has been decided which is the x variable and which the y variable, it is essential to plot the data with the y variable on the vertical axis and the x variable on the horizontal axis. In this way we can easily see if the variables are linearly related and the degree of variability about the straight line. This step should never be omitted. The OD data are clearly linearly related with little scatter (*Figure 2a*). The child data are very scattered (*Figure 2b*) and from this plot it is not really clear whether there is any significant linear relationship or not. The enzyme data are non-linear and show two clear curves (*Figure 2c*) as velocity (v) reaches a maximum value with increasing substrate concentration (s); this appears to be a typical Michaelis–Menten relationship. The rotenone data are also non-linear, showing a clear sigmoidal relationship (*Figure 2d*). All the plots in *Figure 2* are made with simple text-based output and illustrate that this style of plot is quite sufficient for most purposes during routine regression analysis. It is only necessary to use higher-resolution graphics output for special purposes (e.g. for confidence intervals and lines of best fit) or for final presentation of the data.

Protocol 1. Route through a bivariate regression analysis

1. Decide which variable is to be y and which is to be x (NB y is predicted from x).

Protocol 1. *Continued*

2. Plot data; y as vertical axis, x as horizontal axis. If line looks curved rather than approximately linear go to *Protocol 3*.
3. Check evenness of x and y variables with
   - boxplots
   - letter value displays
   - histograms
4. Transform x and/or y if not even; use ladder of powers to find suitable transformation (e.g. x^2, $\sqrt{y}$, $\log_{10}y$, $1/x$) or the transformation plot for symmetry (see Section 2.1).
5. Compute regression, save residuals, fitted y values ($\hat{y}$) and influence statistics (leverage, Cook's D and Dfits), calculate Durbin–Watson statistic if data are in a logical order.
6. Plot studentized deleted or standardized residuals against
   - fitted values, $\hat{y}$
   - x variable
   - the sequence of observations, if in a logical order

   Examine residual plots for outliers, data points a long way from the rest. Consider rejection of outliers with studentized deleted or standardized residuals > 2 and return to step 5.
7. Compare influence statistics with critical values
   - leverage $> 2p'/n$
   - Cook's $D > F_{0.5(p',n\text{-}p')}$ or $4/n$
   - Dfits $>$ absolute value of $\sqrt{p'/n}$

   Where p' = the number of parameters in the model ($b_o = 1$ parameter; $b = 1$ parameter) and n = number of data points in the regression. If two or more influence statistics are greater than the critical values consider rejecting points and return to step 5.
8. If outliers or leverage points seem a problem and all the data are accurate consider using a robust regression method
   - three-group resistant line
   - linear regression using least absolute residuals or minimized χ^2

1.5 Assumptions

The basic assumptions upon which the calculations done by the standard least squares regression analysis available in most statistical packages depend are:

- x and y are linearly related by equation (1)
- x and y are measured for each of n observations

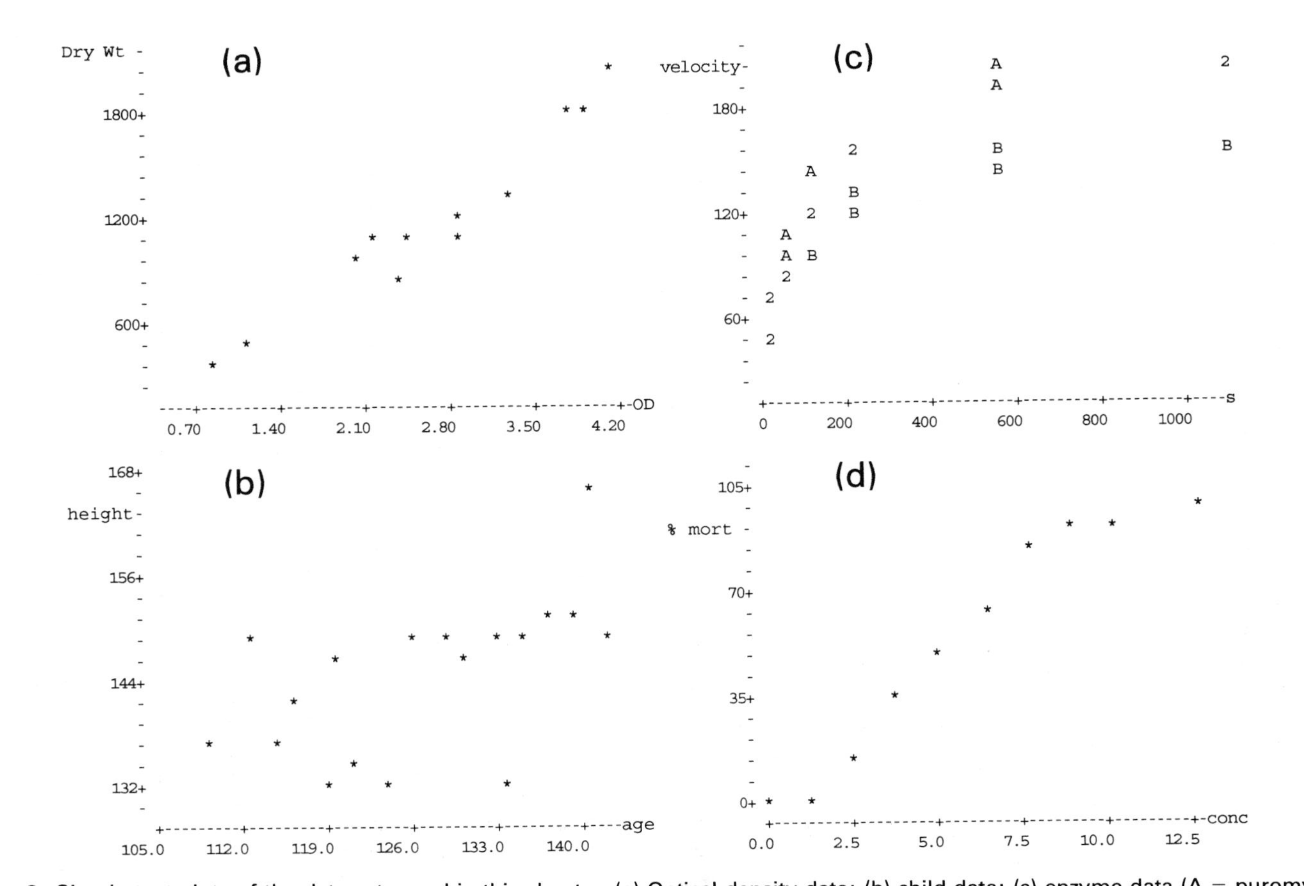

Figure 2. Simple text plots of the data sets used in this chapter. (a) Optical density data; (b) child data; (c) enzyme data (A = puromycin treated; B = untreated; 2 = two points plotted in one character position); (d) rotenone data.

- x is measured without error
- y is a set of random observations measured with error
- the variance of the y observations is constant
- the errors (ε) of y are normally distributed
- the errors of y are mutually independant

Most computer packages will produce output from data with missing x or y values. It can sometimes be useful to provide extra x values without corresponding y values. If this is done, the data with both x and y values will be used for calculating the basic regression statistics, such as the line of best fit and the residuals. However, $\hat{y}$, some influence statistics (e.g. leverage—see Section 2.3.3), and the confidence intervals will be calculated for all x values.

In theory only y should be measured with error: if x also has error then the regression calculations will be wrong. Although it is possible to perform the regression calculations when x has error (2) this will not be discussed here. However, provided the errors of y are much greater than the errors of x few problems are likely to be encountered. I will describe later (Section 2.3.1) how to check for non-constant variance. The assumption of normality of errors is only required when significance tests are done on the regression statistics, confidence or prediction intervals are calculated, or when regression lines are compared. The errors do not need to be normally distributed to calculate a line of best fit nor to calculate predicted values from this line.

Another important point is that almost all standard regression procedures calculate regression statistics for the model with one y value for every x value. If there are replicate y values for the x values (e.g. enzyme data) the line of best fit is calculated in the same way, but some of the regression statistics can be calculated differently to give more information (see Section 2.6).

2. Least squares linear regression

Almost all standard regression commands in computer packages perform least squares regression as the main, primary procedure. In this type of regression the residuals are optimized by minimizing the sum of the squares of the residuals, and so the line of best fit calculated by this method is very sensitive to extreme data points. Although other methods are more robust (see Section 4), least squares regression is a very powerful approach from which a lot of useful information can be calculated which cannot be estimated using the more robust approaches. Hence it is probably the best method to try first.

2.1 Evenness of *x* and *y*

Regression analysis is far more likely to calculate an accurate line of best fit if the values of x and y are evenly spread through the range. This is easily tested

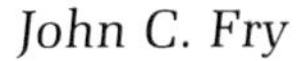

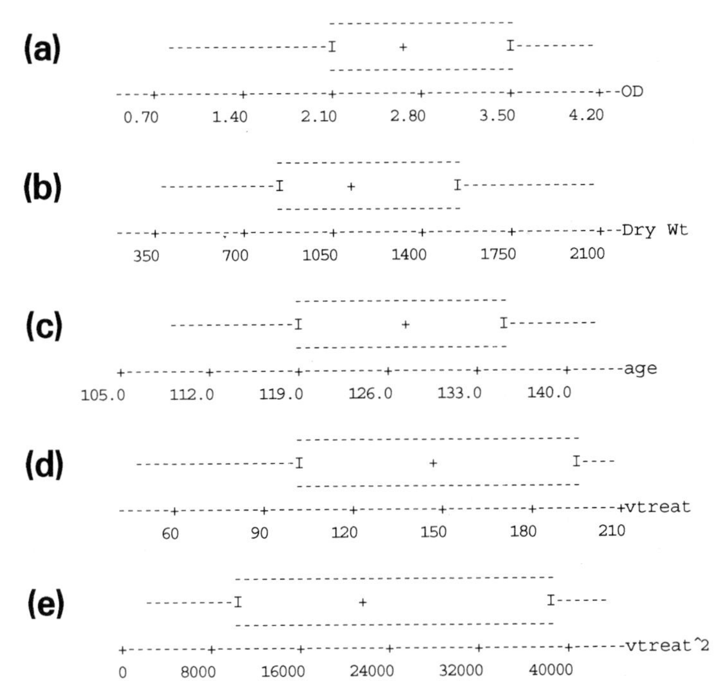

Figure 3. Boxplots from untransformed (a–d) and transformed (e; square transformation) x and y variables from the example data sets.

with simple graphical procedures (*Protocol 1*) like boxplots (Chapter 1, Section 3.2) and histograms. Letter value displays (Chapter 1, Section 4.3) can also be used, in which the midsummaries should be equal in a perfectly symmetrical distribution. *Figure 3a–d* shows boxplots of some variables from the example data sets. All are acceptably even.

If a variable was very uneven with several outside and/or far outside values on one side of the boxplot only (see Chapter 1, *Figure 5a* and Chapter 4, *Figure 4b*) then transformation might be necessary. Power transformations from the ladder of powers (Chapter 1, *Table 4*) can be used and the best one found by trial and error, moving along the ladder according to the shape of the distribution obtained. Data skewed to the right (with a long right tail) will use lower powers and left skewed data (with a long left tail) will need higher powers.

Emerson and Soto (7) describe a useful method for choosing a power transformation that will make data symmetrical. This is an exploratory data analysis technique and uses letter value displays. It is called the transformation plot for symmetry and is described below.

From the upper (L_U) and lower (L_L) letter values and the median (M) of the variable, two sets of statistics are calculated for each letter value. These are then plotted against each other with

$$\frac{L_L + L_U}{2} - M$$

on the vertical axis and

$$\frac{(L_U - M)^2 + (M - L_L)^2}{4M}$$

on the horizontal axis. These calculations are given in *Table 1* for the puromycin treated velocities for the enzyme data (which is slightly skewed left; *Figure 3d*) and the plot is in *Figure 4*. The slope (b) of the transformation plot is -1.37 and the appropriate power (p) transformation is calculated by

$$p = 1 - b,$$

which in this case is 2.37 ($p = 1 + 1.37$). This is close to the square transformation ($y^{2.37} \simeq y^2$) which gives an almost perfectly symmetrical boxplot (*Figure 3e*). This plot works better and is more useful with larger data sets.

Table 1. Calculations for the transformation plot for symmetry using the puromycin treated velocity from the enzyme data

Letter value	L_L	L_U	$\frac{L_L + L_U}{2} - M$	$\frac{(L_U - M)^2 + (M - L_L)^2}{4M}$
H	102	195.5	3.25	7.55
E	76	201	−7.0	13.59
D	47	207	−18.5	23.17
$M = 145.5$				

2.2 Performing regression and interpreting the output

The x and y variables must be put in separate columns for regression analysis with most packages. However, the method of defining the analysis to be done is very varied. I will give some examples for the child data where the y variable is called 'height' and the x called 'age', as in *Appendix 3.1*, in which it is intended to predict height from age. With *Minitab* the variables are defined by name or column number (assume 'age' in column 2 and 'height' in column 1) and the number of x variables must also be specified; hence the command is one of the following:

```
REGRESS 'HEIGHT' 1 'AGE'
REGRESS C1 1 C2
```

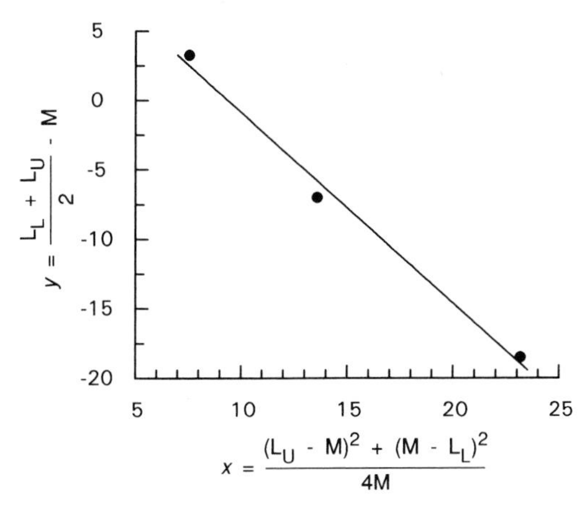

Figure 4. The transformation plot for symmetry with the puromycin treated velocities from the enzyme data.

With *Systat* the regression model is specified in a similar form to the regression equation; hence the command is

MODEL HEIGHT = CONSTANT + AGE

which is part of the MGLH commands. Alternatively, equivalent boxes can be filled in the menu mode of the program. *Statgraphics* relies entirely on filling in boxes for dependent variable (y) and independent variable (x) and toggling the model box to linear. With *SPSS/PC+* the corresponding command line would be

REGRESSION VARIABLES = AGE, HEIGHT/DEPENDENT = HEIGHT.

As can be seen in *Protocol 1* it is useful to save the residuals, y values and influence statistics (leverage, Cook's D, and Dfits). This is normally done in the same command set as the basic regression definition, with subcommands and/or command line extensions.

Figure 5 gives the standard output from *Minitab* with the regression line defined earlier. This is fairly typical of the output from several packages, so the key features of this output will be described.

The first two lines after the command line give the regression equation for calculating new values of height ($\hat{y}$) from age, so the intercept (b_0) is 79.7 and the slope (b) is 0.511. These values are also given in the coefficient column (Coef) below. The next column gives the standard errors of the two coefficients (called Stdev here; s_b for b and s_{b_0} for b_0). From these the 95% confidence intervals of the coefficients can be calculated by multiplying by $t_{0.05(n\text{-}2)}$ from *Appendix B.6*. Note that the number of degrees of freedom for these data is 16. More generally n-2 is derived from $n - p'$, where p' is the number of regression coefficients. In this case $p' = 2$, the coefficients being

```
MTB > regress 'height' 1 'age'

The regression equation is
height = 79.7 + 0.511 age

Predictor        Coef        Stdev     t-ratio        p
Constant        79.70        21.25        3.75    0.002
age            0.5113       0.1670        3.06    0.007

s = 7.029       R-sq = 36.9%     R-sq(adj) = 33.0%

Analysis of Variance

SOURCE        DF          SS          MS          F        p
Regression     1      462.83      462.83       9.37    0.007
Error         16      790.43       49.40
Total         17     1253.26

Unusual Observations
Obs.       age     height         Fit  Stdev.Fit   Residual    St.Resid
 13        134     133.20      148.21       2.04     -15.01      -2.23R
 17        141     165.30      151.79       2.89      13.51       2.11R

R denotes an obs. with a large st. resid.
```

Figure 5. *Minitab* output for the child data using the standard regression command to predict height from age.

the intercept and the slope. So in this case the coefficients and their 95% confidence intervals are

$$b \pm s_b t_{0.05(16)} = 0.5113 \pm (0.167 \times 2.12) = 0.5113 \pm 0.354;$$
$$b_0 \pm s_{b_0} t_{0.05(16)} = 79.70 \pm (21.25 \times 2.12) = 79.70 \pm 45.05.$$

The large range in these intervals reflects the wide variation observed in the original plot (*Figure 2b*). The *t*-ratios for the coefficients and their *P* values are in the next two columns and these indicate whether the coefficients are significantly different from zero, $P < 0.05$ indicating significance. Thus for these data both the intercept and slope are significant. This is sensible, as we all know that children grow taller as they get older and are not born at zero height!

On the next line, s is the estimated standard deviation of the errors in y and represents the deviation about the regression line. R-sq is more commonly called R^2 which is the coefficient of determination and indicates the percentage of the variation in the data explained by the straight line relationship. The square root of R^2 is the linear correlation coefficient (r), which in this case when expressed as a proportion is 0.607 (i.e. $\sqrt{36.9/100}$). This figure can be compared with table values (*Appendix B.9*) as the absolute value of the coefficient. Here $r_{table} = 0.468$ ($n = 18$), which is greater than the calculated value and so there is significant linear correlation between age and height. The adjusted R^2 can be ignored.

The analysis of variance table follows for the regression model used (i.e. bivariate linear regression). This is similar to the one-way ANOVA table

(Chapter 1, Section 2). The first line gives the F and corresponding P value for the overall fit of the regression model, again significant. The error mean square (49.4) is the variance about the regression line and will be designated MS_{rerror} here. Note $\sqrt{MS_{rerror}}$ ($\sqrt{49.4} = 7.029$) is the same as s defined earlier in the output.

The unusual observations are given as warnings of points that are possibly extreme outliers or have a strong influence on the line and will be discussed later.

2.3 Analysing residuals

2.3.1 Residual plots and outliers

Examination of residuals is essential for checking that the linear model assumed by the regression calculations and other assumptions are valid for the data set being analysed. Three types of residuals are commonly provided by computer packages:

- ordinary residuals
- standardized residuals
- studentized residuals

All will give the same pattern of points in the residual plots. The ordinary residuals are expressed in the original y units whilst the other two are in units of standard deviation. It is normally best to examine the studentized residuals, although the standardized residuals are a good substitute (but are more conservative for outlier detection). Studentized residuals are sometimes called studentized deleted or just deleted residuals (see Chapter 4; Section 4.1.2). The ordinary residuals should be examined to see the magnitude of the errors in the original units; this is particularly useful for calibration curves (e.g. the OD data; 8).

The studentized or standardized residuals should be plotted against the

- fitted values, $\hat{y}$
- x variable
- the sequence of the observations if they are in a logical order

These plots are then examined along with the absolute magnitude of the ordinary residuals. A well fitted model will give a random distribution of residuals around zero. Several of the common patterns of deviation from this ideal are given in *Figure 6*. Outliers with studentized or standardized residuals $> +2$ or < -2 (*Figure 6a*) should be considered for rejection (see Chapter 4; Section 4.1.2 for a more accurate test). When considering points for rejection it is important to

- examine the residual plots to ensure that they are not just the extreme values of an unusually variable data set

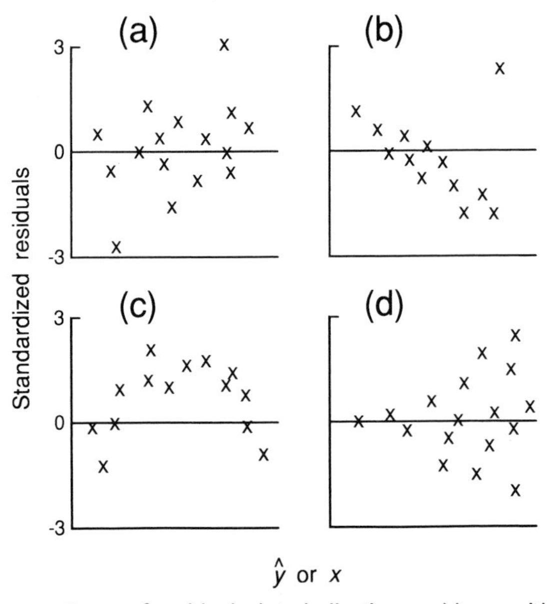

Figure 6. Common patterns of residual plots indicating problems with the regression model being used. The problems are (a) extreme outliers, (b) poorly fitted slope due to one extreme outlier, (c) curved pattern indicating non-linear data, and (d) non-constant variance.

- examine laboratory records and field note books to see if there are any basic problems with the recording of the data, the experimentation or whether a transcription error has occurred

Exclusion of data points from the analysis that are not real errors is very dangerous. Extreme outliers may tell you something important about the data. For example if the outlier is the highest value of x or y it might indicate a region of non-linearity just outside the range of observations (the OD data has an example of this).

Figure 6b shows what will be observed if one or a few data points have excessive influence on the slope of the regression line, this is easily spotted as a sloping line of residuals. Fitting a linear model to a curve is evident from a sweeping arc of residuals (*Figure 6c*). This is evident even if the magnitude of the ordinary residuals is very small in relation to the y values (8). Violation of the assumption of constant variance is seen by a funnel shaped pattern (*Figure 6d*). This is best corrected by transformation of y by square root, $\log_{10}$, or reciprocal.

As an example, one residual plot is given (*Figure 7*) for the child data analysed previously. The other two residual plots are not shown because they give essentially the same pattern. This shows that two points (children 13 and 17 when counted from the top in *Appendix 3.1*) are possible outliers (ringed in *Figure 7*) and were also flagged as unusual observations in *Figure 5*. There

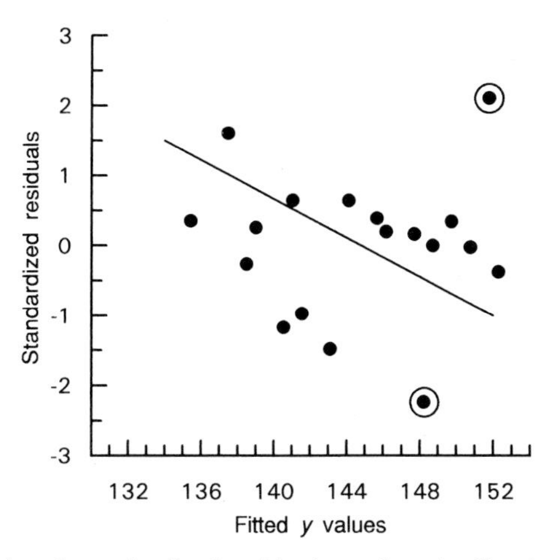

Figure 7. Residual plot of standardized residuals against the fitted *y* values for the child data; possible outliers circled and possible trend marked with a line.

is a possibility of a poorly fitted line, indicated by the slope on the remaining residuals. There is also the suspicion of funnelling, with low variance for younger children (low $\hat{y}$) and high variance for older children (high $\hat{y}$). This funnelling, however, is probably due to the outliers, and so can be discounted.

2.3.2 The Durbin–Watson test

This test is commonly available in computer packages and tests for the significance of autocorrelation between residuals. Hence, it will pick out as significant the problems identified in *Figure 6b* and *6c*. It should only be used if the data are in a logical order. Thus it can be done on the child data, which are ordered by age, but the OD data would need sorting by OD before the result would be meaningful. The Durbin–Watson statistic (DW) for the child data is 2.21. This is compared with table values (*Appendix B.10*). For the child data the table values (n = 18, k = 1) are d_L = 1.158 and d_U = 1.391; hence there is no doubt, as 2.21 > d_U and so there is no significant autocorrelation in the residuals.

2.3.3 Influence statistics

There are statistics which test whether data points have a large influence on the slope of the regression line. The most common statistics of this type calculated by statistical packages are leverage (also called HI in *Minitab*, and LEVER in *SPSS/PC+*), Cook's D, and Dfits. Leverage (h_{ii}) is the diagonal of the hat matrix and is very useful for the calculation of confidence and prediction intervals (see Section 2.5). All three statistics should be calculated and compared with critical values (see *Protocol 1*, step 7; *Table 2*). It is

Table 2. Values of the influence statistics for the child data with their critical values; influential points above the critical values are underlined

Child number		Leverage	Cook's *D*	Dfits
1		0.235	0.019	0.191
2		0.164	0.253	0.751
3		0.135	0.005	−0.099
4		0.122	0.005	0.093
5		0.090	0.068	−0.373
6		0.082	0.019	0.189
7		0.075	0.038	−0.275
8		0.060	0.070	−0.390
9		0.056	0.012	0.153
10		0.058	0.005	0.094
11		0.061	0.001	0.049
12		0.077	0.001	0.046
13		0.085	0.230	−0.791
14		0.093	0.000	−0.001
15		0.114	0.007	0.119
16		0.139	0.000	−0.010
17		0.169	0.452	1.083
18		0.185	0.016	−0.176
critical value	(i)	0.222	0.222	0.667
	(ii)		0.724	
Formula[a]	(i)	$>2p'/n$	$>4/n$	$>2\sqrt{p'/n}$
	(ii)		$>F_{05(p',n-p')}$	

[a] p' = the number of parameters in the model (b_o = 1 parameter; b = 1 parameter); n = number of data points in the regression; for Dfits the absolute value must be compared with the critical value, so the sign is ignored

common for several different data points to be identified as having high influence by these statistics. Thus at least two of the statistics should be above the critical value before they are considered as truly influential. Once identified, such influence points should be considered carefully for possible exclusion. The same cautionary notes as given earlier for elimination of points with high residuals (Section 2.3.1) apply equally here. The words of Rawlings (3) summarize well the purpose of looking for points of influence:

> The purpose of the diagnostic techniques is to identify weaknesses in the regression model or the data. Remedial measures, correction of errors in the data, elimination of true outliers, collection of better data, or improvement of the model, will allow greater confidence in the final product.

The values for the three influence statistics from the child data are given in *Table 2* and points above the critical values are indicated. No data point is identified by all the statistics, but the points for children 13 and 17 are identified for the lower critical value of Cook's D and for Dfits as well. These points are clearly suspicious because they were identified as outliers from the residuals earlier. Additionally, the point for child 2 is indicated by two of the statistics and so is a possible influence point. The point for child 1 is only high for leverage and was not an outlier, so it is not considered further. Note also that for these data the two critical values which have been suggested for Cook's D give different results. The value for $4/n$ will almost always be lower than that for $F_{0.5(p',n-p')}$. So the latter statistic will only indicate points that are very strongly influential.

This is quite a large number of influence points and outliers for such a small data set. So we should be suspicious, and in the real world probably collect more data. However, without that option the line of best fit is probably best described by a more robust type of regression (*Protocol 1*: see Section 4).

2.4 Regression through the origin

With some data sets it is known with certainty that the regression line must pass through the origin ($y = 0$; $x = 0$). The OD data is an example where a zero OD must mean there were no bacterial cells in the culture, or at least a vanishingly small number on a linear scale.

Forcing the regression line through the origin is straightforward in most computer packages. *Minitab* uses the NOCONSTANT command placed before the REGRESS statement, *SPSS/PC+* uses the NOORIGIN subcommand and *Systat* uses a modified regression model statement:

```
MODEL DRYWT = OD
```

For the OD data the regression equation with a constant is

```
DRYWT = −89.7 + (472 × OD)
```

and without a constant (i.e. line forced through origin) is

```
DRYWT = 442 × OD
```

Without the constant, R^2 is not calculated but all the other regression statistics are given. It is clear from the equations above that the slope in the model without a constant is modified to allow the line of best fit to go through the origin. The model without a constant also gives point 9 (OD = 4.13; DRYWT = 2050; see *Figure 2a*) as influential with all three statistics. This indicates possible lack of linearity at the extremes of the data, so more data in this region are required to test this possibility further.

Care should be taken when forcing regression lines through the origin. For example, if the true model is curved or changes slope close to the origin, the normal regression equation will probably be more appropriate. The chance of this problem occurring undetected can be minimized if data points are collected very close to zero. The residuals should also be examined for any sign of curvature so that departures from linearity can be spotted. The Durbin–

Watson test for autocorrelation must be modified for regression through the origin and different tables for DW are required (9, 10).

2.5 Confidence and prediction intervals

Most packages allow calculation of confidence and prediction intervals and some allow these values to be stored for subsequent use in graphs (e.g. *Statgraphics*). If they are not stored they are easily calculated from the leverage values (h_{ii}) which are more commonly available as stored variables. The formulae for these intervals are given in *Table 3*. These formulae can be applied to all x values in the regression and the result stored as a column for plotting. *Figure 8* gives the result of the *Minitab* PREDICT subcommand for all x values for the whole OD data with a constant term. Note that in this example the column called Stdev.Fit contains the $s_{\hat{y}}$ values used to calculate the two types of confidence intervals for $\hat{y}$ given in *Table 3*. Also the 95% confidence and prediction intervals in *Figure 8* (called CI and PI respectively) are those based on t (CI_t, PI_t) and so only properly apply to one $\hat{y}$. It is better to use the F or Scheffé's intervals (CI_F, PI_F) which apply to all $\hat{y}$ values (3) and so are wider. These four intervals have been calculated with the *Minitab* macro provided in *Appendix 3.2* and are plotted with the line of best fit in

Table 3. Formulae for standard errors, confidence, and prediction intervals for linear regression

Statistic	Symbol for standard error	Formula for standard error[a]	Formula for interval
Confidence intervals			
Regression coefficient, b	s_b	—[b]	$s_b t_{P(n-p')}$
Intercept, b_0	s_{b_0}	—[b]	$s_{b_0} t_{P(n-p')}$
One estimated $\hat{y}$ from a given x, CI_t	$s_{\hat{y}}$	$\sqrt{MS_{rerror} h_{ii}}$	$s_{\hat{y}} t_{P(n-p')}$
All $\hat{y}$ values, CI_F			$s_{\hat{y}} \sqrt{p' F_{P(p',n-p')}}$
Prediction intervals			
One new value of $\hat{y}$ from a new x value, PI_t	$\hat{s}_y$	$\sqrt{MS_{rerror}(1 + h_{ii})}$	$\hat{s}_y t_{P(n-p')}$
All new values of $\hat{y}$ from any number of new x values, PI_F			$\hat{s}_y \sqrt{p' F_{P(p',n-p')}}$

[a] MS_{rerror} = mean square from the regression ANOVA; h_{ii} = leverage values (one h_{ii} value for each x value)

[b] These standard errors are usually on the standard regression output (*Figure 5*) and are explained in Section 2.2

Fit	Stdev.Fit	95% C.I.	95% P.I.
1758.7	65.5	(1612.7, 1904.8)	(1413.3, 2104.2)
1447.5	47.4	(1341.9, 1553.2)	(1117.1, 1778.0)
947.7	44.7	(848.2, 1047.2)	(619.2, 1276.2)
853.4	48.6	(745.0, 961.8)	(522.1, 1184.7)
1042.0	41.9	(948.6, 1135.4)	(715.3, 1368.7)
306.4	84.6	(117.9, 494.9)	(-59.0, 671.9)
1249.5	41.2	(1157.6, 1341.4)	(923.2, 1575.8)
452.6	73.7	(288.3, 616.9)	(99.0, 806.2)
1857.8	72.5	(1696.2, 2019.3)	(1505.5, 2210.1)
1070.3	41.4	(978.2, 1162.5)	(744.0, 1396.7)
1277.8	41.7	(1184.8, 1370.8)	(951.2, 1604.4)
1702.2	61.8	(1564.5, 1839.8)	(1360.2, 2044.2)

Figure 8. Output from the *Minitab* PREDICT command for the whole OD data, calculated with a constant term for all x values.

Figure 9. It can be seen that they are biconcave about the mean values of x and y. This indicates greater certainty for $\hat{y}$ near the middle of the data and less certainty close to the extremities. When presenting data graphically with confidence and prediction intervals it is better to use the wider F intervals, as a continuous line implies all possible points have been considered.

The shape of these intervals when the line is forced through the origin is different (*Figure 10*). In this case the confidence intervals converge towards the origin as the error at this point must be zero if it is known with certainty.

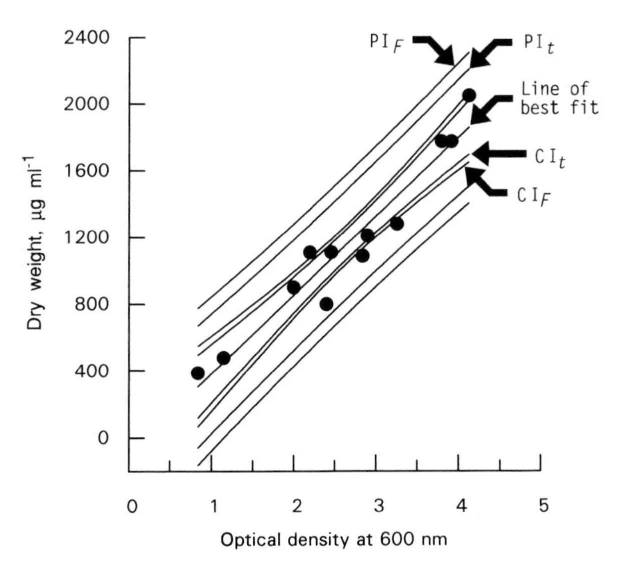

Figure 9. Confidence (CI) and prediction (PI) intervals for the OD data with a normal regression model. CI_t, PI_t = t based intervals which apply to only one predicted y value; CI_F, PI_F = Scheffé's intervals based on the F statistic and which apply to all predicted y values.

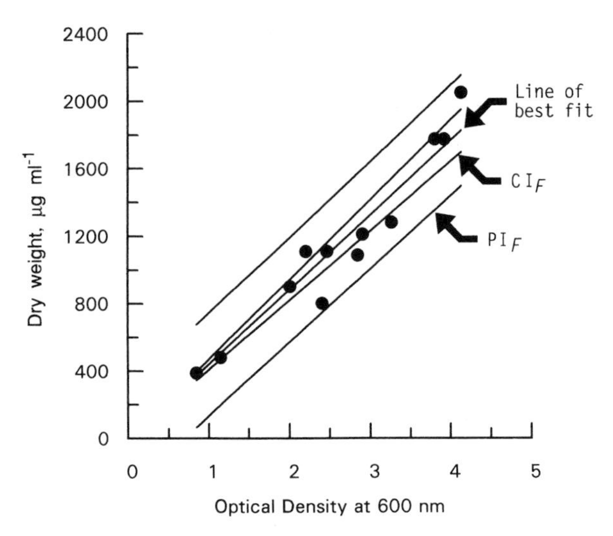

Figure 10. Confidence and prediction intervals for the OD data with the regression forced through the origin; abbreviations as *Figure 9*.

2.6 Regression with more than one *y* for each *x*

This can be thought of as regression with replicates of the *y* values. The replicates provide extra information about the errors in the data. Thus there are now two sources of information valuable for regression analysis, which are

- the standard regression ANOVA table
- the one-way ANOVA table calculated with the replicates of *y* for each *x* assigned to a different group

The one-way ANOVA provides the MS_{error} which is an estimate of the average variance of the replicate *y* values. This has been called the pure or experimental error. The differences between the degrees of freedom and the sums of squares between the error lines in the two ANOVA tables provide information for a lack of fit test for the linear regression model. This test has also been called a test for deviations from regression and misspecification of the regression model. Most authors suggest comparison of the regression mean square with the pure error mean square (MS_{error} from the one-way ANOVA). This is certainly the best test for the significance of the regression when the lack of fit test is significant. However, when lack of fit is not significant (i.e. when the linear model is acceptable), it is often better to use the ordinary regression error mean square (MS_{rerror} from the standard regression ANOVA), which usually has more degrees of freedom and so is a more accurate estimate of the variance (11). These tests allow a corrected regression ANOVA table to be constructed. Unfortunately few statistical packages allow this table to be calculated. *Minitab*, however, does give the *F* and P values for the lack of fit test with the PURE subcommand. For these reasons *Protocol 2* explains how to calculate the complete, corrected table.

Protocol 2. Calculation of the full, corrected ANOVA table for regression of more than one y value for every x value

1. Calculate a one-way ANOVA table with the replicate y values in each group. This will normally involve labelling the groups with integers (see Chapter 1, Section 2). Note that the number of replicate y values need not be the same for each x value. Assign letters[a] to the different parts of the ANOVA table as below:

Source	df	SS	MS	*F*
Between groups	a	b	c	d
Within groups	e	f	g	
Total	h	i		

2. Calculate a standard regression ANOVA table (see Section 2.2). Assign letters[a] to the different parts of the ANOVA table as below:

Source	df	SS	MS	*F*
Regression	A	B	C	D
Error	E	F	G	
Total	H	I		

3. Construct a corrected regression ANOVA table as below:

Source	df	SS	MS	*F*
Between groups of y	a	b	c	d
Linear regression	A	B	C	$\frac{C}{g}$ or $\frac{C}{G}$
Lack of fit	$E–e = Z$	$F–f = Y$	$\frac{Y}{Z} = X$	$\frac{X}{g}$
Pure error	e	f	g	
Total	H	I		

4. Test for lack of fit as follows:
   - if $F_{table} < F_{calc}$ (X/g) then lack of fit is significant
   - if $F_{table} > F_{calc}$ (X/g) then lack of fit is not significant

   (i.e. the model is acceptably linear).
5. Test for linear regression as follows:
   - use C/g when lack of fit is significant
   - use C/G when lack of fit is not significant and $E \gg e$.

[a] symbols used in the ANOVA tables in this protocol do not apply elsewhere.

Table 4. The corrected ANOVA table for the lack of fit test for Hane's plot (*s*/*v* against *s*) for the puromycin treated enzyme data and the one-way ANOVA and regression ANOVA tables used to calculate it (see *Protocol 2*)

One-way ANOVA table

Source	df	SS	MS	*F*	*P*
Between groups	5	37.041520	7.48304	895.87	⩽0.001
Within groups	6	0.05012	0.00835		
Total	11	37.46532			

Standard regression ANOVA table

Source	df	SS	MS	*F*	*P*
Linear regression	1	37.388	37.388	4863.08	⩽0.001
Error	10	0.077	0.008		
Total	11	37.465			

Corrected regression ANOVA table

Source	df	SS	MS	*F*	*P*
Between groups of *y*	5	37.415	7.483	895.87	⩽0.001
Linear regression	1	37.388	37.388	4477.6	⩽0.001
Lack of fit	4	0.0269	0.00673	0.805	>0.5
Pure error	6	0.05012	0.00835		
Total	11	37.46532			

The puromycin treated enzyme data are of this type, although they are not linear. The Hane's plot of such data obeying Michaelis–Menten kinetics is the best linearization (12; Section 5.4). This splots s/v (where s is the substrate concentration and v is the reaction velocity) as the y variable against s as the x variable. The enzyme data is acceptably linear when plotted in this way ($R^2 = 99.8$; residuals random). So the corrected ANOVA table and those from which it was calculated are in *Table 4*. The between groups of y line shows there are significant differences between the replicate y values. The linear regression line shows the overall linear model is highly significant. The lack of fit line shows that none of the points deviate significantly from a straight line.

The confidence and prediction intervals for regressions with replicate y values are calculated as usual. Most authors are agreed on this; however, Sokal and Rohlf (2) give different formulae for these intervals with replicate ys, but as they are in a minority the formulae in *Table 3* are satisfactory.

3. Comparison of regression lines

This is a common requirement amongst biologists, and analysis of covariance is best used for this, which works for any number of lines and is not affected by replicated y values. Most packages use model specifications for this type of

Table 5. The form of the Hane's plot (s/v against s) modification of the full enzyme data, treated and untreated, for use in analysis of covariance to compare regression lines

x	*y*	lines
20	0.26326	1
20	0.42553	1
60	0.61856	1
60	0.45075	1
110	0.89431	1
110	0.79137	1
220	1.38365	1
220	1.44737	1
560	2.93194	1
560	2.78607	1
1100	5.31401	1
1100	5.50000	1
20	0.29851	2
20	0.39216	2
60	0.71429	2
60	0.69767	2
110	1.12245	2
110	0.95652	2
220	1.67939	2
220	1.77419	2
560	3.88889	2
560	3.54430	2
1100	6.87500	2

$x = s$, substrate concentration
$y = s/v$, substrate concentration divided by velocity
lines = labels for the two regression lines (treated = 1, untreated = 2)

analysis. I will again use *Minitab* as the example here, with the Hane's linearization of the enzyme data described earlier. The data are organized as in *Table 5*. The *Minitab* command used to carry out the analysis is

```
GLM Y = LINES | X;
COVARIATE X.
```

and the output is given in *Figure 11*. Note that in this *Minitab* command Y, LINES, and X are column names (see *Table 5*). The three top lines in the ANOVA table are interpreted from their P values as follows

(a) lines: significance of the differences between the intercepts

(b) x: whether the slopes, if parallel, are significantly different from zero

(c) lines*x: significance of difference between the slopes

```
MTB > glm y=lines|x;
SUBC> covariate x.

Factor    Levels Values
lines          2      1      2

Analysis of Variance for y

Source      DF       Seq SS       Adj SS       Adj MS         F        P
lines        1        0.042        0.002        0.002      0.18    0.672
x            1       76.543       77.202       77.202   7260.43    0.000
lines*x      1        1.281        1.281        1.281    120.42    0.000
Error       19        0.202        0.202        0.011
Total       22       78.067


Term           Coeff       Stdev   t-value        P
Constant     0.32644     0.02871     11.37    0.000
x           0.005309    0.000062     85.21    0.000
x*lines
       1   -0.000684    0.000062    -10.97    0.000
```

Figure 11. *Minitab* output from analysis of covariance to compare the slopes of two regression lines. The data used is the Hane's plot modification of the enzyme data as given in *Table 5*.

In this case the intercepts are not significantly different, but the slopes are significantly different from each other and zero. If the intercepts and/or the slopes are not significantly different, then their common values are given as the coefficients for constant and x in the table below the ANOVA table. So for these data the common intercept is 0.326, but the two separate slopes must be obtained from two separate regression analyses, one for each line.

If many regression lines need to be compared, then an overall test should be done first, followed by multiple tests comparing separate pairs of lines until it is clear which lines are different. For such multiple tests the acceptable level of significance needs to be reduced, because with multiple comparisons the chance of an error increases. A suitable significance level can be calculated by using Bonferroni's approximation (α/m), where α is the normally acceptable probability and m is the number of comparisons made. Thus for making 5 comparisons from 10 lines the significance level used should be $P < 0.05/5 = 0.01$.

4. Robust linear regression

When there are severe problems with large residuals or influence statistics it could be considered better to use a robust regression method which is less susceptible to extreme data points than the least squares method. Some methods of robust regression are discussed below.

4.1 The three-group resistant line

This technique is perhaps the most resistant method to outliers and influence points. It has been described in detail, in a very readable form for biologists, elsewhere (7, 13). Basically, the method divides the data points into three groups and takes the median of each group and then calculates a straight line to fit through these medians. *Minitab* calculates the slope and intercept (called level) by this procedure with the RLINE command which has a similar form to the REGRESS command. As with least squares regression, residuals and fitted values can be calculated, stored and examined to check the efficacy of the model, as described previously (Section 2.3). *Table 6* illustrates the

Table 6. Regression coefficients for the child data with and without outliers and influence points[a] calculated by least squares and three-group resistant-line methods

	Data set used			
Method and coefficients	**Full**	**Without influence points**	**Without outliers**	**Without outliers and influence points**
Least squares				
slope	0.5113	0.4757	0.4563	0.5525
intercept	79.70	82.72	86.69	73.90
R^2	36.9	40.2	45.1	60.1
Resistant line				
slope	0.4286	0.4269	0.4333	0.4333
intercept	91.01	91.12	90.40	90.37

[a] Points for children 2 and 17 were considered influence points, whilst those for children 13 and 17 were considered outliers

robustness of this form of regression, which compares the slope and intercepts for both least squares and resistant line methods for the child data with outliers and influence points removed. It can be seen that the coefficients hardly vary with the resistant line, but they vary greatly for the least squares calculations. Also these latter values never quite reach those for the resistant line, despite large increases in the R^2 value, indicating improved fit.

4.2 Least absolute residuals and minimum χ^2

These two methods use approaches other than least squares to minimize the distance between the data points and the line of best fit. The values minimized are the absolute value of $y - \hat{y}$ for the least absolute residuals (LAR) method and χ^2, which is

$$\frac{(\text{observed} - \text{expected})^2}{\text{expected}} \text{ or } \frac{(y - \hat{y})^2}{\hat{y}}$$

for the minimum χ^2 method. Many statistical packages cannot do this type of calculation, and of the four used here only *Systat* was capable of doing such regressions. *Systat*'s non-linear regression procedure (NONLIN) must be used, because with this it is possible to minimize any function with the LOSS statement. The regression model must also be given, which in this case is the normal regression equation $y = b_0 + bx$. However, it was not possible to find a non-linear solution for the child data set with the algorithms used in *Systat*, so I use the OD data in the following examples.

The commands needed for LAR regression were

```
MODEL DRYWT = CONSTANT + B1 * OD
LOSS = ABS(DRYWT - ESTIMATE)
ESTIMATE/SIMPLEX
```

and for the minimum χ^2 method were

```
MODEL DRYWT = CONSTANT + B1 * OD
LOSS = ((DRYWT - ESTIMATE)^2)/DRYWT
ESTIMATE/QUASI
```

In these command sets I have chosen to call b_0 CONSTANT and b B1, but $\hat{y}$ must be called ESTIMATE. The variables are called DRYWT and OD as before. Both these methods produced results different from the least squares regression approach, as did the three-group resistant line procedure from *Minitab* (*Table 7*). However, for these data and regression methods the differences betwen the lines of best fit and the residuals were small. Hoaglin *et al.* (7) give detailed arguments about the robustness of several different

Table 7. Regression coefficients for the full OD data calculated by four different methods

	Regression method used			
Coefficient	**Least squares**	**Least absolute residuals**	**Minimum χ^2**	**Three-group resistant line**
Intercept	−87.7	−11.5	−23.9	−36.1
Slope	472	456	441	464
R^2	93.0	—	—	—

— = R^2 not calculated

regression methods. They conclude that the three-group resistant line method is best, followed by the LAR and least squares methods, in that order. They do not consider the χ^2 method. Thus only with data having very extreme outliers or influence points would it be worthwhile considering the LAR or χ^2 approaches when the three-group resistant line method is available.

5. Curved regression lines

If the initial plot of y against x looks curved or there is a curved pattern to the residual plots and a significant Durbin–Watson statistic, then linear regression is inappropriate and another method is needed. There are several methods suitable for curvilinear regression and these are outlined in *Protocol 3* and described in more detail afterwards.

Protocol 3. Regression methods for curved lines

1. Select the most appropriate approach from the following guidelines:
  (a) polynomial regression (step 2)
    - use as a purely empirical method of fitting a curve
    - gives no idea of functional relationships

  (b) transformations (steps 3 and 4)
    - use for known relationships (e.g. $\log_{10}y$ against x) or when a knowledge of the relationship is required

  (c) direct non-linear solutions (go to step 5)
    - use when an equation relating y and x is known from theory

2. Perform polynomial regression as follows:
  (a) transform x to $x^2, x^3, x^4 \ldots x^k$ as required to make a set of predictor variables
  (b) pick best set of predictor variables to fit a polynomial equation (NB see Chapter 4, Section 6, for methods; the *Minitab* BREG command works well)

3. Transformations for 'one-bend' curves:
  (a) use the power transformations (see Chapter 1, *Table 4*) for y and/or x.
  (b) choose powers based on:
    - theory
    - shape of curve (see *Figure 14*)
    - comparisons of plots selected from a correlation matrix of y^p against x^p, where $p = 3$ to -2

4. Transformations for 'two-bend' curves
Choose appropriate transformation from the following:
- logit $y = \log_e (y/(1 - y))$
- generalized 'two bend' $y = \log_e (y/(K - y))$
- probit y

Protocol 3. *Continued*

5. Direct non-linear solutions
Use correct equation from biological theory as regression model.

6. Calculate regression statistics and check regression diagnostics carefully as in *Protocol 1* (steps 5–7). (NB Durbin–Watson test and influence statistics are not applicable to non-linear regression.)

7. Calculate and plot confidence and prediction intervals as required (see *Table 3*; not applicable to non-linear regression).

5.1 Polynomial regression

This type of regression analysis is simply a mutiple regression of y against a suitable set of powers of x, so readers with no knowledge of multiple regression should read Chapter 4 before attempting polynomial regression. The basic polynomial equation is

$$y = b_0 + b_1x + b_2x^2 + b_3x^3 \ldots b_kx^k,$$

which is simply a logical extension of the normal bivariate regression equation. There are still only two variables, as x^2, x^3, and x^k are all transformations of x. First, a set of transformed x variables are calculated: I will call these predictors. Then the best set of predictors is chosen by a suitable variable selection procedure. It is rarely necessary to exceed x^4 and beyond this collinearity is often a problem. I find the BREG command in *Minitab* to be the best selection method for polynomial regression. The best set of predictors is simply indicated by the lowest value for Mallows' C_p, which is normally very close to the number of predictors. With the puromycin treated enzyme data a three predictor model is clearly optimal (*Figure 12*), although in this case collinearity prevented predictors past x^3 being used. After selecting the predictors the regression constants are calculated, giving the following prediction equation

$$\text{vtreat} = 56.28 + 0.717\text{s} - 0.00116\text{s}^2 + 0.00000057\text{s}^3.$$

This provides a reasonable fit (*Figure 13*), particularly at lower substrate concentrations (see Section 5.4 for discussion of the fit). With this solution all predictors were significant, $R^2 = 96.0$, and the residuals were random, with no outliers nor important influence points.

5.2 Transformations

This approach to fitting curves is best treated in two parts. 'One-bend' curves are simple, with essentially only one curve (e.g. enzyme data; *Figure 2c*), whilst 'two-bend' curves are more complex, showing two distinct parts to the curve, and are often sigmoidal in shape (e.g. rotenone data; *Figure 2d*). The

```
MTB > BReg 'vtreat' 's' 's^2' 's^3' 's^4' 's^5'
* ERROR * Predictor columns are highly correlated.
* ERROR * Use REGR command to find correlated vars.
* ERROR * Completion of computation impossible

MTB > BReg 'vtreat' 's' 's^2' 's^3'

Best Subsets Regression of vtreat

                                                s s
              Adj.                              ^ ^
Vars   R-sq   R-sq    C-p          s        s 2 3

   1   69.1   66.0   53.0     30.898        X
   1   48.3   43.1   93.9     39.944          X
   2   90.8   88.7   12.2     17.808        X X
   2   88.1   85.4   17.5     20.237        X   X
   3   95.9   94.4    4.0     12.514        X X X
```

Figure 12. Output from the *Minitab* BREG command used to select the best predictor variables for a polynomial regression of the puromycin treated enzyme data. The predictors used are s, s^2 (s^2), s^3 (s^3), s^4 (s^4), and s^5 (s^5); where the *Minitab* column name is given in brackets.

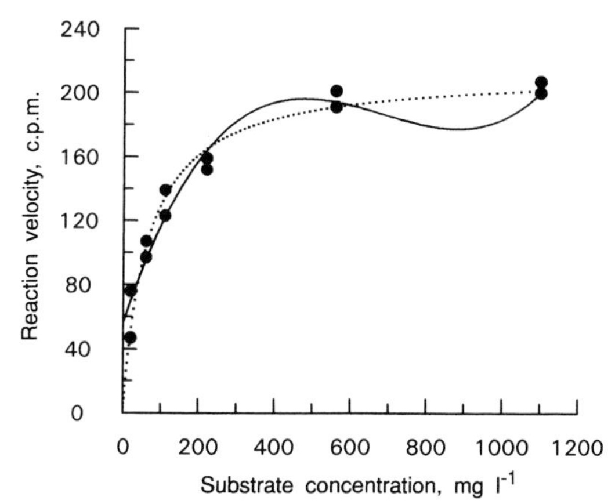

Figure 13. Lines of best fit drawn through the puromycin treated enzyme data from polynomial regression (______) and non-linear regression by *SPSS/PC+* using the Michaelis–Menten equation (· · · · · ·).

use of transformations for the linearization of curved relationships has been discussed frequently and many different approaches have been suggested (1, 3, 7, 14). Here I will describe only those methods that I have found most useful.

5.2.1 'One-bend' curves

The series of power transformations from the ladder of powers (Chapter 1, *Table 4*) provide an excellent series for 'one-bend' curves. Either y or x or both can be transformed as necessary. It is not a trivial problem to select the best transformations for linearization and all the effective approaches take considerable time and effort. Hoaglin *et al.* (7) describe a transformation plot for straightness, which is similar to the transformation plot for symmetry (Section 2.1). However, despite the attractiveness of such a simple procedure, I have not found this very useful. I describe three approaches for selecting suitable power transformations for linearity. Whichever method is used, plots of the transformations must be examined to check their efficacy.

i. Theoretical considerations

The analyst might know that a certain transformation can be expected to give a straight line from biological theory. For example, populations grow logarithmically and so a plot of change in numbers of an animal (y) with time (x) might be best analysed as $\log_{10}y$ against x whilst the population is growing exponentially. The enzyme data would be expected to follow Michaelis–Menten kinetics; hence the best simple pair of power transformations for linearization should be the reciprocals of y and x, as this is the well known Lineweaver–Burk plot ($1/v$ against $1/s$; 12).

ii. Curve shape

This second approach aims to guess the power required from the shape of the curve. Some authors recommend this method (e.g. 3, 15). However, a great deal of experience is required before powers can be guessed effectively. Hence for the beginner this normally results in large numbers of plots having to be examined before a good straight line is obtained. Possible powers are selected as outlined in *Figure 14*. A large arrow is drawn on the plot pointing in the direction of the bulge in the curve. Two vectors are then drawn against the diagonal arrow. One vector is horizontal, parallel to the x-axis, and one is vertical, parallel to the y-axis. When the vectors point to increasing values a higher power transformation is suggested and vice versa. Thus for a curve like the puromycin treated enzyme data (*Figure 2c*) an arrow and vectors like those in *Figure 14a* indicate increasing the power for y and decreasing it for x. Appropriate guesses of powers can then be made and the resulting plot examined. If it is still markedly curved the steps are repeated until an approximately linear graph results. *Figure 14b–c* gives the rules for other shaped curves. It should be noted that this is a crude method and provides only an indication of what powers might be suitable.

iii. Correlation matrix method

This involves calculating a correlation matrix of the possible power transformations of both y and x. The largest absolute correlation coefficient should give the best pair of transformations. This will be illustrated with the puromycin treated enzyme data. The correlation matrices from the full data with replicate y values and from the data with only the mean y values are given in

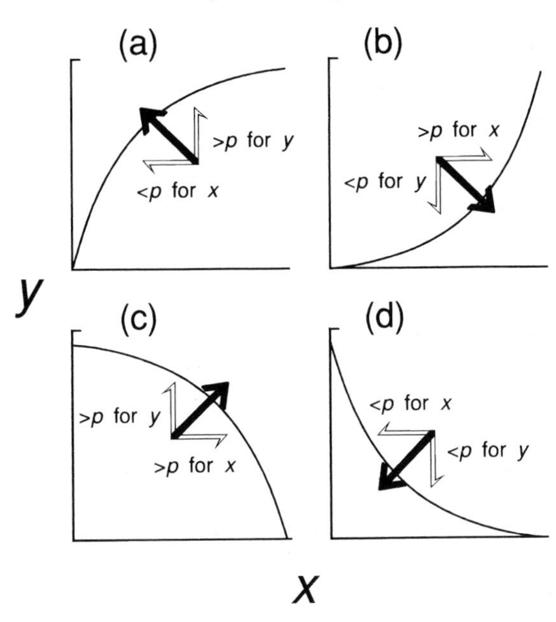

Figure 14. Guide for choosing power transformations (p) from the shape of a curved relationship between y and x.

Table 8. The full data give lower absolute values for the correlation coefficients because of the extra variability introduced by the replicate y values. The highest correlation coefficient for the full data was for y against $\log_{10} x$ (0.982) and for the mean y data was $1/y^2$ against $1/x$ (1.000). Note that this latter transformation pair is very similar to the best theoretical simple power transformation ($1/y$ against $1/x$, the Lineweaver–Burk plot), as are the others with the very highest absolute correlation coefficients (>0.995 or <−0.995) in the mean y correlation matrix (*Table 8b*). Inspection of the plots (using the full data) for the two pairs of 'best' transformations from the correlation matrices (*Table 8a* and *8b*) shows a great difference in the spread of variability (*Figure 15a,b*). The replicates in *Figure 15a* are much more evenly spaced than in *Figure 15b*. This is because use of the whole data set suggested transformatiuons which were a compromise between even variability of replicates and linearity, whilst with the mean y data the suggested transformation ignored variability in favour of linearity. It is well known that the Lineweaver–Burk transformation (*Figure 15c*) emphasizes variability at low substrate concentration and minimizes variability at high substrate concentration (12), so it is not surprising that the similar transformation suggested from the mean y correlation matrix did the same (*Figure 15b*). These general points should be carefully considered when selecting transformations with replicated data.

The ideal compromise would be a transformation that gave a straight line and had even variability. The Hane's plot used earlier in the comparison of

Table 8. Correlation matrices for the power transformations in the ladder of powers for y and x using the puromycin treated enzyme data (y = treatment velocity; vtreat; x = substrate concentration, s); with (a) both y replicates (full data) and (b) mean values of y

Power and transformation for y		Power and transformation for x							
Power	**Transformation**	**3** x^3	**2** x^2	**1** x	**0.5** $\sqrt{x}$	**0** $\log_{10}x$	**−0.5** $\frac{1}{\sqrt{x}}$	**−1** $\frac{1}{x}$	**−2** $\frac{1}{x^2}$
(a) Full data (n = 12)									
3	y^3	0.734	0.807	0.922	0.973	0.962	−0.858	−0.730	−0.585
2	y^2	0.690	0.764	0.891	0.961	0.981	−0.910	−0.801	−0.668
1	y	0.623	0.695	0.831	0.922	0.982	−0.956	−0.878	−0.766
0.5	$\sqrt{y}$	0.578	0.647	0.786	0.887	0.968	−0.968	−0.910	−0.813
0	$\log_{10}y$	0.525	0.591	0.729	0.839	0.941	−0.968	−0.930	−0.852
−0.5	$1/\sqrt{y}$	−0.468	−0.529	−0.664	−0.779	−0.898	0.952	0.936	0.878
−1	$1/y$	−0.409	−0.465	−0.595	−0.712	−0.845	0.921	0.925	0.886
−2	$1/y^2$	−0.308	−0.353	−0.467	−0.582	−0.727	0.833	0.868	0.861
(b) Mean y data (n = 6)									
3	y^3	0.739	0.812	0.928	0.980	0.969	−0.866	−0.737	−0.592
2	y^2	0.694	0.768	0.896	0.967	0.989	−0.918	−0.809	−0.675
1	y	0.630	0.703	0.841	0.933	0.994	−0.967	−0.888	−0.775
0.5	$\sqrt{y}$	0.590	0.661	0.802	0.904	0.987	−0.985	−0.924	−0.825
0	$\log_{10}y$	0.546	0.615	0.757	0.869	0.971	−0.996	−0.955	−0.872
−0.5	$1/\sqrt{y}$	−0.500	−0.566	−0.708	−0.827	−0.949	0.999	0.978	0.912
−1	$1/y$	−0.455	−0.517	−0.657	−0.782	−0.920	0.994	0.992	0.944
−2	$1/y^2$	−0.376	−0.431	−0.565	−0.696	−0.858	0.969	1.000	0.982

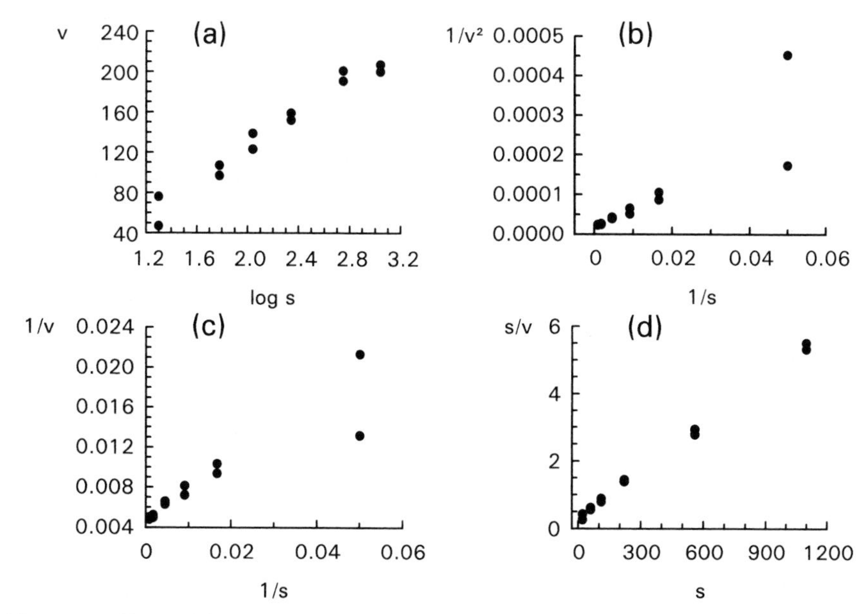

Figure 15. Plots of four pairs of transformations for v (reaction velocity, vtreat) and s (substrate concentration) for the puromycin treated enzyme data. The transformations are (a) v against $\log_{10}s$; (b) $1/v^2$ against $1/s$; (c) the Lineweaver–Burk linearization, $1/v$ against $1/s$, and (d) the Hane's plot, s/v against s,

lines example (Section 3) provides this compromise and is clearly satisfactory (*Figure 15d*). However, it is not a simple power transformation and so could not have been found by any of the methods described in this section.

5.3.2 'Two-bend' curves

When there are two bends in a curve the power series will not linearize the relationship and special transformations are needed. Mortality, survival, and dose–response curves are often sigmoidal. In these mortality, survival, or response is on the y-axis and concentration, dose, or time is on the x-axis. These are typical 'two-bend' curves and the rotenone data (*Appendix 3.1*; *Figure 2d*) will be used as an example in this section.

Apart from the commonly used 'two-bend' transformations discussed below (and in *Protocol 3*) the arcsine transformation (Chapter 1, Section 4.1.3) can also be used to linearize 'two-bend' curves (3).

i. Logit method

The logit transformation is derived from the logistic equation (1, 3) and essentially fits a logistic model to the data. To do this with the rotenone data the $\log_{10}$ of concentration is used as the x variable and the logit of the proportion killed (y) is used as the y-axis, where

$$\text{logit } y = \log_e\left(\frac{y}{1-y}\right).$$

With this type of data the mortality values at the extremes are often poorly estimated by experiment because the tails of the distribution are very flat (*Figure 2d*) and so it is hard to get accurate values when relatively small numbers of animals are tested. For this reason, the mortality values at 0% and 100%, which are closest to the centre of the data, should be recalculated (1) as indicated in *Table 9* (footnote *a*). The results of these calculations are shown in *Table 9*. Some of the regression output for logit y against $\log_{10}$ rotenone concentration and the plotted data with the line of best fit are shown in *Figure 16*. The linear model fits these data fairly well as R^2 was high and both t ratios and the F-value were highly significant; also there was no significant autocorrelation in the residuals ($DW = 2.2; d_U - d_L = 0.824 - 1.320$, $n = 9$, $k = 1$; *Appendix B.10*). Despite this, two of the three influence statistics highlighted both the extreme values as possible influence points and the standardized residual of the 100% mortality point was >2.0. Hence it is possible that the calculated values at these extremities were poor approximations and so were unreasonably affecting the regression. This problem has

Table 9. Results for the initial calculations required before linear regression can be done on the rotenone data by the logit and probit methods

Rotenone concentration (mg/l)	Percentage mortality	Proportion killed[a]	$\log_{10}$ rotenone concentration	Logit proportion killed[b]	Probit proportion killed[c]
12.7	100	0.99[a]	1.104	4.595	7.326
10.2	88	0.88	1.009	1.992	6.175
9.0	92	0.92	0.954	2.442	6.405
7.7	86	0.86	0.886	1.815	6.080
6.4	66	0.66	0.806	0.663	5.412
5.1	52	0.52	0.708	0.080	5.050
3.8	33	0.33	0.580	−0.708	4.560
2.6	12	0.12	0.415	−1.992	3.825
1.2	0	0.01[a]	0.079	−4.595	2.674
0.0[d]	0	0.00	*	*	*

[a] To include extreme data points (0% and 100% values for percentage mortality) the proportion killed has been recalculated (1) as $1/(2n_1)$ for the 0% point and $1 - 1/(2n_1)$ for the 100% point, where n_1 is the number of individuals tested at the concentration for which the proportion killed is being recalculated. A maximum of one 0% point and one 100% point should be included

[b] Logit transformation = $\log_e (y/(1 - y))$ where y is the proportion killed

[c] See text for an explanation of the probit transformation

[d] The control data without rotenone cannot be included as $\log_{10}0.0$ is incalculable

```
MTB > Regress 'logit-m' 1 'lg-conc'.

The regression equation is
logit-m = - 5.46 + 8.17 lg-conc

Predictor      Coef     Stdev   t-ratio       p
Constant    -5.4596    0.4629    -11.79   0.000
lg-conc      8.1685    0.5870     13.92   0.000

s = 0.5391     R-sq = 96.5%   R-sq(adj) = 96.0%

Analysis of Variance

SOURCE      DF        SS        MS         F       p
Regression   1    56.296    56.296    193.67   0.000
Error        7     2.035     0.291
Total        8    58.330
```

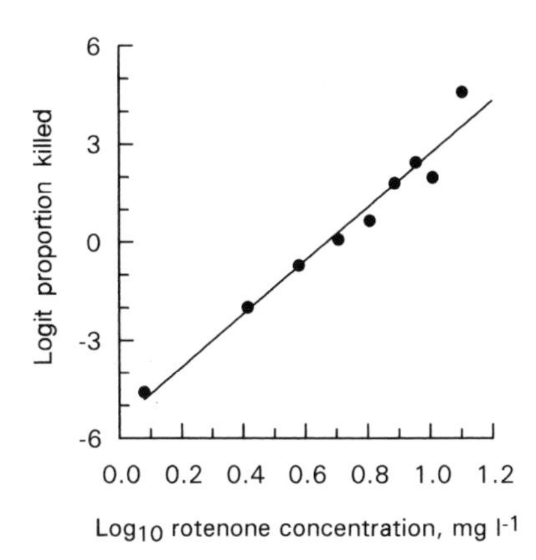

Figure 16. Some of the *Minitab* regression output and the line of best fit drawn through the data points for the logit method on the rotenone data (y = logit proportion killed; x = $\log_{10}$ concentration) with recalculated extreme values (see Section 5.3.2, *Table 9*).

prompted some authors to recommend careful comparison of regressions, with and without the inclusion of the extreme points, before any decision to use them is made. The regression without the extreme points gave similar results, but in this case the 88% mortality point was identified as a possible influence point. This was not unexpected as it looks a bit lower than the other points on the plotted data (*Figure 16*).

Some authors recommend weighted least squares regression with the logit method as the variances are not equal at all x values (1). If required this is simply done by using a column of weights (w), one for each data point. These are calculated as

$$w = n_1 y(1 - y),$$

where n_1 is the number of individuals tested for that data point and y is the proportion killed. In *Minitab* this type of regression is done by referring to the column containing the weights in the WEIGHTS sub-command of the REGRESSION statement.

ii. A generalized 'two-bend' transformation

There is a widely suggested, more universally applicable, transformation for 'two-bend' curves. This is similar to the logit method and is defined as

$$\text{transformed } y = \log_e\left(\frac{y}{K - y}\right),$$

where K is unknown and must be estimated before the transformation can be applied. This is best done by non-linear regression (see Section 5.3 for information on this topic). However, plotting the transformed y against x with a variety of values for K will also prove satisfactory. With practice K can be estimated crudely from the shape of the untransformed relationship.

iii. Probit analysis

As the culmulative curve of the normal distribution is sigmoidal in shape, normal density functions can be used as the basis for another 'two-bend' linearizing transformation. The popular probit transformation is based on this idea because probits are normal equivalent deviates with a mean of 5.0 and a standard deviation of 1.0. Finney (6, 16) extensively discusses the application of the probit method to dose–response curves and these texts should be consulted for more details. The *Minitab* command to obtain probits is

```
INVCDF C3 C4;
NORMAL 5 1.
```

where C3 contains the values for the proportion killed and C4 is where the probits for these proportions are stored. The same rules for extreme values as suggested for the logit method can also be used here and the values for the probit transformation on the rotenone data are also given in *Table 9*. The regression is then straightforward with the probits as the y variable and $\log_{10}$ rotenone concentrations as the x variable. Some authors have suggested using a minimized χ^2 regression technique (see Section 4.3) in place of least squares for probit analysis. However, as was discussed earlier the three-group resistant line method would almost certainly be better as a robust technique to minimize the effect of outliers (Section 4.3).

iv. Calculating a predicted x *from* y *and its confidence intervals*

Biologists often want to calculate the dose or concentration giving a 50% response together with the confidence interval for this value. To do this it is necessary to predict a new value of x from a specific y value; the logit and probit values for 50% are 0.0 and 5.0 respectively. As this is the reverse of the normal way in which predictions are made (Section 2.5) another approach is needed (*Protocol 4*).

Protocol 4. Calculation of confidence intervals for a new, predicted value of x ($\hat{x}$) from a new value of y (based on a method given in Sokal and Rohlf (2))

1. Calculate $\hat{x}$ from y:

$$\hat{x} = \frac{y - b_0}{b}.$$

2. Calculate statistics used later

- mean of all the y values, $\bar{y}$

- mean of all the x values, $\bar{x}$
- sum of squares of all the $x - \bar{x}$ values, $\Sigma(x - \bar{x})^2$

3. Calculate the first intermediate statistic, D:

$$D = b^2 - (t^2_{P(n\text{-}2)}\, s^2_b).$$

4. Calculate the second intermediate statistic, H:

$$H = \frac{t_{P(n-2)}}{D}\left[\mathrm{MS}_{\mathrm{rerror}}\left\{D\left(1 + \frac{1}{n}\right) + \frac{(y - \bar{y})^2}{\Sigma(x - \bar{x})^2}\right\}\right]^{½},$$

or when y is known:

$$H = \frac{t_{P(n-2)}}{D}\left[\mathrm{MS}_{\mathrm{rerror}}\left\{D\left(\frac{1}{n}\right) + \frac{(y - \bar{y})^2}{\Sigma(x - \bar{x})^2}\right\}\right]^{½}.$$

5. Calculate the third intermediate statistic, J:

$$J = \bar{x} + \frac{b\,(y - \bar{y})}{D}.$$

6. Calculate confidence intervals:

$$\mathrm{CI_U} = J + H;$$
$$\mathrm{CI_L} = J - H.$$

7. Apply confidence intervals to $\hat{x}$:

$$\mathrm{CI_L} \leqslant \hat{x} \leqslant \mathrm{CI_U}.$$

Note that the confidence intervals are not symmetrical about $\hat{x}$.

As an example of this method I will apply the calculations given in *Protocol 4* to the regression of the rotenone data using the logit method with the inclusion of the recalculated extreme mortality values (*Table 9*). Some of the regression statistics needed for this are in *Figure 16*. In this case $\hat{x}$ is the lethal concentration for 50% of the aphids (LC50) and the confidence intervals calculated will be the 95% intervals for the LC50. Hence, we need to find $\hat{x}$ when logit $y = 0.0$ (mortality = 50%).

First the predicted x value, the mean x and y values, and the $\Sigma(x - \bar{x})^2$ are calculated, which for these data are

$$\hat{x} = \frac{0.0 + 5.460}{8.169} = 0.668;$$
$$\bar{y} = 0.477;$$
$$\bar{x} = 0.727;$$
$$\Sigma(x - \bar{x})^2 = 0.8437.$$

Then the three intermediate statistics, D, H, and J, must be calculated sequentially:

$$D = (8.1685)^2 - \{(2.365)^2(0.587)^2\} = 64.797.$$

The LC50 is known by definition, so in this case we use the second formula for H in step 4 of *Protocol 4*:

$$H = \frac{2.365}{64.797}\left[0.291\left\{64.797\left(\frac{1}{9}\right) + \frac{(0.0 - 0.477)^2}{0.8437}\right\}\right]^{1/2} = 0.0539;$$

$$J = 0.727 + \frac{8.169(0.0 - 0.477)}{64.797} = 0.667.$$

So the confidence interval for $\hat{x}$ (0.668) is

$$0.613 \leqslant 0.668 \leqslant 0.721,$$

as $CI_L = 0.667 - 0.0539 = 0.613$ and $CI_U = 0.667 + 0.0539 = 0.721$, which, converted into the original units, is

$$4.10 \leqslant 4.66 \leqslant 5.26.$$

v. Comparison of the logit and probit methods

The logit and probit methods normally produce very similar results. They both work well for the dose–response type of data discussed above and other data with a symmetrical 'two-bend' curve. Finney (16) discusses these methods in relation to the analysis of the age of the onset of menstruation with data from 3918 Warsaw girls and concludes that the models fit the data well and give almost identical results. *Table 10* summarizes regression results from both methods with and without the recalculation of extreme points. It is clear that the two approaches give very similar results. Only the logit method with the extreme points gives an outlier > 2.0, but this is probably not a significant difference as all the other statistics are very similar. The three-group resistant line method had only a very slight effect on the regression statistics, further indicating that neither outliers nor the extreme points have an important effect on the regression solution for these data. The intercept and slope values appear different, but this is due to the logits and probits having means of 0.0 and 5.0 respectively. Although the results are not given here, all the regressions give highly significant t ratios for slope and intercept ($P < 0.001$) and F values from the regression ANOVA ($F > 140$; $P \ll 0.001$). The LC50 values are consistently slightly higher for the regressions without extreme values, but this difference is probably of minor significance as the 95% confidence intervals are much larger than this difference. So we can conclude that for these data it makes no practical difference whether the logit or probit method is used; this conclusion is probably generally applicable to most examples of this type of data.

Table 10. Summary statistics from *Minitab* for logit and probit regression of the rotenone data with and without inclusion of the recalculated extreme data points in the regression

Regression method[a]	Extreme values[b]	b_0	b	R^2 (%)	Most extreme standardized residual[c]	LC50 (mg/l)
Logit	+	−5.46	8.17	96.6	2.27	0.668
	−	−5.07	7.43	96.5	−1.63	0.683
Probit	+	2.12	4.35	97.4	1.93	0.663
	−	2.01	4.38	96.9	−1.70	0.684
Probit, robust	+	1.84	4.78	—[d]	−1.80	0.661
	−	2.03	4.33	—	1.46	0.686

[a] All regressions were of transformed proportions killed against the $\log_{10}$ rotenone concentration. Robust indicates the three-group resistant line method, all other results were for least squares regression

[b] + = extreme values included (n = 9); — = extreme points excluded (n = 7)

[c] Values for the three-group resistant line method were calculated by dividing the residuals by their standard deviation

[d] Values not calculated by *Minitab*

5.3 Direct non-linear solutions

Non-linear regression provides a method of estimating a line of best fit directly from accepted, biologically useful equations (5). This means that the empirical regression equations do not have to be used and biologically important constants can be directly estimated. The disadvantages of non-linear regression are that the calculation of confidence intervals and regression diagnostics is not as well developed as for the linear, least squares, methods. *Systat, SPSS/PC+*, and *Statgraphics* can all do non-linear regression, but *Minitab* cannot. I will confine my discussions to *Systat* and *SPSS/PC+*, and will use the puromycin treated enzyme data as an example.

In the equations and commands which follow, the variable names will be as used previously (*Appendix 3.1*) and the constant names will be VMAX = V_{max} = maximum reaction velocity and KM = K_m = Michaelis or half saturation constant. The Michaelis–Menten equation

$$v = \frac{V_{max}\, s}{K_m + s}$$

where v = reaction velocity (vtreat), must be used as the regression model. The commands needed to execute this non-linear regression in *Systat* are

```
NONLIN
MODEL VTREAT = (VMAX * S)/(KM + S)
ESTIMATE/QUASI
```

and for *SPSS/PC+* are

```
MODEL PROGRAM VMAX = 1 KM = 1.
COMPUTE PRED = (VMAX*S)/(KM + S).
NLR VTREAT WITH S.
```

Note that for *Systat* there is no LOSS statement, so the loss function will default to least squares, whilst with *SPSS/PC+* only least squares is available. Also, starting values of 1.0 are used by default in *Systat*, but must always be defined in *SPSS/PC+*. Sometimes more realistic starting values are required and should be roughly estimated directly from the data. In this case they could be estimated directly from the graph (*Figure 2c*), sensible guesses being $V_{max} = 200$ and $K_m = 100$; but the use of starting values other than 1.0 does not effect the answers here. The calculation procedures are iterative and with both packages the key results at each step are printed, followed by some statistics for the final solution. These statistics are an ANOVA table, R^2, value and the estimates of VMAX and KM with their standard errors and 95% confidence intervals. *Figure 17* gives this *SPSS/PC+* output using the larger starting values discussed above; output with starting values of 1.0 was similar but had more iterations. As expected, this solution fits the original data well (*Figure 13*). The algorithms for these two packages gave slightly different results. The constants given by *Systat* were VMAX = 204.9 and KM = 59.04, both being well within the *SPSS/PC+* confidence limits. Such differences between packages are not unexpected for non-linear regression.

5.4 The best method

It is clear that there are normally several approaches that can be used for regression analysis where the relationship between y and x is curved. Choosing the best approach is not always straightforward. *Table 11* gives a summary of the regression results for the puromycin treated enzyme data. It is clear that the Lineweaver–Burk method and $1/v^2$ against $1/s$ were the least satisfactory; they both had the lowest R^2 values and strongest outliers, and did not have normally distributed residuals. All the other regressions gave acceptable and fairly similar results. Thus, if a purely empirical prediction equation is required they would all be satisfactory. However, if values of the biologically important constants (V_{max} and K_m in this example) were required, only the non-linear methods or Hane's plot could be used. Neither the polynomial solution nor v against $\log_{10}s$ could provide estimates of these constants. Hane's plot depends on a knowledge of the rearranged Michaelis–Menten equation (*Table 11*), so it is likely that non-linear regression provides the most generally useful approach when the underlying biological equation is known. When a suitable equation is not known, it is likely that polynomial regression would be both easier and less prone to problems, such as uneven variances, than the methods which select suitable power transformations by examining curve shape (Section 5.2.1.*ii*) or by studying correlation coefficients (Section

```
Iteration  Residual SS        VMAX          KM

    1      7964.185201  200.000000  100.000000
    1.1    1593.159441  212.023790  54.2873641
    2      1593.159441  212.023790  54.2873641
    2.1    1201.034526  211.772798  62.3244628
    3      1201.034526  211.772798  62.3244628
    3.1    1195.508871  212.563259  63.9264826
    4      1195.508871  212.563259  63.9264826
    4.1    1195.449383  212.671588  64.1022790
    5      1195.449383  212.671588  64.1022790
    5.1    1195.448820  212.682567  64.1194489
    6      1195.448820  212.682567  64.1194489
    6.1    1195.448814  212.683630  64.1211054

Run stopped after 12 model evaluations and 6 derivative evaluations.
Iterations have been stopped because the relative reduction between
successive residual sums of squares is at most SSCON = 1.000E-08

Nonlinear Regression Summary Statistics     Dependent Variable VTREAT

  Source                   DF  Sum of Squares  Mean Square

  Regression                2   270213.55119   135106.77559
  Residual                 10     1195.44881      119.54488
  Uncorrected Total        12   271409.00000

  (Corrected Total)        11    30858.91667

  R squared = 1 - Residual SS / Corrected SS =     .96126

                                              Asymptotic 95 %
                            Asymptotic      Confidence Interval
  Parameter   Estimate      Std. Error      Lower          Upper

  VMAX      212.68362994  6.947090658 197.20454734 228.16271255
  KM         64.121105356  8.280753406 45.670436968 82.571773744
```

Figure 17. Non-linear regression output from *SPSS/PC+* for the puromycin treated enzyme data using the Michaelis–Menten equation as the regression model.

5.2.1.*iii*). However, polynomial regression does have its own problems. *Figure 13* shows that the polynomial solution gives an unlikely dip in the fitted line between the data points at substrate concentrations of 560 and 1100 mg/ml. Also, the y values below the lowest substrate concentration soon became negative and those over the highest concentration rapidly became unnaturally high. Such problems can be minimized by using more evenly spaced x values and never extrapolating outside the limits of the data.

Readers should not be tempted to try to find an arbitrary transformation of the data where the dependent variable, y, is calculated from the predictor

Table 11. Comparison of regression statistics calculated from the puromycin treated enzyme data[a] using several of the regression methods for curved lines

Regression method	R^2 (%)[b]	Most extreme standardized residual[c]	Correlation coefficient of normal scores and standardized residuals[d]	V_{max} (counts/min)	K_m (mg/ml)
Polynomial[e]	95.9	−2.27	0.975*	—[f]	—
Lineweaver-Burk[g]	85.6	−3.10	0.859	195.8	48.4
Hane's plot[h]	99.8	−1.77	0.977*	216.2	67.9
v against $\log_{10}s$	96.5	−1.94	0.986*	—	—
$1/v^2$ against $1/s$	75.3	3.12	0.802	—	—
Non-linear by *Systat*	99.5	1.97	0.977*	204.9	59.0
Non-linear by *SPSS/PC+*	99.3	2.36	0.959*	212.7	64.1

[a] v = reaction velocity, vtreat; s = substrate concentration
[b] Uncorrected value given; calculated from sums of squares, where

$$R^2 = \left(\frac{SS_{regression}}{SS_{total}}\right) \times 100$$

Note that because y varies in the different regression methods the R^2 values are not strictly comparable
[c] Values for non-linear regression were calculated by dividing the ordinary residuals by their standard deviation; the ordinary residuals themselves were calculated from the predicted values of v, obtained from the non-linear regression estimates of V_{max} and K_m and the Michaelis–Menten equation
[d] Critical value (*Appendix B.4*) = 0.927; * = residuals normally distributed, $P < 0.05$; see Chapters 1 and 4 for further details
[e] Obtained by multiple regression of v against s, s^2, and s^3
[f] Not easily calculable from these regressions
[g] $1/v$ against $1/s$; V_{max} and K_m calculated from slope and intercept, where $1/v = (1/V_{max}) + (K_m/V_{max})(1/s)$ (12)
[h] s/v against s; V_{max} and K_m calculated from slope and intercept, where $s/v = (K_m/V_{max}) + (1/V_{max})\, s$ (12)

variable, x. When this is done it can sometimes happen that an apparent, but spurious, relationship can be demonstrated purely because y was calculated from x. The Hane's plot used here is satisfactory because it is derived from a good theoretical basis.

References

1. Chatterjee, S. and Price, B. (1977). *Regression analysis by example.* John Wiley, New York.
2. Sokal, R. R. and Rohlf, F. J. (1981). *Biometry.* W. H. Freeman, San Francisco.
3. Rawlings, J. O. (1988). *Applied regression analysis: A research tool.* Wadsworth and Brooks, Pacific Grove, California.
4. Greenberg, B. G. (1953). *Am. J. Public Health,* **43,** 692.
5. Bates, D. M. and Watts, D. G. (1988). *Nonlinear regression analysis and its applications.* John Wiley, New York.

6. Finney, D. J. (1947). *Probit analysis: A statistical treatment of the sigmoid response curve*. Cambridge University Press, Cambridge.
7. Hoaglin, D. C., Mosteller, F., and Tukey, J. W. (1983). *Understanding robust and exploratory data analysis*. John Wiley, New York.
8. Fry, J. C. (1989). *Binary–Computing in Microbiology,* **1,** 83.
9. Farebrother, R. W. (1980). *Econometrica,* **48,** 1553.
10. Johnston, J. (1984). *Econometric models*. McGraw-Hill, New York.
11. Gunst, R. F. and Mason, R. L. (1980). *Regression analysis and its applications*. Marcel-Dekker, New York.
12. Cornish-Bowden, A. (1979). *Fundamentals of enzyme kinetics*. Butterworth, London.
13. Velleman, P. F. and Hoaglin, D. C. (1981). *Applications, basics and computing of exploratory data analysis*. Duxberry Press, Boston.
14. Daniel, C. and Wood, F. S. (1980). *Fitting equations to data*. Wiley Interscience, New York.
15. Ryan, B. F., Joiner, B. L., and Ryan, T. A. (1985). *Minitab handbook*. PWS-Kent Publishing, Boston.
16. Finney, D. J. (1971). *Probit analysis*, 3rd edn. Cambridge University Press, Cambridge.

Appendix 3.1. Contents of file REGRESS.DAT[a]

Optical density		**Child**		**Enzyme**			**Rotenone**	
Dry Wt	**OD**	**age**	**height**	**s**	**vtreat**	**v-untr**	**conc**	**mort**
1775	3.92	109	137.6	20	76	67	12.7	100
1280	3.26	113	147.8	20	47	51	10.2	88
1110	2.20	115	136.8	60	97	84	9.0	92
900	2.00	116	140.7	60	107	86	7.7	86
800	2.40	119	132.7	110	123	98	6.4	66
388	0.84	120	145.4	110	139	115	5.1	52
1088	2.84	121	135.0	220	159	131	3.8	33
480	1.15	124	133.0	220	152	124	2.6	12
2050	4.13	126	148.5	560	191	144	1.2	0
1110	2.46	129	148.3	560	201	158	0.0	0
1210	2.90	130	147.5	1100	207	160		
1775	3.80	133	148.8	1100	200			
		134	133.2					
		135	148.7					
		137	152.0					
		139	150.6					
		141	165.3					
		142	149.9					

[a] The file is organized in 19 rows. The top row contains the variable labels for the data and may have to be deleted before the file will be acceptable to some packages. The first two columns are the optical density data (Dry Wt: dry weight of bacteria, μg/ml; OD: true optical density at 660 nm). The child data (age, months; height, cm) are from Greenberg (4). The enzyme data (s: substrate concentration, mg/ml; vtreat: reaction velocity when treated with puromycin, counts/min; v-untr: untreated reaction velocity, counts/min) are from Bates and Watts (5). The rotenone data (conc: rotenone concentration, mg/l; mort: mortality, %) are modified from Finney (6). The columns in the file have all been made to equal length by adding asterisks (*); this makes the file readable by *Minitab* once the first row has been deleted, but the asterisks might need to be removed for some packages

Appendix 3.2. Listing of *Minitab* macro (REG-CIPI.MTB) for calculating and plotting confidence and prediction intervals for linear bivariate regression analysis

To run this macro the file must be present in the directory being used by *Minitab*. The *x* values must be put in C99 and the *y* values in C98; the macro uses columns C82–C99 and constants K94–K97, with some being used twice. The macro adds about 50 evenly spaced new *x* values to give smoother plots of the intervals and produces two ASCII files containing the results. All values calculated are kept in the worksheet as labelled columns at the end of the macro. TINT.DAT contains the *t*-intervals and FINT.DAT the *F*-intervals; both files also contain the original data and the line of best fit. This macro was written for *Minitab* release 8.2 and might need modification for other releases.

```
note REG-CIPI.MTB
noecho
note
note Minitab macro; calculates t and F type 95% confidence &
note prediction intervals (CI, PI) for simple bivariate regression.
note
note Gives high resolution Minitab plot of data, line of best fit
note and intervals. Produces ASCII files for plotting data with
note other packages; see full macro text for list of
note column contents.
note
note To use with line forced through origin type NONCONSTANT before
note running. To obtain a results file type OUTFILE 'filename'
note before running macro (N.B. results in filename.lis).
note
note Written by J.C. Fry 1991 for Minitab release 7.1 & 8.
note ************************************************************************
note *            Put data in c99 (x-values) and c98 (y-values)            *
note ************************************************************************
note Uses columns c82-c99 and constants k94-k97 (some used twice).
#
# 1.  Adding a range of new x values to x variable to allow
#     smoother intervals when plotted
name c99 'x-vals' c98 'y-vals'
name c97 'sresidu' c96 'y-fits'
maximum c99 k97                         # k97=largest x value
minimum c99 k96                         # k96=smallest x value
let k95=(k97-k96)/50                    # k95=interval size for 50
                                        # values of x-variable
set c94
k96:k97/k95
end
count c94 k94                           # k94=number of extra
                                        # x-vals calculated
set c93
k94('*')
end
count c98 k95                           # k95=number of yx points; n
stack (c99 c98) (c94 c93) (c99 c98)     # new x-var and y-var
sort c99 c98 c99 c98                    # data sorted for smooth lines
#
```

Appendix 3.2. (*contd.*)

```
# 2.  Basic regression and stats needed for further calculations
regress c98 1 c99 c97 c96;
mse k98;                                # k98=MSerror
hi c95;
coefficients c94.
name c94 'coeffs' c95 'hii'
# Calculation: F and t values for subsequent calculations (P=0.05)
count c94 k94                           # k94= number of coefs; p'
let k95=k95-k94                         # k95=n-p'
invcdf 0.95 k97;                        # k97=F value; df=p',n-p'
f k94 k95.
invcdf 0.975 k96;                       # k96=t value; df=n-p'
t k95.
#
# 3.  Calculation of confidence and prediction intervals
#       (i) Basic intervals
name c93 'CIt' c92 'CIf' c91 'PIt' c90 'PIf'
let c93=(sqrt(k98*c95))*k96                     # c93=CIt
let c92=(sqrt(k98*c95))*(sqrt(k94*k97))         # c92=CIf
let c91=(sqrt(k98*(1+c95)))*k96                 # c91=PIt
let c90=(sqrt(k98*(1+c95)))*(sqrt(k94*k97))     # c90=PIf
#       (ii) Upper and lower intervals (yhat + or - CI or PI)
name c98 'PIf-low' c88 'PIf-up'
name c87 'PIt-low' c86 'PIt-up'
name c85 'CIf-low' c84 'CIf-up'
name c83 'CIt-low' c82 'CIt-up'
let c89=c96−c90                         # PIf
let c88=c96+c90
let c87=c96−c91                         # PIt
let c86=c96+c91
let c85=c96−c92                         # CIf
let c84=c96+c92
let c83=c96−c93                         # CIt
let c82=c96+c93
#
# 4.  Plotting high resolution graph
gplot c98 c99;                          # points; white
lines 1 2 c96 c99;                      # line of best fit; red
lines 4 3 c89 c99;                      # PIf; green
lines 4 3 c88, c99;
lines 4 4 c87 c99;                      # PIt; blue
lines 4 4 c86 c99;
lines 2 6 c85 c99;                      # CIf; magenta
lines 2 6 c84 c99;
lines 2 7 c83 c99;                      # CIt; yellow
lines 2 7 c82 c99.
#
# 5.  Output ASCII files for plotting results with another package.
#         Data are old x & y variables with about 50 new x values
#         added for smoother plotting. Data ordered by x-values
#         and contain asterisks for missing values in last column
```

Appendix 3.2. (*contd.*)

```
#          which contains the original y-values only. Files are
#          TINT.DAT and FINT.DAT which contain the t-intervals and
#          F-intervals respectively.  (N.B. Some packages might not
#          read the last column accurately)
#            Data in columns of ASCII files are as follows
#                col 1 - new and old x values
#                col 2 - line of best fit
#                col 3 - CI upper
#                col 4 - CI lower
#                col 5 - PI upper
#                col 6 - PI lower
#                col 7 - old y values
#
write 'tint' c99 c96 c82 c83 c86 c87 c98
write 'fint' c99 c96 c84 c85 c88 c89 c98
note ****************************************************************
note *   Macro finished; results in TINT.DAT and FINT.DAT   *
note ****************************************************************
echo
```

4

Multiple regression

TERENCE C. ILES

1. Introduction

The previous chapter covers methods of fitting equations to data where there is just one predictor variable x for the dependent variable y. Sometimes data are collected on two or more different predictor variables $x_1, x_2, \ldots, x_k$ and an equation is sought to calculate y from the set of measurements of $x_1, x_2, \ldots, x_k$. This chapter describes the fitting and interpretation of linear equations with such data sets. The choice of the variables that should be included in the prediction equation, and the possible transformation of variables, will also be discussed. The calculations required for multiple regression are usually too time-consuming to be done by hand so it is necessary to use a computer. Fortunately, most statistical packages have regression routines and these give the user a wide choice of statistics that help in finding suitable prediction equations. Many of these diagnostic statistics are most easily interpreted by the use of plots, so a package with built-in plotting routines should be used.

There are three main uses of multiple regression:

- finding a prediction equation for y
- investigating the variables x that influence y
- demonstrating a physical law

Multiple regression is a very widely-used analytical technique and many books have been written on the subject, some dealing only with special aspects. Chatterjee and Price (1) is a particularly useful text for a reader unfamiliar with the subject. Another book giving much helpful guidance on regression techniques, with the data analyst in mind, is Gunst and Mason (2). Another helpful text, though written for statisticians and scientists with some experience of analysing their data, is by Atkinson (3). A text on regression diagnostics is by Cook and Weisberg (4), but in this book it is assumed that the reader is familiar with the mathematical theory of regression methods.

1.1 Data structure

Multiple regression equations are calculated from measurements made on a representative sample of n individuals from a population. For each individual in this sample, values are recorded of k predictor variables $x_1, x_2, \ldots, x_k$ and the dependent variable y that will appear on the left-hand side of the equation.

As a first simple illustrative example, the loblolly pine data given in *Table 2* of Chapter 2 will be used to show how a polynomial equation can be fitted to a set of data. *Figure 10* of Chapter 2 suggests the possibility of fitting a parabola to predict the number of seedlings with the date of sowing. The dependent variable y is the number of seedlings. There are two predictors: the date of sowing x_1, represented as 1–6 inclusive, and the squares of these numbers x_2. The data set for this regression therefore occupies three columns. The data, sorted by date of sowing, are presented here as *Table 1*.

Table 2 is the data set that will be used in this chapter to illustrate multiple regression analysis techniques in detail. The data are in exactly the format used by *Minitab*. The aim in collecting the data was to establish the nature of the variables influencing the breeding of British dippers, thrush-sized birds living mainly in the upper reaches of rivers. They feed on benthic invertebrates by probing the river bed with their beaks. Measurements were made of 8 variables at 22 stretches of river inhabited by dippers (see *Table 2* for details). Multiple regression will be used to derive an equation to predict the breeding density of dippers with some or all of the seven other variables used as predictors, possibly after suitable transformations have been made.

A third data set will be used to describe the techniques of fitting different equations to subsets of a bivariate data set by using dummy variables and the methods of multiple regression. The data are in the first two columns of *Table 3*; the other columns will be described in Section 7. These data are derived from surveys of the numbers of O-group plaice in Swedish and Dutch coastal waters, and the calculated mortality rate assumes an exponential rate of decline in the numbers of fish. The scatter plot of these data in *Figure 1* suggests that one possibility to describe the relationship between these two variables is a constant mortality up to a threshold maximum density, then a straight line relationship of mortality with log density. A curve is another possibility, but this will not be investigated here (see Chapter 3, Section 5 for details about fitting curves).

Where the regression equation is used for the demonstration of a physical law or for prediction, care should be exercised in generalizing from the sample to populations that have not been studied, however similar to the survey sample these populations are believed to be. It is particularly dangerous to extrapolate from the equation beyond the range of measurement of the variables. If interrelationships between variables are studied, it should be borne in mind that the establishment of a linear relationship between variables does not necessarily imply causation. The two variables in question may be linked by a third, unmeasured, variable.

As in bivariate regression, it is desirable that the distribution of the variables should be even. Equations derived from data mainly concentrated at one end of the scales of measurement are usually heavily influenced by the

Table 1. Numbers of seedlings produced by loblolly pine seeds sown on six dates and contents of file LOBLOLL2.DAT[a]

Row	seedling	date	date-sq
1	900	1	1
2	880	1	1
3	810	1	1
4	1100	1	1
5	760	1	1
6	960	1	1
7	1040	1	1
8	1040	1	1
9	880	2	4
10	1050	2	4
11	1170	2	4
12	1240	2	4
13	1060	2	4
14	1110	2	4
15	910	2	4
16	1120	2	4
17	1530	3	9
18	1140	3	9
19	1160	3	9
20	1270	3	9
21	1390	3	9
22	1320	3	9
23	1540	3	9
24	1080	3	9
25	1970	4	16
26	1360	4	16
27	1890	4	16
28	1510	4	16
29	1820	4	16
30	1490	4	16
31	2140	4	16
32	1270	4	16
33	1960	5	25
34	1270	5	25
35	1670	5	25
36	1380	5	25
37	1310	5	25
38	1500	5	25
39	1480	5	25
40	1450	5	25
41	830	6	36
42	150	6	36
43	420	6	36
44	380	6	36
45	570	6	36
46	420	6	36
47	760	6	36
48	270	6	36

[a] The file does not contain the row numbers or headings. These data are essentially the same as in Chapter 2, *Tables 2* and *5*, with numbers of seedlings ordered by date; date-sq = date squared

Table 2. Data[a] from a survey of dippers in file DIPPER.DAT[b]

ROW	Alt	W Hard	Gradient	Caddis	Stonefly	Mayfly	Other In	Br. Dens
1	259	12.20	10.90	9	188	0	3	3.60
2	198	22.00	14.70	17	76	29	4	4.30
3	251	26.30	6.90	43	186	338	3	3.80
4	184	22.50	4.60	82	188	313	3	3.40
5	145	29.50	1.91	24	45	246	2	3.80
6	145	39.90	5.00	50	133	313	20	4.50
7	198	42.80	6.20	38	77	214	3	4.30
8	160	59.60	14.30	83	564	0	18	5.00
9	251	69.25	4.60	43	223	124	12	4.50
10	159	68.00	3.30	85	33	415	31	3.40
11	160	85.28	15.80	230	76	534	144	4.50
12	145	84.18	5.90	133	505	484	33	6.90
13	214	89.00	5.70	91	92	277	317	3.50
14	191	103.90	7.60	60	30	705	873	3.60
15	167	90.90	17.40	52	281	972	130	4.70
16	244	95.10	6.10	37	165	523	29	4.00
17	83	153.90	2.88	16	20	364	338	2.90
18	175	150.50	12.80	35	325	273	2	6.40
19	107	15.50	4.90	48	120	431	71	4.00
20	305	115.80	26.20	254	520	520	24	8.46
21	152	130.70	8.50	224	166	742	733	5.00
22	277	90.00	19.00	383	889	696	14	8.00

[a] The first column (ROW) contains row numbers, each of which represent separate sites on the River Wye and its tributaries in Wales; the next three columns are environmental variables (Alt = site altitude, m above sea level; W Hard = water hardness, mg $CaCO_3$/l; Gradient = gradient or slope of the river bed, m/km); the following four columns are abundancies of invertebrates in riffles and marginal areas expressed as numbers from 2 × 3 min kick samples (Caddis = caddis fly larvae; Stonefly = stonefly larvae; Mayfly = mayfly larvae; Other In = all other invertebrates collected); and the last column (Br. Dens) is the number of breeding pairs of dippers per 10 km of river. Data provided by Dr S. J. Ormerod

[b] The file does not contain row numbers or headings

rare extreme data, and are not therefore truly representative. However, predictor variables are frequently interrelated, and it is then not possible to obtain data covering all combinations of values of the variables. If two predictors are approximately linearly related then few individuals in the sample will be found with a combination of these variables any distance from the approximate straight line. This is a fact of life, and has to be accepted by the analyst. It is preferable that the scales of measurement of the predictor variables be roughly commensurable (similar numerical orders of magnitude). Rounding error in calculations can otherwise be a problem in multiple regression, and the extent to which computer packages can deal with non-commensurable variables depends on the way the numerical methods of calculation are programmed.

Table 3. Data from surveys of O-group plaice

ROW	M	log Dmax	Zone	x1	x2
1	0.01052	5.09987	2	1	0.00000
2	0.00889	5.25227	2	1	0.00000
3	0.00697	5.30827	2	1	0.00000
4	0.01376	5.69373	2	1	0.00000
5	0.00745	5.76832	2	1	0.00000
6	0.01013	6.21461	2	1	0.00000
7	0.00850	6.25190	2	1	0.00000
8	0.01310	6.26340	1	0	6.26340
9	0.01265	6.39693	1	0	6.39693
10	0.01082	6.68461	1	0	6.68461
11	0.02087	7.20042	1	0	7.20042
12	0.03474	7.78322	1	0	7.78322
13	0.05147	7.90101	1	0	7.90101

[a] The first column, after the row number (ROW), is the daily mortality rate (M; d^{-1}) and the second is the natural logarithm of the maximum density (numbers per thousand square metres). The other columns are explained in Section 7. Each row of the table gives data for a year-class of a particular sub-population of plaice. This short data set is not provided in a file

1.2 The model and assumptions

The form of relationship between y and x variables assumed in multiple regression is:

$$y = \beta_0 + \beta_1 x_1 + \beta_2 x_2 + \ldots \beta_k x_k + \varepsilon. \tag{1}$$

The assumption is made that the form of this equation is a correct model: that all relevant predictors are included on the right-hand side of the equation. We assume also that they are measured on a scale such that their effect on the dependent variable y is additive. If all measurements of $x_2, x_3, \ldots, x_k$ are fixed, a unit increase in x_1 causes an increase of β_1 units in y. Values of the

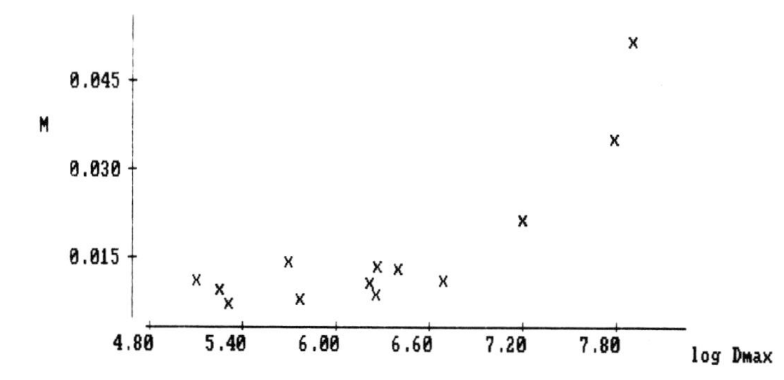

Figure 1. Scatter plot of mortality against log maximum density for O-group plaice.

constants $\beta_0, \beta_1, \ldots, \beta_k$ are not known. A sample of n observations of $y, x_1, x_2, \ldots, x_k$ is used to obtain estimates of these constants. If n is less than $k + 1$ it is not possible to estimate all the constants and, preferably, n should be much greater than $k + 1$. The problem addressed by multiple regression is that no values for the constants can be found that make the equation fit precisely for all n sets of observations. A compromise solution has to be sought that makes the errors ε as small as possible. The statistical justification for the usual compromise, minimizing the sum of the squares of the errors, relies on five further assumptions:

- the *x*s are not random variables, and are measured without error
- the errors ε have a mean of zero
- the errors are independent
- the errors have the same variance, σ^2
- the errors are normally distributed

Various extensions of the simple theory can be made to relax these assumptions, but these will not be described in detail in this chapter. It is rarely practicable to assume that the *x*s are error-free and that all errors are in the measurement of y alone. A multiple regression equation based on *x*s measured with error is then only valid on the assumption that it is conditioned on those fixed values of x actually obtained. Details of the theory of fitting linear equations to data with errors in both y and x where there is only one predictor x can be found in Miller (5). Very little has been written on multiple regression with errors in the x variables. A rather mathematical description is given by Kendall and Stuart (6, pp. 408–10).

If the errors are not independent the model has to include correlated errors. Some details of these models are given by Chatterjee and Price (1, Chapter 6). Non-constant error variances can be allowed for, either for transforming the variables (this will be discussed in Section 4.3) or by weighted regression. Details of the latter approach are in Chatterjee and Price (1, Chapter 5).

The assumption that the errors are normally distributed is used to establish procedures for statistical testing and the derivation of confidence intervals. The estimation procedure itself does not depend on this assumption since it can be justified using purely geometrical arguments. Nevertheless, an alternative approach is to use a technique of robust estimation. Further details of these methods in the context of multiple regression are given in Hoaglin *et al.* (7, Chapter 7). Procedures using these methods are not yet available in commonly used statistical packages. Another possibility is to use a model called the general linear model. This is described by McCullagh and Nelder (8). The essence of this approach is that some function of the linear combination of the predictor variables is supposed to model the average value of the dependent variable, and the errors are assumed to be some member of a family of distributions called the exponential family. The method should not be confused with so-called general linear model commands in packages such as *SAS* or *Minitab*. These commands are for multiple regression, analysis of variance, and analysis of covariance models. A special package called *GLIM* is available to fit the general linear model (See *Appendix A* for details of this package.)

2. Estimation and interpretation of the regression equation

The procedure outlined in *Protocol 1* of Chapter 3 needs little modification for multiple regression; however, the modified procedure is presented here as *Protocol 1*. Because there are now several potential predictor (x) variables, there are more plots to examine to decide the scale of measurement to be used and whether transformations should be applied. However crude the initial indications for transformations are, I recommend that these plots be examined at the outset of the analysis, since the alternative is to fit a multiple regression equation to the raw data, omitting steps 1 and 2 of *Protocol 1*, and use the diagnostic statistics to identify appropriate transformations. My experience suggests that this is just as time-consuming a procedure, and a more refined model is a better starting-point for an examination of the data. A major advantage of an initial scanning of the data is that obvious errors can be rectified from the start and anomalous data may be identified.

Protocol 1. Initial fitting and checking of multiple regression equations

1. Plot y against each x variable in turn. Curvature indicates the need for transformations. Linear plots indicate important predictors.
2. Check for evenness in variables using boxplots, letter value displays, and histograms.
3. Plot y against the index i[a] or time of collection of data (if known). Any relationship indicates an unsuspected lurking variable.
4. Fit the regression equation, after transformation if necessary. Save the studentized deleted residuals, leverages, and Cook's D. Calculate the Durbin–Watson statistic, particularly if the data are in time order.
5. Assess the significance of the relationship using the F-ratio (see Section 3). If the F-ratio is small, good predictions are not possible except, possibly, after transformation or inclusion of extra variables (x^2, x^3, etc.).
6. Perform diagnostic checks (*Protocol 2*).
7. Check for multi-collinearity (see Section 5, *Protocol 3*).
8. Investigate the possibility of reducing the number of predictor variables (see Section 6, *Protocol 4*).

Protocol 1. *Continued*

9. When an optimum regression equation is obtained, assess its value for the purposes for which it was intended. If it is used for prediction, calculate confidence intervals or prediction intervals (see Section 3 and the guidance on Bonferroni and Scheffé intervals, in Section 3.3).

[a] The index i is the order in which the data sets are entered in the data file. Use a logical ordering where such is available.

2.1 The loblolly pine seedling data

As a first example, just to show how a regression equation is obtained from a set of data, the loblolly pine data of *Table 1* will be used. The regression equation is calculated using the REGRESSION command in *Minitab*. The dependent variable, number of seedlings y, is in column C1 and the two predictors, date x and $(\text{date})^2$ x^2 are in columns C2 and C3 respectively. The command

```
REGRESS C1 2 C2 C3
```

calculates the required regression equation. Notice the necessity for specifying the number of predictors, in this case 2, with the *Minitab* REGRESS command. The regression equation is given in the *Minitab* output (*Figure 2*), and is

$$y = -19 + 914\,x - 133\,x^2.$$

A detailed description of the interpretation of the remainder of the output from the REGRESS command will be left to the illustrative example using the dipper data, but two points are worth making here. Firstly, the F-ratio testing the hypothesis that both regression coefficients are zero is 29.98 with 2 and 45 df, and a P-value less than 0.0005. There is no doubt here that the hypothesis of zero coefficients is decisively rejected. Secondly, attention is automatically drawn to unusual observations. This is a most useful feature of the REGRESS command in *Minitab*. Details of diagnostic checking are given in Section 4 of this chapter. *Figure 3* is a plot of the data together with the fitted equation. This also was obtained using *Minitab*.

A comparison of the analysis of variance section of the output given in *Figure 2* and the two-way crossed ANOVA given in *Figure 9* of Chapter 2 is instructive. The total sum of squares, 9 339 648 with 47 df, is the same in both cases. In *Figure 2* the explained variation in the data is the regression line with SS 5 335 739 and 2 df. *Figure 9* of Chapter 2 gives the explained variation due to dates, for a model in which a separate mean is fitted for each date, as 7 500 086 with 5 df. The simpler parabola model has explained a substantial proportion of the variation due to differences in the dates. In this example no account is taken of the method of preparation of ground, the 'burning' factor

```
MTB > regress c1 2 c2 c3

The regression equation is
seedling = - 19 + 914 date - 133 date-sq

Predictor        Coef          Stdev      t-ratio         p
Constant        -18.9          188.7        -0.10     0.921
date            913.9          123.4         7.40     0.000
date-sq       -133.10          17.26        -7.71     0.000

s = 298.3        R-sq = 57.1%       R-sq(adj) = 55.2%

Analysis of Variance

SOURCE         DF           SS           MS           F         p
Regression      2      5335739      2667870       29.98     0.000
Error          45      4003908        88976
Total          47      9339648

SOURCE         DF       SEQ SS
date            1        44464
date-sq         1      5291275

Unusual Observations
Obs.      date  seedling        Fit  Stdev.Fit  Residual    St.Resid
 31       4.00    2140.0     1507.1       64.3     632.9       2.17R
 33       5.00    1960.0     1223.0       58.4     737.0       2.52R

R denotes an obs. with a large st. resid.
```

Figure 2. Multiple regression to fit a parabola to the graph of loblolly pine seedling numbers against date of sowing. Output from *Minitab* REGRESS command.

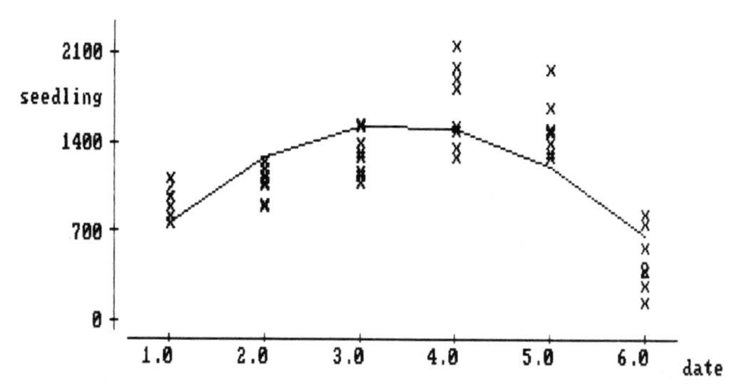

Figure 3. Scatterplot of loblolly pine seedling numbers against date of sowing, together with the fitted parabola.

of *Figure 9* of Chapter 2. This can be incorporated into regression models using the analysis of covariance, but this subject is outside of the scope of this book.

2.2 The dipper data

For the dipper data of *Table 2* the dependent variable y is the breeding density, or some transformation thereof. There are seven potential predictors and there is insufficient space here to print all the plots and charts suggested in *Protocol 1* steps 1 and 2 for the initial data scrutiny. *Figure 4a* is a boxplot

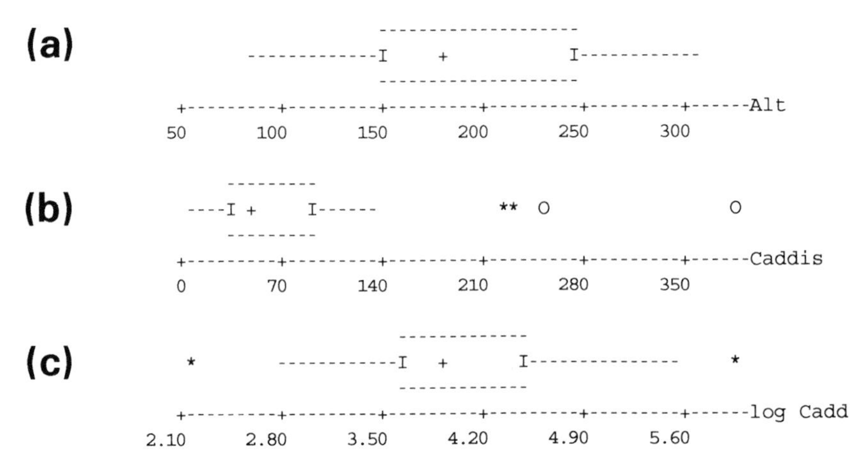

Figure 4. Boxplots of predictor variables for breeding density of dippers from data in *Table 2*: (a) altitude; (b) caddis fly numbers; (c) $\log_e$ (1 + caddis fly number).

of the altitude data, and this indicates a symmetric distribution so that no transformation of this variable is needed. *Figure 4b* is a plot of the caddis fly numbers and these data are clearly highly skewed, with two extreme outliers. *Figure 4c* shows the boxplot of the same data after a logarithmic transformation has been used. This results in a symmetric distribution, so this transformation will be used for the initial model for these daa. Similar transformations are indicated for all four of the variables measuring invertebrate numbers. Because of the zero counts of mayfly at two sites the straight $\log_e$ transform cannot be used, so the $\log_e(1 + x)$ transformation is used instead. The two transformations $\log_e x$ and $\log_e(1 + x)$ differ greatly only for small values of x (less than about 10), and for large values are virtually indistinguishable. For the sake of consistency the same $\log_e(1 + x)$ transformation has been used for all four variables measuring invertebrate numbers. In the initial model no transformation is used for the other predictors, altitude, water hardness, and gradient. *Figure 5* shows the scatterplot of stonefly numbers against breeding density and $\log_e$(1 + stonefly number) against $\log_e$ (breeding density) respectively. There is perhaps slightly less evidence of a scatter from a straight line in the plot of the transformed data, and the data are more evenly spaced. Thus $\log_e$ (breeding density) will be used to fit the model.

The next stage in *Protocol 1* is to fit the regression line and store the diagnostic statistics for subsequent checking. *Figure 6* gives the output from *Minitab* using the REGRESS command. *SAS* and *SPSS/PC+* give very similar output, though with a slightly different layout. On the command line in *Minitab*, the first column (C18) is where the logarithm of breeding density, the dependent variable, is located. The number 7 refers to the number of predictor variables and these are in C1 to C3 (untransformed altitude, water hardness, and gradient) and C14 to C17 (the transformed invertebrate

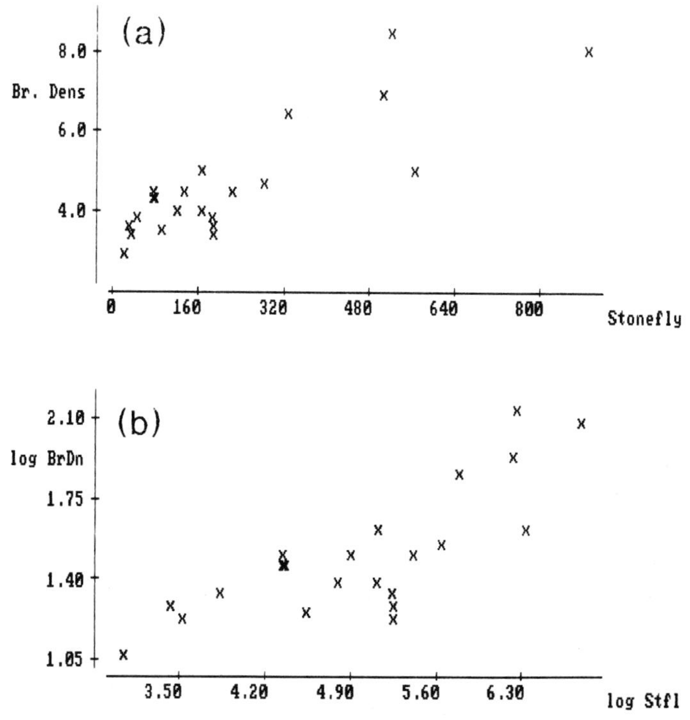

Figure 5. Scatter plots of data on breeding density of dippers from *Table 2*: (a) breeding density against stonefly numbers; (b) $\log_e$ of breeding density against $\log_e$ (1 + stonefly number).

numbers). The following sub-command lines will be discussed in subsequent sections. All the output down to the line 'R denotes an obs. with a large st. resid.' is obtained in exactly the same form if the sub-commands are not invoked.

The first four lines of output give the prediction or regression equation. This is the best equation to predict y in the sense of having the smallest sum of squares of errors. It is rather difficult to interpret an equation involving so many predictors. The multipliers of the predictor variables, which will be denoted by $b_1, b_2, \ldots, b_k$, are called the partial regression coefficients. The size of these coefficients is not necessarily a reliable indication of the importance of the predictor variables in the prediction equation, since they depend on the scale of the xs. Multiplication of a predictor by a constant factor simply divides the corresponding partial regression coefficient by the same factor. It is not possible to plot this equation because of the large number of dimensions. Even with only two predictors a three-dimensional plot is needed. A further difficulty of interpretation stems from the possibility of interrelationships between the predictors. The magnitude of a partial

```
MTB > regress c18 7 c1-c3 c14-c17;
SUBC> xpxinv m1;
SUBC> predict 85 12 2 3 3 0 1;
SUBC> predict 189.5 72.58 9.33 4.122 4.977 5.33 3.332;
SUBC> predict 300 150 25 6 6 6 6;
SUBC> tresid c21;
SUBC> cookd c22;
SUBC> hi c23.

The regression equation is
log BrDn = 0.440 -0.000606 Alt + 0.00159 W Hard + 0.0152 Gradient
           + 0.0705 log Cadd + 0.134 log Stfl + 0.0216 log Mayf
           - 0.0472 log OInv

Predictor        Coef         Stdev     t-ratio        p
Constant       0.4402        0.2271        1.94    0.073
Alt        -0.0006062     0.0006611       -0.92    0.375
W Hard      0.0015877     0.0009272        1.71    0.109
Gradient     0.015152      0.006688        2.27    0.040
log Cadd      0.07049       0.05128        1.37    0.191
log Stfl      0.13428       0.04657        2.88    0.012
log Mayf      0.02162       0.02133        1.01    0.328
log OInv     -0.04725       0.02464       -1.92    0.076

s = 0.1347       R-sq = 84.7%      R-sq(adj) = 77.1%

Analysis of Variance

SOURCE        DF          SS          MS         F        p
Regression     7     1.40763     0.20109     11.08    0.000
Error         14     0.25408     0.01815
Total         21     1.66171

SOURCE        DF      SEQ SS
Alt            1     0.23906
W Hard         1     0.20079
Gradient       1     0.42897
log Cadd       1     0.15212
log Stfl       1     0.29181
log Mayf       1     0.02815
log OInv       1     0.06675

Unusual Observations
Obs.      Alt   log BrDn        Fit  Stdev.Fit   Residual    St.Resid
  4       184     1.2238     1.5083     0.0637    -0.2845      -2.40R

R denotes an obs. with a large st. resid.

     Fit  Stdev.Fit          95% C.I.            95% P.I.
  1.0051     0.1518   ( 0.6794, 1.3309)   ( 0.5696, 1.4406) X

  1.4986     0.0287   ( 1.4370, 1.5603)   ( 1.2031, 1.7941)

  1.9502     0.1046   ( 1.7258, 2.1746)   ( 1.5843, 2.3161)

X  denotes a row with X values away from the center


MTB > print m1
 MATRIX M1

 2.84119 -0.00310  0.00130  0.02860  0.04799 -0.37963 -0.08153 -0.13324
-0.00310  0.00002  0.00000 -0.00009 -0.00005 -0.00022 -0.00004  0.00021
 0.00130  0.00000  0.00005 -0.00009  0.00049 -0.00043 -0.00039 -0.00061
 0.02860 -0.00009 -0.00009  0.00246 -0.00454 -0.00405  0.00205 -0.00017
 0.04799 -0.00005  0.00049 -0.00454  0.14491 -0.07074 -0.03205 -0.03200
-0.37963 -0.00022 -0.00043 -0.00405 -0.07074  0.11951  0.01725  0.02850
-0.08153 -0.00004 -0.00039  0.00205 -0.03205  0.01725  0.02506  0.00337
-0.13324  0.00021 -0.00061 -0.00017 -0.03200  0.02850  0.00337  0.03345
```

Figure 6. Multiple regression to predict breeding density of dippers using the data in *Table 2* with the transformations discussed in the text. Output from *Minitab* REGRESS command.

regression coefficient for a variable depends on which other predictors are included in the equation.

The potential difficulties of interpretation are illustrated by the artificial example plotted in *Figure 7*. Clearly the trend is for y to increase with x_1, so in a bivariate regression of y on x_1 alone the slope of the regression line is positive. However, for any fixed x_2, either $x_2 = 2$, 4, 6, or 8, it is clear that y decreases with x_1 so that the slope of a regression line for any of these four subsets of the data would be negative. If a multiple regression is done of y on

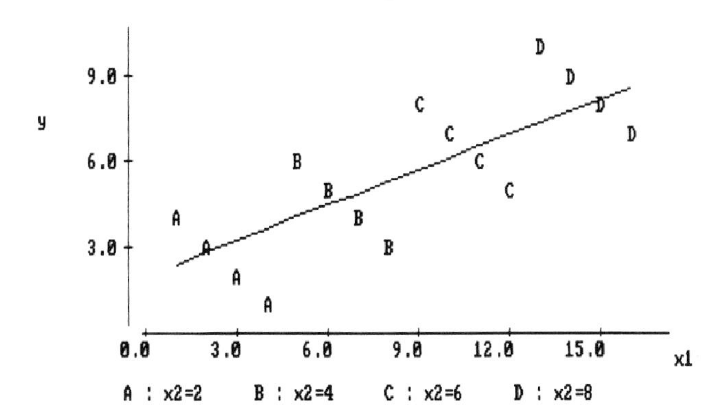

Figure 7. Scatter plot to show the potential difficulty of interpretation of partial regression coefficients. For an explanation see text.

x_1 and x_2 then it would be seen that the partial regression coefficient b_1 for the variable x_1 is negative, despite the apparent positive slope indicated by the scatterplot of *Figure 7*. The reason for this apparent anomaly is that b_1 is the change in predicted y resulting from a unit change in x_1 adjusted for the linear relationship between x_1 and the other predictor x_2. Once adjustment is made for x_2 with these data the trend is clearly for y to decrease with x_1.

If the model is correctly specified the partial regression coefficients are unbiased estimates of the unknown constants $\beta_1, \beta_2, \ldots, \beta_k$ in the model given in equation (1). The word unbiased in this context means that the theoretical average value of b_j over imagined repetitions of the survey is equal to β_j. However, if the model is misspecified by exclusion of predictors that genuinely should be included in the linear relationship, then the coefficients are biased. This fact should be borne in mind in interpreting models used to investigate interrelationships between variables.

Around the middle of *Figure 6*, just above the analysis of variance table, the statistic $s = 0.1347$ is printed. This is the estimate of the standard deviation σ of the error terms ε in the linear model of equation (1). This is the square root of the value of MS_{error} of 0.018 15 in the middle of the analysis of variance table itself. MS_{error} is an estimate of the error variance σ^2. Although s is the estimate of the standard deviation of the error terms it is misleading to interpret this as a measure of dispersion or variance of observations from the predicted values. These predicted values are calculated using the partial regression coefficients and they are themselves calculated from the observations and are therefore estimated with error. This complicates the expression for the variance of a prediction.

The matrix referred to in *Minitab* as XPXINV is used in the calculation of the partial regression coefficients. This matrix is printed at the foot of *Figure 6* and was calculated by invoking the XPXINV subcommand. Its usefulness to the practitioner is that when all of its elements are multiplied by the estimate of the error variance s^2, the result obtained is a matrix of variances and covariances of the coefficients $b_0, b_1, \ldots, b_k$. The element on the jth diagonal of this matrix, counting from 0, is the variance of b_j. The element in the jth row and lth column, again counting from 0, is the covariance between b_j and b_l. If this covariance is divided by the square root of the product of the variances of b_j and b_l the correlation coefficient between b_j and b_l is obtained. Thus the leading diagonal element 2.841 19, when multiplied by 0.018 15, gives 0.051 57 as the variance of the constant term b_0. The square root, 0.2271, is the standard deviation of b_0. The element in the sixth row (row 5 counting from 0) and last column, 0.028 50, gives, on multiplication by 0.018 15, $5.172\,78 \times 10^{-4}$ as the estimated covariance between b_5 and b_7. The correlation coefficient between these two coefficients is obtained by dividing by $\sqrt{(0.119\,51 \times 0.018\,15) \times (0.033\,45 \times 0.018\,15)}$ or $1.147\,56 \times 10^{-3}$. This gives a correlation coefficient of 0.450 76, indicating a strong interrelation between the estimates of these coefficients. The matrix XPXINV, after multiplication by s^2, is called the estimated variance–covariance matrix of b_0, b_1, $b_2, \ldots, b_k$.

3. Tests and confidence intervals in multiple regression

3.1 Overall tests of significance for the regression coefficients

As has been mentioned already, the criterion for determining the optimum multiple regression equation is to make the sum of squares of the errors as small as possible. Thus the error sum of squares is a direct measure of the efficacy of the equation in predicting the observed values of the dependent variable y, but its value depends on the scale of measurement of y and it cannot therefore be interpreted in isolation. The principle of multiple regression modelling is to include in the equation those predictors that significantly decrease the error sum of squares. The simplest model is that the y values are randomly scattered about their overall mean $\bar{y}$, in which case the error sum of squares would be $\Sigma(y - \bar{y})^2$. This is called the total sum of squares. The difference between the error sum of squares with a regression model fitted and the total sum of squares thus measures the gain in explained variation obtained by using the regression equation. This is called the regression sum of squares. A formal comparison of the regression and error sum of squares is made by first dividing the sums of squares by their degrees of freedom to get the mean squares, then calculating the ratio of these mean squares. Standard F tables are used to assess the significance of the ratio of the mean squares. This formal test depends on the assumption that the errors in the measurement of y are normally distributed, but the F-test can be relied upon except where this assumption is badly wrong. The formal statistical hypothesis tested by the F-ratio is that all of the coefficients $\beta_1, \beta_2, \ldots, \beta_k$ are equal to zero. A large F-ratio suggests that this hypothesis should be rejected and that at least one, but not necessarily all, of the coefficients is non-zero. In the output of *Figure 6* the F-ratio is 11.08, with 7 and 14 df, and the associated P-value is less than 0.0005, indicating that the hypothesis is decisively rejected. The initial indications are that some linear prediction equation is tenable.

A related measure of the effectiveness of a multiple regression equation is the coefficient of determination or squared multiple correlation coefficient. This is designated R^2 (or R-sq in *Minitab*) and is calculated as the ratio of regression sum of squares to total sum of squares. It is often expressed as a percentage by multiplication by 100. Thus R^2 measures the proportion of variation, as measured by sum of squares of errors, explained by the prediction equation. When an additional predictor variable is included in the regression equation R^2 always increases, and an adjusted R^2, defined as

$$R^2_{\mathrm{ADJ}} = 1 - (1 - R^2)(n - 1)/(n - p'),$$

where p' is the number of constants in the model, including the constant β_0 (so $p' = 1 + k$). Since the adjusted R^2 does not have the simple definition as a proportion of explained variability, it is more difficult to interpret practically than the simple R^2. The overall significance of the multiple regression equation can also be found from the multiple correlation coefficient ($R = \sqrt{R^2}$) for which critical values are in *Appendix B.9*. As a measure of the effectiveness of a multiple regression equation R^2 has the defect that it is relatively insensitive, particularly where it is used in variable selection. This will be discussed further in Section 6. Thus although the R^2 value given in *Figure 6* is high, 84.7%, this value should be treated with some caution. The overall significance of a multiple regression equation depends very much on the use to which it will be put.

The output from the REGRESS command enables the overall significance of the multiple regression equation to be judged. It does not give unequivocal guidance on the variables to include in the regression equation. This will be discussed in Section 6. However, the next subsection shows how significance tests and confidence intervals can be calculated for individual regression coefficients.

3.2 Significance tests and confidence intervals for individual regression coefficients

The table underneath the analysis of variance in *Figure 6* gives the sequential sums of squares for the variables in the regression equation. The values of these in *Minitab* will usually be different if the order in which the predictor variables are included in the command line is changed. (The only exception is where the predictor variables are orthogonal, that is, mutually uncorrelated.) Thus the regression sum of squares for the variable altitude in a simple bivariate regression is 0.239 06, with 1 df. The regression sum of squares for altitude and water hardness together is 0.239 06 + 0.200 79 = 0.439 85, with 2 df. The regression sum of squares for water hardness alone cannot be derived from the data in *Figure 6*. To obtain this sum of squares, water hardness has to be the first predictor variable included in the command line. The sum of squares for water hardness alone is 0.165 36 and then the extra due to altitude is 0.274 48. Notice that these also add to 0.439 85 (apart from rounding error), with 2 df. The sum of all seven of the sequential sums of squares is equal to the overall regression sum of squares of 1.407 63.

If the errors are normally distributed, and the x variables are assumed not to be random variables, then the partial regression coefficients are also normally distributed. The mean of b_j is β_j and the variance is σ^2 times the jth diagonal element of the matrix called in *Minitab* XPXINV. This enables hypotheses to be tested and confidence interals constructed for the unknown constants β_j. In *Minitab* the coefficients are tabulated together with their estimated standard deviations in the table after the regression equation in *Figure 6*. The t-ratio, also printed here, is the standard Student's t test statistic for the hypothesis that $\beta_j = 0$. The associated P-value of this statistic is printed alongside. Thus only in two cases in this analysis is the hypothesis of a zero constant β_j rejected, the two being gradient with $t = 2.27$ and $P = 0.0\,40$ and $\log_e(1 + \text{stonefly})$ with $t = 2.88$ and $P = 0.012$. The lack of significance of the remaining t-ratios should not, however, be taken as conclusive evidence that the remaining variables should be excluded from the regression equation. Because the sum of squares associated with any predictor variable depends on the other variables in the equation, the t-ratios will be different if the multiple regression is done again with one or more predictors omitted. In a regression with fewer predictors included, it may well be that another of the t-ratios is significant. If a confidence interval for an individual constant β_j is required, this is readily calculated from the formula

$$b_j \pm t\sqrt{\text{Var}(b_j)},$$

where t is a percentile of Student's t distribution with $(n - p')$ df and $\text{Var}(b_j)$ is the estimated variance of b_j already described. The square root of this variance is the standard deviation of b_j, often called the standard error of the coefficient. For a 95% confidence interval the two-tailed critical value with $P = 0.05$ is needed. For the dipper data $n = 22$ and $p' = 8$, so the df are 14. The two-tailed critical value of Student's t with 14 df and $P = 0.05$ is given in *Appendix B.6* and is 2.145. Thus a 95% confidence interval for the constant β_0 is

$$0.4402 \pm 2.145 \times 0.2271,$$

or

$$0.4402 \pm 0.4871.$$

This procedure is analogous to that used in bivariate regression (see Chapter 3, Section 2.2, *Table 3*).

3.3 Confidence intervals for predictions from the regression equation

The mean prediction $\hat{y}$ for the dependent variable at the set of values x_1, x_2, . . ., x_k is obtained from the equation

$$\hat{y} = b_0 + b_1x_1 + b_2x_2 + \ldots + b_kx_k.$$

The formula for the estimate of the variance of $\hat{y}$ is

$$\mathrm{Var}(\hat{y}) = s^2/n + \sum_1^k (x_j - \bar{x}_j)\ \mathrm{Var}(b_j)^2 + 2 \sum_{j<l}\sum (x_j - \bar{x}_j)(x_l - \bar{x}_l)\ \mathrm{Cov}(b_j, b_l).$$

Thus the formula for the confidence interval is calculated by multiplying the square root of this variance by a percentile of Student's t. In most packages confidence intervals for predictions can be printed directly so this rather complicated formula is not needed.

Where the leverages h_{ii} (discussed in Section 4.2 of this chapter and Section 2.3.3 of Chapter 3) are calculated by the package, the formulas given in *Table 3* of Chapter 3 and described there in Section 2.5 can be used for confidence intervals. The formula for the confidence interval of a prediction $\hat{y}$ is $\hat{y} \pm t\sqrt{s^2\ h_{ii}}$. To illustrate the use of this formula, a 95% confidence interval for the single prediction corresponding to the first row of data of *Table 2* will be worked out. Recall that the last four predictor variables, those giving invertebrate numbers, were transformed by $\log_e(1 + x)$ in deriving the regression equation given in *Figure 6*. The values of the seven predictors used in this equation are (259, 12.2, 10.9, 2.302 59, 5.241 75, 0, 1.386 29). Substitution of these values into the regression equation given in *Figure 6* gives the prediction $\hat{y}_1$ as 1.2684. The correct t-value is the two-tailed $P = 0.05$ point of Student's t given in *Appendix B.6* and is 2.145, whilst s^2 is the error mean square ($\mathrm{MS}_{\mathrm{rerror}}$) from *Figure 6* and is 0.018 15. The value of the leverage, h_{11}, for the first observation, was calculated using the HI subcommand of the *Minitab* REGRESSION command. *Figure 6* shows how this was done: the values of the leverages were stored in column C23; h_{11} is the first tow of column C23 and its value is 0.557 926. Thus the 95% confidence interval for the single prediction is

$$1.2684 \pm 2.145\ \sqrt{0.018\,15 \times 0.557\,926} = 1.2684 \pm 0.2159.$$

Sometimes it is useful to be able to calculate confidence intervals at other sets of values of the predictor variables than those used in the regression calculations. In *Minitab* this can be done using the PREDICT sub-command of the REGRESSION command. These are the second, third, and fourth sub-commands of *Figure 6*. The first set of values of predictor variables for which a prediction and confidence interval is obtained in *Figure 6* is at approximately the minimum for the data. Notice that a warning is printed that these values are away from the centre; some of the specified values are smaller than the minima. The second set of values is at the mean and the last set is at approximately the maxima. Notice also that the standard deviation of the fit, and hence the width of the confidence intervals, is much narrower for the central values than it is for the extremes. This is a general rule for confidence intervals for predictions in multiple regression. The final column of intervals, labelled P.I. for prediction interval, are 95% intervals for a further imaginary observation taken at the specified set of values of the predictor values. The formula for the variance of the prediction intervals differs from that of the confidence intervals for the mean predicted $\hat{y}$ in that the standard error is $\sqrt{s^2\,(1 + h_{ii})}$ instead of $\sqrt{s^2 h_{ii}}$. Thus the prediction intervals are somewhat wider, representing the scatter of further observations about the mean prediction $\hat{y}$. In *Minitab* if an interval other than 95% is required, it should be calculated using the leverage, h_{ii}, as outlined in *Table 3* of Chapter 3. For a 99% interval the value of Student's t with 14 df is 2.977, from *Appendix B.6*, so the 99% prediction interval at the mean is $1.4986 \pm 2.977 \times \sqrt{0.018\,15\,(1 + 0.045\,38)}$ or (1.0885, 1.9087).

In these confidence intervals the standard deviation is multiplied by the $100(1 - \alpha/2)$ percentile of Student's t with $(n - p')$ df to give the $100(1 - \alpha)\%$ confidence interval. These values are tabulated as $P = \alpha$ in *Appendix B.6*. Thus for a 95% confidence interval, the multiplier is the 97.5th percentile tabulated under $P = 0.05$. The confidence coefficient is at the stated level only if one such interval is required. If several intervals are required simultaneously, some adjustment is needed to ensure that the confidence intervals are not too narrow. One method of ensuring that the joint confidence coefficient is at least equal to $100(1 - \alpha)\%$ is to use the Bonferroni adjustment. If c confidence intervals are required simultaneously, the $100\{1 - \alpha/(2c)\}$ percentile of Student's t is used as the multiplier for the standard deviation. The Bonferroni adjustment is an approximate method since the inequality in probability theory on which it is based assumes that the c confidence intervals are independent. In this application they are not independent, since all predictions are calculated from the same partial regression coefficients. Nevertheless they are conservative bands for independent confidence intervals and can be used as an approximate method in regression so long as the c different intervals are calculated for reasonably separated values of the predictor variables, and if the number of intervals c is no bigger than the number of parameters p'.

To illustrate the use of the Bonferroni adjustment, suppose a total of six 95% confidence intervals are to be calculated at different sets of values of the predictor variables, including the first set used in calculating the regression equation. This set was used earlier for illustration of the method of calculation of confidence intervals for a single prediction. The only difference in the calculations is in the value of Student's t used. For a 95% confidence interval $\alpha = 0.05$, so with $c = 6$ the Bonferroni adjustment requires the $100\{1 - 0.05/(2 \times 6)\} = 99.5833$ percentile of Student's t to be used in place of the 95% percentile. With 14 df, this percentile can be found in *Minitab* using the INVCDF command. To do this use 0.995 833 in the INVCDF command with the T subcommand for 14 df as follows:

```
INVCDF 0.995 883;
T 14.
```

The percentile is calculated as 3.0687. Alternatively, interpolation can be used in *Appendix B.11* between the values of 3.276 85 with 10 df and 3.036 28 with 15 df, but this is less accurate because the values of t percentiles given there are not linear in the error df. The Bonferroni-adjusted confidence interval is

$$1.2684 \pm 3.0687 \sqrt{0.018\,15 \times 0.557\,926} = 1.2684 \pm 0.3088$$

A selection of Bonferroni-adjusted Student's t values is given in *Appendix B.11*. All are for 95% confidence intervals with different numbers of intervals c and different degrees of freedom $(n - p')$.

Another method of ensuring the confidence coefficient is at least equal to $100(1 - \alpha)\%$ is to use Scheffé's method (see also Chapter 3, Section 2.5, *Table 3*), and this can be used for any number c of intervals. The multiplier for Scheffé's method is $\sqrt{(p' F_{p', n-p'})}$ where F is the $100(1 - \alpha)$ percentile of the F distribution with p' and $(n - p')$ df. *Appendix B.12* gives some of these multipliers, for various values of the number of predictors and degrees of freedom, but all are for a 95% confidence coefficient. This procedure is conservative; it gives intervals that are too wide for the stated confidence coefficient, so the Bonferroni method should be used for a small number of intervals if it gives narrower intervals. In the example used to illustrate the Bonferroni adjustment, the adjusted t multiplier of 3.0687 is replaced by $\sqrt{8 \times 2.699} = 4.6467$. The 95th percentile of the F distribution with 8 and 14 df, 2.699, is obtained from *Appendix B.1*.

4. Diagnostic checking

Protocol 2 outlines the steps followed in diagnostic checking. Reference should be made to the subsequent text for explanation of technical details.

Protocol 2. Diagnostic checking in multiple regression

1. Check for autocorrelation using the Durbin–Watson test (see Section 4.1.1).
2. Check the studentized deleted residuals for outliers, constant variance, and indications that transformations are needed. Use index plots and plots against predictor variables (see Sections 4.1.2 and 4.1.3).

Protocol 2. *Continued*

3. Check for normality using studentized deleted residuals plotted against corresponding normal scores (see Section 4.1.3):
- a straight line indicates normality
- non-linearity indicates a need to transform the y variable

4. Check for unusual values of x variables using index plots of leverages h_{ii}.
- check data if $h_{ii} > 3p'/n$ (see Sections 4.2.1 and 4.2.3).

5. Check for leverage using index plots of Cook's D_i:
- check data if $D_i > F_{.5,p',n\text{-}p'}$ (see Sections 4.2.2 and 4.2.3)
- an alternative check is if $D_i > 4/n$

6. Plot the partial residuals against the x variables (see Section 4.3.2). Curvature indicates the need for transformations of the x variables.

4.1 Checks on residuals

One way of assessing the effectiveness of a multiple regression equation in predicting the dependent variable is to make a simple comparison of the observations y with the predictions $\hat{y}$. The differences between them are called the raw residuals, and any large residual is an indication of an unusual value of y. A statistic based on the raw residuals is the sum of their squares, the error sum of squares. This is used in the analysis of variance procedure as a measure of variation not explained by the model. Modified residuals, described later in this section, are more sensitive for checking for unusual y values.

4.1.1 Checks on autocorrelation

One diagnostic test that is based on the raw residuals is the Durbin–Watson test for serial autocorrelation in the residuals. This is described in Chapter 3, Section 2.3.2. The formula for the Durbin–Watson test statistic is

$$\Sigma(r_{i+1} - r_i)^2/\Sigma r_i^2$$

where r_i is the ith raw residual. A tendency for residuals of similar size and sign to be clustered together in the sequence of i results in a low test statistic and indicates a positive association in the error of one observation with the error of the next. This can be an indication that there is a missing variable in the model, or it may be that there is some genuine autocorrelation in the errors and the assumption of independent errors is untenable.

If the data are in the order of increasing value of a predictor variable x, a significant value of the Durbin–Watson test statistic may result from curvature in the relationship between y and x. A transformation of the y variable, or inclusion of powers of x as well as x as predictors, may be enough to obtain independent residuals. So that time-dependent correlations are picked up by the Durbin–Watson statistic it is necessary for the data to be entered row by row in order of measurement in time.

4.1.2 Standardized residuals and studentized deleted residuals

One reason for the insensitivity of the raw residuals is that their variance is not constant over the range of measurement of the predictor variables. The variance in the dependent variable y is assumed to be constant and y is equal to the prediction plus the residual. As was pointed out in Section 3.2, the variance of the predictions is greatest at the margins of the predictor variables, so the variance of the residuals is least. Conversely, the variance of residuals close to the mean of the predictor variables is greatest. Allowance can be made for this non-constant variance when standardizing the raw residuals by dividing them by their estimated standard deviations. In *Minitab* these are called standardized residuals, but other authors refer to them as studentized residuals. Another refinement recognizes the fact that an extreme outlier may influence the estimates of the partial regression coefficients and also the error variance. This approach calculates the residual by subtracting from the observed y the prediction using the data with the ith individual omitted, and standardizing by division by the estimated standard deviation from this depleted data set. These are called in *Minitab* studentized deleted residuals, and are accessed by the TRESIDUALS sub-command of the REGRESSION command. They are also called externally studentized residuals and deletion residuals by other authors, so some care has to be exercised in reading different accounts of this subject. I recommend the use of the studentized deleted residuals for diagnostic checking where these are automatically calculated by the package, since they are most sensitive in checking for outliers.

4.1.3 Procedures for checking residuals

There are three procedures to follow in checking the residuals:

- checks for outliers
- checks for non-constant variance and the wrong form of predictor by plots
- checks for normality by normal score plots.

A simple check for outliers is to consider all data with a studentized deleted residual exceeding 2 in absolute magnitude as an indication of an unusual y value. A more refined procedure is based on the fact that these residuals are distributed as Student's t with $(n - p' - 1)$ df. (p' is the number of constants, including β_0, so $p' = k + 1$.) For a significance level of α and a two-tailed test a simple comparison with the $100(1 - \alpha/2)$ percentile of Student's t is likely to lead to false declaration of outliers, since with n residuals a multiple test procedure is needed to test for the significance of the maximum. An approximation is to use the Bonferroni correction and compare the magnitude of the extreme studentized deleted residual with the $100\{1 - \alpha/(2n)\}$ percentile of Student's t with $(n - p' - 1)$ df. Standard tables are rarely extensive enough to provide these percentiles, but packages such as *Minitab* and *SAS* allow them to be easily calculated with a computer. A worked example follows.

Plots of the studentized deleted residuals against the index number of the data i defined in the footnote of *Protocol 1* or the time order in which data are collected are valuable in that any relationship may indicate a lurking variable, some missing predictor from the model. Plots against the predictions are also useful in this regard. Plots against the predictor variables $x_1, x_2, \ldots, x_k$ may indicate by curved relationships the need for transformations of these variables or the inclusion of extra terms such as quadratic terms, with x^2 as well as x.

Another use of these plots is as a rough check on the assumption of constant variance. If the variance increases as x_1 increases, say, then the plot of the residuals against x_1 will be wedge-shaped (see Chapter 3, *Figure 6d*), with larger residuals towards the right-hand side of the plot. If the model is correct, all the plots should exhibit a random scatter of residuals.

The assumption of normality can be checked by plotting the studentized deleted residuals against the normal scores or on normal probability paper. The former technique, using *Minitab*, was described in earlier chapters (Chapter 1, Section 3.2). A straight line indicates agreement with normality. Unfortunately this check can be unreliable for small sample sizes because of a property called supernormality. The predictions can be written as a linear combination of the data, and the central limit theorem shows that these will tend to be normally distributed even when the errors are not normal. If n is large the first term y in the residual will dominate, and supernormality is not so much of a problem.

4.1.4 Illustrative examples

In *Figure 6*, the output from the multiple regression for the dipper data, the 4th observation is indicated by *Minitab* as an outlier because the standardized residual is -2.40, thus greater than 2 in absolute magnitude. The more refined Bonferroni-corrected t-test, with a significance level of 0.05, uses as a critical value the $100(1 - 0.05/44) = 99.89$ percentile of Student's t with $(22 - 8 - 1) = 13$ df. In *Minitab* this can be done with the INVCDF command, as described in Section 3.3. The critical value is obtained as 3.8018, and the studentized deleted residual for the 4th observation is smaller than this in absolute magnitude (it is -3.01), so the observation is not judged on this more conservative test for identification of an outlier. There is probably no reason therefore to exclude observation 4 from the equation at this stage.

The plots for the studentized deleted residuals are illustrated by a typical example given in *Figure 8a* where they are plotted against $\log_e$ (1 + stonefly). There is no pattern indicating an incorrect relationship or non-constant

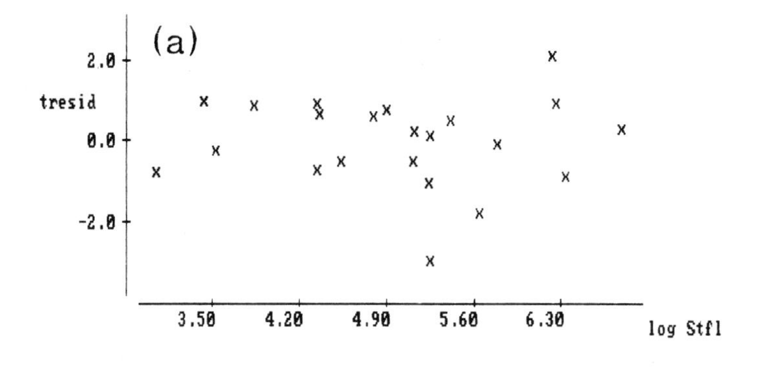

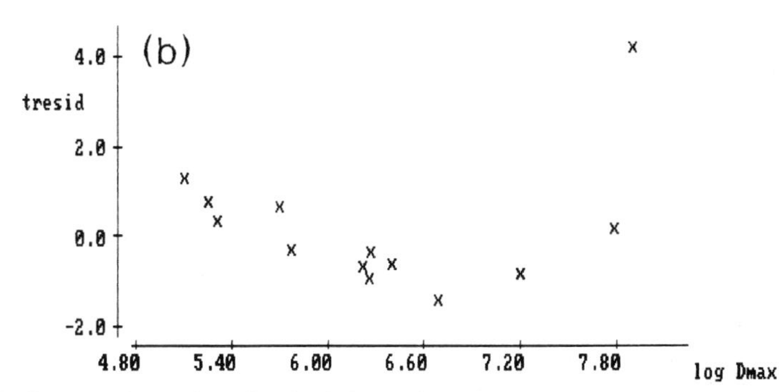

Figure 8. Scatter plots of studentized deleted residuals against predictor variables. (a) Multiple regression given in *Figure 6*; (b) simple linear regression for the scatter plot of *Figure 1*.

variance, though the suspected outlier stands out as the lowest residual. *Figure 8b* gives an example of a patterned set of residuals. These are the studentized deleted residuals from a regression of the mortality on log density for the data given in *Table 3*. It is obvious from *Figure 1* that a straight line is not an adequate model for these data and the residual plot shows this clearly.

Figure 9 is a plot of the studentized deleted residuals against their normal scores for the dipper data. This is not a straight line, and the indication is therefore that some further transformation of the dependent variable, y, the breeding density of dippers, should be investigated, or the model should be further refined. This will be followed up in Section 4.3.

4.2 Checks on influential data

4.2.1 Leverages

The residuals described above indicate anomalies in the dependent variable, but do not identify observations with unusual values of the predictor variables. Statistics designed to do this are based on the diagonal elements of a matrix called the hat matrix, and denoted by h_{ii} (HI in *Minitab*). They are

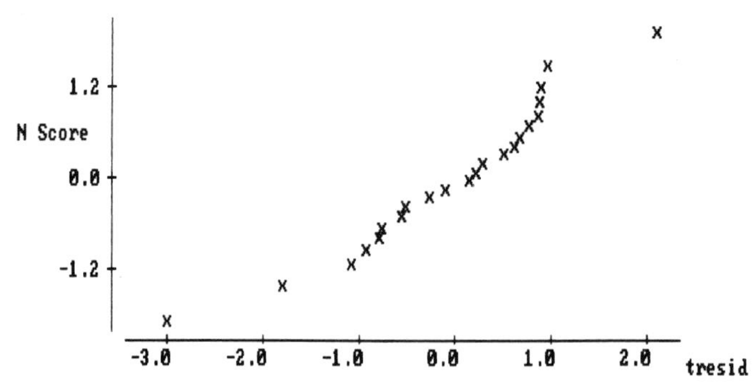

Figure 9. Scatter plot of the studentized deleted residuals against their normal scores for the multiple regression given in *Figure 6*.

called the leverages, and there are n of them, one for each individual. As well as appearing in the formulae for standardized and studentized deleted residuals their relevance is that they measure the joint influence of the predictors by a standardized distance of the ith observation to the other $n - 1$. The leverages are constrained to lie between 0 and 1 (between $1/n$ and 1 if a constant β_0 is included in the model) and their sum is equal to p'. A rough indication of an unusual observation is a leverage exceeding $3p'/n$, though $2p'/n$ has also been suggested. *Minitab* uses $3p'/n$ as the criterion for automatically displaying an unusual observation, but clearly the advice of Chapter 3 (*Protocol 1*) to check when h_{ii} exceeds $2p'/n$ is a prudent precaution against errors.

4.2.2 Cook's *D* and Dfits

A disadvantage of the leverages is that they do not distinguish between high leverage points that are influential in the calculation of partial regression coefficients and those that are not. A measure that is more sensitive to such influential points is Cook's D. The idea behind this measure is to compare the estimates of the regression coefficients from the full data set with those obtained when the ith observation is omitted, so a large value indicates an influential point. Cook's D can be calculated from the ith studentized deleted residual t_i and the ith leverage h_{ii} by the formula

$$D_i = h_{ii} (1 - h_{ii})^{-1} t_i^2 p',$$

so the measure combines residuals and leverages. An indication of a large value of D_i is where it exceeds the 50th percentile (median) of the F distribution with p' and $(n - p')$ df. Values for a range of degrees of freedom are given in *Appendix B.1*. Another, but cruder, criterion is to check observations if D_i exceeds $4/n$, and this is the more cautious (see also Chapter 3, Section 2.3.3).

Another idea in diagnostic checking is to compare the predictions $\hat{y}_i$

obtained from the full data set with those obtained when the ith observation is omitted. The difference between these, when divided by the estimated standard deviation of $\hat{y}_i$, is a measure called Dfits. In fact, though, this measure is the square root of p' times Cook's D with the sign of the studentized deleted residual attached so the two measures are essentially the same.

4.2.3 Plots based on influence statistics

As well as the indications already mentioned for h_{ii} and Cook's D_i that an observation may need checking, it is useful to plot these statistics against the index number i. This may indicate an unusual sequence of data that the rough checks do not identify. Another check for normality is to plot the square root of Cook's D_i, with the sign of the studentized deleted residual attached, against the normal scores. The commands needed to do this in *Minitab* for the analysis of the dipper data are

```
LET C25 = SQRT (C22) * SIGN (C21)
NSCORE C25 C23
```

Reference to *Figure 6* shows that the studentized deleted residuals were stored in column C21, by using the TRESID sub-command and the Cook's D statistics in column C22 using the COOKD sub-command. The plot against the normal score (*Figure 10*) is less of an indication of departure from normality than is the residual plot of *Figure 9*. The plot of signed Cook's D_i against normal scores is suggested by Atkinson (3). It is not yet clear whether it is more or less sensitive than the residual plot for detecting departures from normality.

The two plots in *Figure 11* are respectively the index plots of the leverages h_{ii} and Cook's D. The bunched up appearance of the latter is because Cook's D is always positive. No unusual leverage is identified, the largest value of Cook's D is 0.3899, and comparison with the median of the F distribution with 8 and 14 df given in *Appendix B.1* (0.964) shows that this is not an

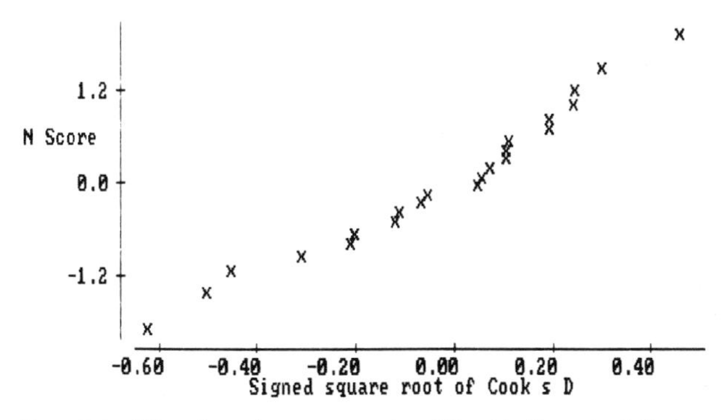

Figure 10. Scatter plot of the signed square roots of Cook's D against their normal scores for the multiple regression given in *Figure 6*.

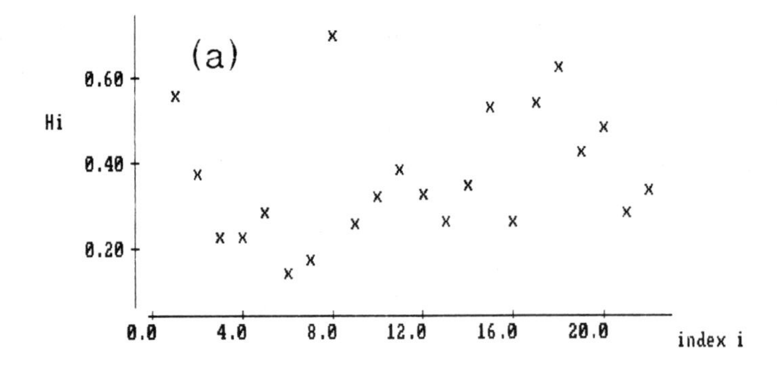

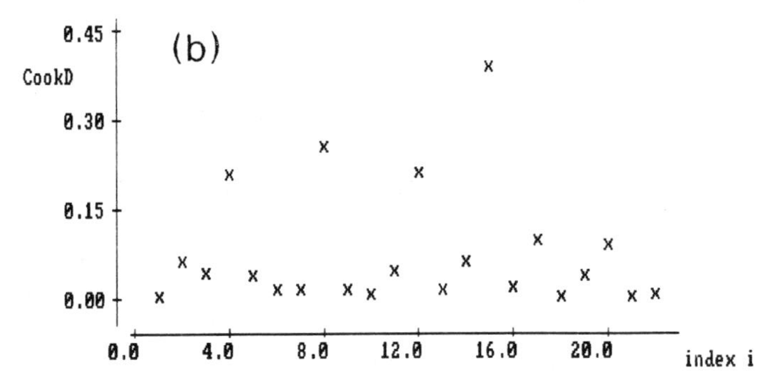

Figure 11. Index plots of (a) the leverages, (b) Cook's D for the multiple regression given in *Figure 6*.

unusually high value. None of the values of h_{ii} exceed $3 \times 8/22$ because this number is greater than 1, and all h_{ii} have to be less than or equal to 1. However, none exceed the less conservative criterion of $2 \times 8/22 = 0.7273$ either. So influential points are not a problem with this regression.

4.3 Transformations

In Chapter 3, Section 5.2, some guidance was given in seeking transformations of the data to allow straight lines to be fitted. It has not proved possible to give a rigorous strategy for determining transformations that linearize the data in the multivariate case. Plots will sometimes indicate the need for transformations, although the precise nature of the optimum transformation is not necessarily obvious. In bivariate regression it is easy to examine a plot of y against x and check for curvature. Comparison can be made with mathematical curves or the ladder of powers can be used to find a suitable linearizing transformation. There are many more plots to examine in multiple regression, and the plot of y against one of the predictors may show considerable scatter even when a regression equation with two or more predictors is a satisfactory model for the data. Some of this scatter is caused by the differing values of the other predictor variables. The detection of curvature in these plots is thus more difficult than in the bivariate case. Nevertheless, an examination of these plots is recommended as a first stage in multiple regression analysis, since they can often point the way to a suitable transformation. In addition, any prior knowledge of the nature of the interrelationships between predictor variables and the dependent variable should be used in determining the form of the variables to be used in the multiple regression equation. If, for example, it is known from scientific principles that y depends additively on the order of magnitude of x then the logarithm of x should be used in the regression equation.

4.3.1 Standardizing variables

Transformation of a predictor variable x_j by dividing each observation of that variable by a constant effects the multiple regression equation only by multiplying the partial regression coefficient b_j by the same constant. Also, the subtraction of a constant from each observation of x_j just adds b_j times the constant to the term b_0 of the multiple regression equation. Thus such transformations have no material effect on the multiple regression calculations. Standardization of the predictor variables, by subtracting the mean and dividing by the standard deviation, is one such transformation, and this is a way of ensuring that the variables are commensurable. Standardization of the dependent variable y is not recommended, however. The division by the standard deviation alters and considerably complicates the results used for tests and confidence intervals outlined in Section 3. The reason is that in the linear model y is assumed to be a normal random variable, but the standardized y is then a t-distribution with $(n - 1)$ df. The predictor variables are assumed to be non-random, so the difficulty does not arise with them. Any scaling or subtraction of constant from y should be done using numbers that are not calculated from the data if the assumptions of the model are not to be compromised.

4.3.2 Partial residual plots

A diagnostic method that has proved useful in the identification of appropriate transformations of the predictor variables is based on another type of residual called the partial residuals. The idea behind these is to eliminate the (linear) effect of all but one of the predictors in calculating residuals and then to plot these against the remaining predictor variable. The calculation of these partial residuals is quite straightforward, based on results from a regression package.

From the prediction equation

$$\hat{y} = b_0 + b_1x_1 + b_2x_2 + \ldots + b_kx_k$$

the prediction of y without using x_j is $\hat{y} - b_jx_j$. So the jth partial residual, which is the residual calculated from the prediction using all predictors excepting x_j, is

$$y - (\hat{y} - b_j x_j) = (y - \hat{y}) + b_j x_j.$$

The term in brackets $(y - \hat{y})$ is the raw residual for the full regression equation. So to calculate the jth partial residual, multiply the column of values of the jth predictor x_j by the partial regression coefficient b_j (obtained from a multiple regression using all predictors) and add the column of raw residuals (again from the full regression equation). This is plotted against x_j. If x_j is important in the model and needs no transformation, the plot will be close to a straight line. This line has slope equal to b_j and is bound to go through the origin, but that is of little practical importance. Any curvature evident in the partial residual plot indicates the need for a transformation, but not the precise form of this transformation. It must be admitted that to do all these calculations, even with a package, is time-consuming. Nevertheless, valuable information may be obtained.

Figure 12 gives three examples of partial residual plots, all based on multiple regressions for the dipper data. *Figure 12a* is the plot for the stonefly partial residual from a regression with $\log_e$ (breeding density) as the dependent variable and all seven predictor variables left untransformed. This is not the regression described in *Figure 6* and discussed earlier. Although there is a lot of scatter in the plot there is a distinct suggestion of curvature, indicating the need for a transformation of the stonefly numbers. *Figure 12b* is the plot of the partial residual for the transformed stonefly data from the regression with all the four invertebrate numbers predictors transformed with the $\log_e (1 + x)$ transformation, the regression described in *Figure 6*. This is much closer to a straight line, indicating that the correct transformation has been found. Finally, *Figure 12c* is an example of a partial residual plot for a variable that is not important in the regression equation. It is for the altitude partial residual, and the scatter in the plot is evident. The slight negative slope evident in this plot is because the partial regression coefficient for altitude is negative.

4.3.2 The ladder of powers

The transformation of the dependent variable that gives the closest agreement with the assumption of normally distributed errors can be found by the method of the ladder of powers. Regression equations are fitted, using the same predictors in each case, for a range of transformations. The transformation is chosen whose normal score plot for the studentized deleted residual most closely follows a straight line. *Figure 13* shows these plots for a range of transformations of breeding density as dependent variable and the same seven predictor variables that were used in the regression described in *Figure 6*. These plots indicate that the y variable should not be transformed, contrary to the indications given by initial plots of the data described earlier. The plot that is closest to a straight line is that corresponding to untransformed y data,

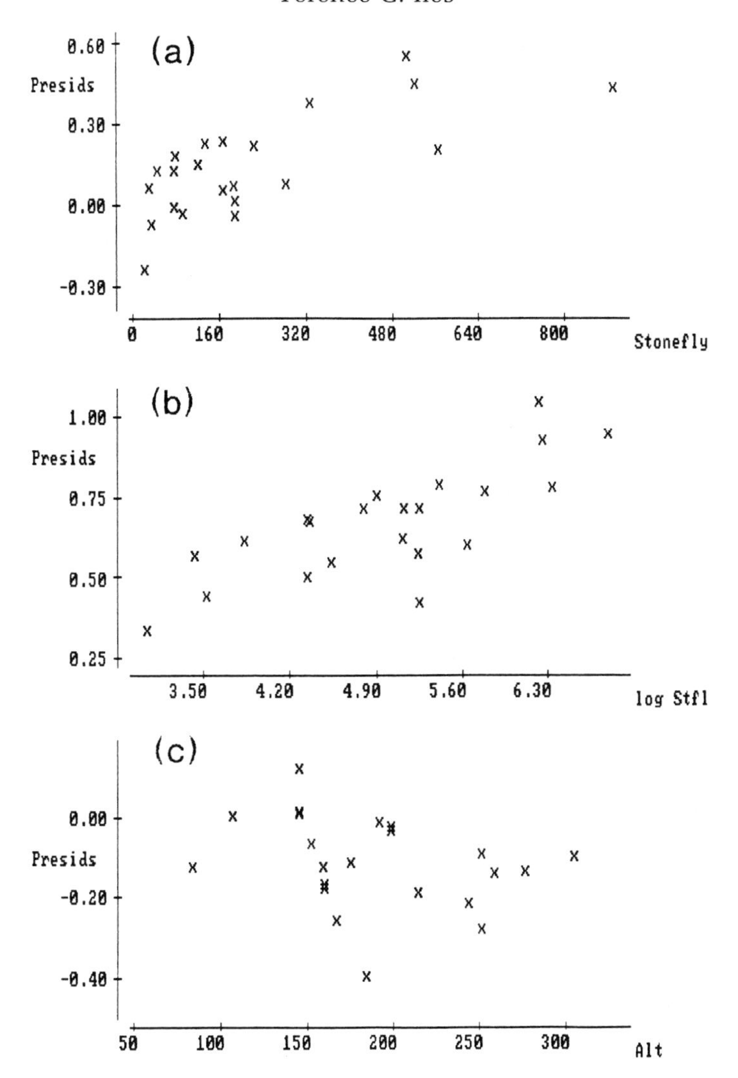

Figure 12. Partial residual plots from the dipper data. (a) Stonefly numbers as a predictor; (b) $\log_e$ (1 + stonefly number) as a predictor; (c) altitude as a predictor. In all three cases, $\log_e$ (breeding density) is the dependent variable.

although there is little to choose between this and the plot for the squared data. The ladder of powers technique is not sufficiently sensitive to identify a precise transformation to use. It merely indicates a range of possibilities.

4.3.3 An appraisal of diagnostic techniques

The difficulty with these investigations is that very often the predictor variables and dependent variable all need different transformations. An optimum

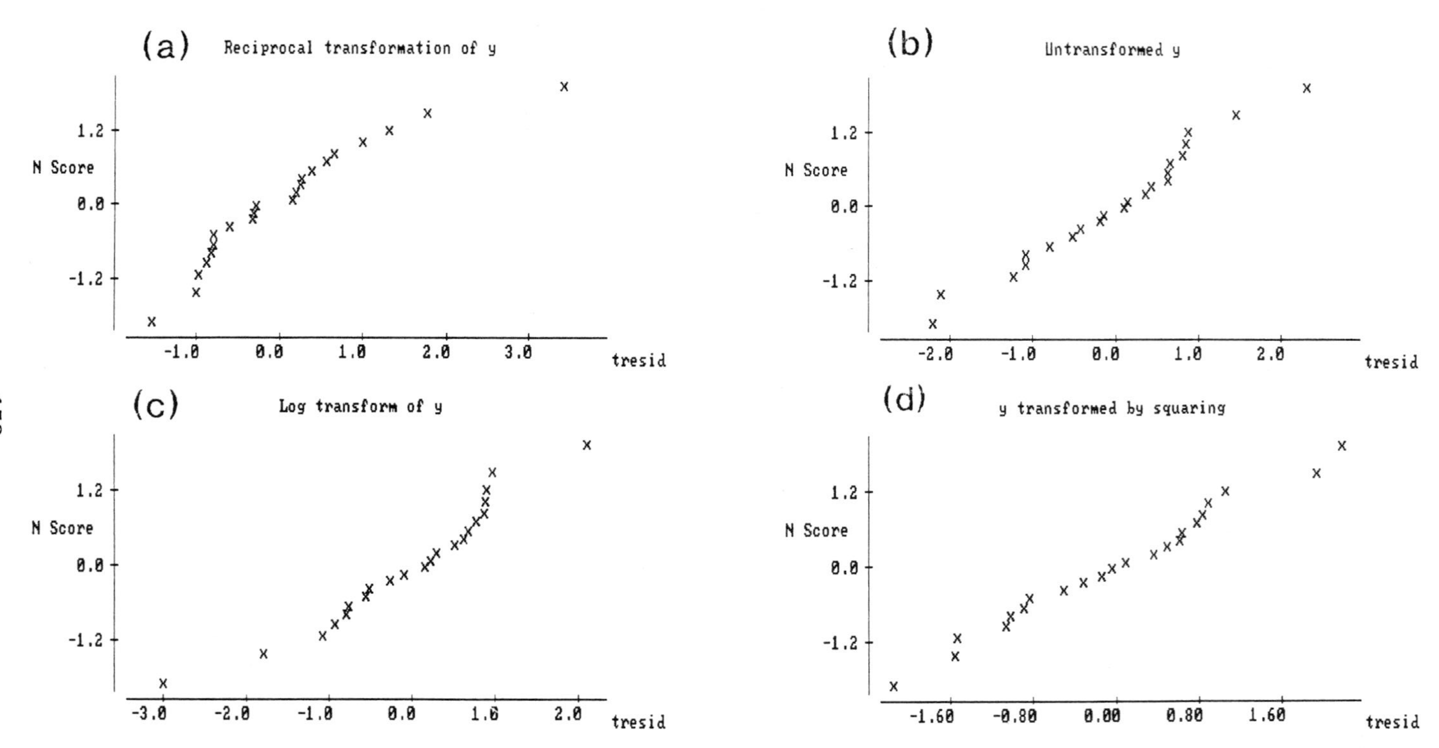

Figure 13. Plots of studentized deleted residuals against their normal scores for different transformations of the dependent variable in multiple regressions to predict breeding density of dippers using (a) reciprocal, (b) no transformation, (c) natural logarithm, and (d) square.

transformation for y with the raw predictors may not be appropriate for transformed predictors. Atkinson (3) discusses the simultaneous transformation of y and x variables and suggests some methods for selecting suitable transformations. The Box–Tidwell approach is used for the predictor variables, and the Box–Cox family of transformations for the dependent variable. I have not given details of these methods here for two reasons. One is that the calculations needed involve considerable extensions to standard packages. The second is that I do not regard these techniques as routine statistical analysis. Atkinson's clearly written account should be consulted by any reader wishing to experiment.

Although the techniques of diagnostic checking outlined in this section are strongly recommended, the user of multiple regression should beware of over-refinement of the regression equation. Only in exceptional circumstances, where a thorough (and time-consuming) analysis is justified, would I recommend an exhaustive use of all the techniques just described. Extensive use of involved transformations and deletion of inconvenient outliers and lever points will often give a convincing multiple regression equation that is highly tailored to the data set used in the calculations. When used on data collected outside the initial survey, the equation performs poorly. One way of guarding against this is deliberately to collect extra data that will not be used in the calculations, but solely to justify the relationships established by the equation.

5. Multicollinearity

Multicollinearity is the presence of near linear relationships amongst some of the predictor variables; that is, one of the predictors is almost equal to a linear combination of the other predictors. From the linear model of equation (1) it is evident that if one of the predictors is exactly equal to a linear combination of some of the others, then it could be removed from the equation and is redundant as a predictor. To take a simple case, if $x_1 = x_2 + x_3$ then equation (1) can be written

$$y = \beta_0 + (\beta_1 + \beta_2)x_2 + (\beta_1 + \beta_3)x_3 + \beta_4 x_4 + \ldots + \beta_k x_k + \varepsilon,$$

and variable x_1 is not needed. If a computer is used to do the calculations, and x_1, x_2, and x_3 are all included as predictors, the multiple regression equation cannot be calculated without first omitting one of the collinear variables. Even if the linear relationship is not exact, close linear interrelationships can cause great difficulties in interpretation though the calculation of the regression equation may then be possible. Thus it is important to recognize multicollinearity and take appropriate steps to eliminate its effects.

The variances of the partial regression coefficients b_j tend to be high for variables x_j that are collinear with other predictors. This has the effect of making the Student's t statistics for the significance of coefficients unreliable.

Moreover the magnitude and sign of the coefficient b_j itself may be grossly misleading. If one of a collinear set of predictors is omitted from the regression calculations, other coefficients may easily change radically in size and even in sign. This can make the techniques of variable selection, to be discussed in Section 6, somewhat erratic. Variables that appear important in some analyses appear unimportant in others.

The effect of the *j*th predictor x_j in the variance of the partial regression coefficient b_j can be assessed by calculating a multiple regression of the standardized values of x_j (standardized by subtraction of mean and division by the standard deviation) on the remaining $(k - 1)$ standardized predictor variables. If the coefficient of determination of this regression is R_j^2, the variance of b_j is inversely proportional to $(1 - R_j^2)$. Thus if R_j^2 is close to 1, indicating a high degree of multicollinearity, then b_j has a high variance. The quantity $(1 - R_j^2)$ is called the variance inflation factor (VIF) and can routinely be calculated in multiple regression packages. *Minitab* calculates the VIF associated with each predictor and automatically drops from the regression any predictor where this is greater than 10^4. When the VIF is greater than 100, a warning of collinearity is printed, but no predictors are excluded.

Although VIF is valuable in identifying that variables are multicollinear, it does not help in finding the nature of the interrelationships. A method that is often useful in this respect is based on a principal components analysis (PCA) of the standardized predictor variables. The use of PCA as an ordination technique is described in Chapter 5, its use to investigate multicollinearity is a somewhat special application of the technique. PCA can be done using standard packages such as *Minitab*, *SAS*, or *SPSS/PC+*. Since standardized values are used, the PCA is done on the correlation matrix. The output from *Minitab*'s PCA of the variables used in the multiple regression of *Figure 6* for the dipper data is printed as *Figure 14*. The row labelled 'eigenvalue' gives the variances of the principal components of the standardized predictors. The sum of these is always equal to the number of predictors. If one or more eigenvalues is small, then collinearity amongst the predictors is indicated. A rough test is to calculate the square root of the ratio of the largest eigenvalue to the smallest to give a number called the condition number. For these data the condition number is 3.69 and the smallest eigenvalue is 0.17. Only if the condition number exeeds about 10 is there any real indication of possible multicollinearity so with these data multicollinearity is not a problem; they were chosen for illustration of multiple regression for that reason.

Another data set is needed to illustrate collinearity. The data are four physical measurements made on 20 soil samples, % sand, % silt, % organic matter, and pH. The complete data set is given in *Table 4*. It may not be readily apparent from a cursory scan of these data that there is a high degree of multicollinearity present, but the PCA in *Figure 15* enables this to be identified. The fourth eigenvalue is small, and the condition number for the

```
MTB > pca c1-c3 c14-c17

Eigenanalysis of the Correlation Matrix

Eigenvalue     2.3765    2.2886    0.7670    0.6017    0.4624    0.3296
Proportion      0.340     0.327     0.110     0.086     0.066     0.047
Cumulative      0.340     0.666     0.776     0.862     0.928     0.975

Eigenvalue     0.1741
Proportion      0.025
Cumulative      1.000

Variable          PC1       PC2       PC3       PC4       PC5       PC6
Alt             0.397     0.317    -0.169     0.666     0.361    -0.374
W Hard          0.242    -0.459     0.421     0.358    -0.542    -0.206
Gradient        0.537     0.101     0.363     0.059     0.141     0.732
log Cadd        0.481    -0.270    -0.323    -0.433     0.256    -0.090
log Stfl        0.503     0.252    -0.038    -0.392    -0.417    -0.340
log Mayf        0.099    -0.479    -0.667     0.270    -0.192     0.291
log OInv        0.033    -0.559     0.334    -0.104     0.529    -0.270

Variable          PC7
Alt             0.004
W Hard          0.298
Gradient       -0.102
log Cadd        0.574
log Stfl       -0.488
log Mayf       -0.348
log OInv       -0.460
```

Figure 14. Principal components analysis of predictor variables used in the multiple regression equation given in *Figure 6*.

Table 4. Data[a] from samples of soil and contents of file SOIL.DAT[b]

ROW	% Sand	% Silt	% Organic matter	pH
1	77.3	13.0	1.5	6.4
2	82.5	10.0	1.5	6.5
3	66.9	20.6	2.3	7.0
4	47.2	33.8	2.8	5.8
5	65.3	20.5	1.9	6.9
6	83.3	10.0	2.2	7.0
7	81.6	12.7	2.9	6.7
8	47.8	36.5	2.3	7.2
9	48.6	37.1	2.1	7.2
10	61.6	25.5	1.9	7.3
11	58.6	26.5	2.4	6.7
12	69.3	22.3	4.0	7.0
13	61.8	30.8	2.7	6.4
14	67.7	25.3	4.8	7.3
15	57.2	31.2	2.4	6.5
16	67.2	22.7	3.3	6.2
17	59.2	31.2	2.4	6.0
18	80.2	13.2	2.0	5.8
19	82.2	11.1	2.2	7.2
20	69.7	20.7	3.1	5.9

[a] The first column (ROW) contains row numbers, each referring to measurements from a separate sample of soil. The other columns contain measurements of % sand, % silt, % organic matter, and pH in the samples.
[b] The file does not contain row numbers or headings

```
MTB > pca c1-c4

Eigenanalysis of the Correlation Matrix

Eigenvalue      2.0229     1.0505     0.9058     0.0209
Proportion       0.506      0.263      0.226      0.005
Cumulative       0.506      0.768      0.995      1.000

Variable           PC1        PC2        PC3        PC4
% Sand           0.684     -0.151      0.151      0.698
% Silt          -0.696      0.086     -0.052      0.711
% OrgMat        -0.215     -0.580      0.781     -0.084
pH              -0.048     -0.796     -0.603      0.005
```

Figure 15. Principal components analysis of the data from soil samples given in *Table 4*.

correlation matrix is $\sqrt{2.0229/0.0209} = 9.84$ and this is close to the critical value of 10. The small eigenvalue indicates that the combination of variables that is the corresponding principal component is almost equal to zero. The advantage of using the standardized variables is that the relative magnitudes of the coefficients of the components can be assessed without having to make reference to the scale of measurement of the variables. Clearly this component is dominated by the coefficients of 0.698 for % sand and 0.711 for % silt and, if z_1 and z_2 are used to denote the standardized values of these variables, the component $0.698\, z_1 + 0.711\, z_2$ is approximately zero. A plot of z_1 against z_2 or equivalently x_1 against x_2 will be close to a straight line. This is confirmed by the plot of *Figure 16*. Thus in any regression either % sand or % silt should be used, but probably not both.

If prediction is the aim of the regression analysis, collinearities should be removed by omitting predictor variables that are highly collinear with others. If the regression is used to construct models to investigate the influential variables on a predictor, collinearities should be detected using *Protocol 3* and care exercised in interpreting the partial regression coefficients. Different

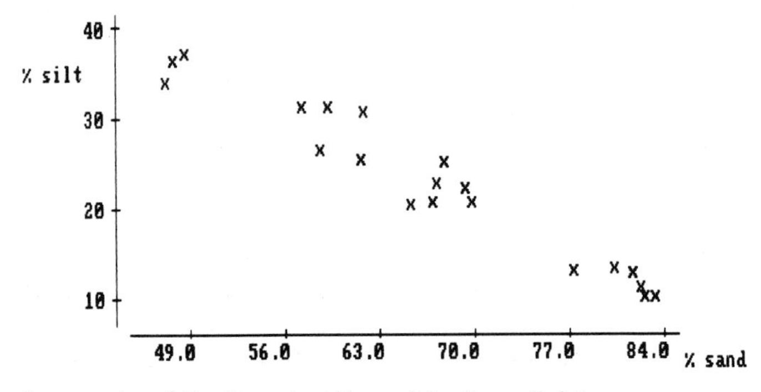

Figure 16. Scatter plot of % silt against % sand for the soil data.

combinations of predictors should be tried, eliminating collinearities using relationships established by the PCA.

Protocol 3. Investigation of muticollinearity

1. Perform a PCA on the correlation matrix calculated from the predictor variables.
2. Calculate the condition number $\sqrt{\lambda_1/\lambda_n}$ where λ_1 and λ_n are respectively the largest and smallest eigenvalues.[a] If this exceeds 30, a high degree of multicollinearity is present. If it exceeds 10, multicollinearity may still need investigation.
3. Examine the coefficients of the eigenvector[b] (or principal component) corresponding to the smallest eigenvalue. Ignore small coefficients. The large coefficients indicate the variables that are collinear, and the coefficients are the multiples of the standardized variables whose sum is approximately zero.

[a] Eigenvalues are sometimes called characteristic values or latent roots.
[b] Eigenvectors are sometimes called characteristic vectors or latent vectors.

Another approach to the investigation of the influence of collinear variables on a dependent variable is to use one of the biased methods of regression. One method is ridge regression. Details are given by Chatterjee and Price (1, Chapter 8) and Gunst and Mason (2, Chapter 10). Other approaches are principal component regression and latent root regression and these are also described in Chapter 10 of Gunst and Mason (2).

6. Selection of variables

The selection of variables in multiple regression is based on the assessment of the variation in the dependent variable, in the sense of sum of squares, explained by the regression. These ideas were discussed in Section 3 on testing for significance. The principle is to include in the regression those variables that markedly decrease the unexplained or error sum of squares. Thus the hypothesis that the regression coefficients of a subset of predictor variables are all zero is tested by comparing the increase in error sum of squares when the subset of variables is left out of the regression calculations with the error sum of squares when all variables are included. It is also possible to test hypotheses that a subset of the regression coefficients are equal to each other. Thus the hypothesis that $\beta_1 = \beta_2$ is tested by comparing a regression with variables $(x_1 + x_2)$, x_3, . . ., x_k with the regression with all variables included. It is not, however, possible to compare a regression of log y on log x_1 with one of y on x_1. *Protocol 4*, outlining the steps of variable selection, is printed at the end of this section.

6.1 Criteria for variable selection

There are three related criteria for the inclusion (or exclusion) of variables in regression, all based on the sums of squares:

- the F-test
- the coefficient of determination R^2
- Mallows' C_p

The formal F-test statistic is based on the difference between $SS_{error,k}$ when all k predictor variables are included in the regression equation and $SS_{error,q}$ when only q of the variables are included. SS_{error} is the sum of squares from the error line of the analysis of variance table for the relevant regression equations (e.g. see *Figure 6* for the full dipper data regression discussed earlier). The F-statistic is calculated by

$$F = \frac{(SS_{error,q} - SS_{error,k})/(k - q)}{SS_{error,k}/(n - k - 1)}.$$

In practice this statistic is sometimes significant, indicating that variables should be included in the regression equation when these variables make no practical difference to the performance of the equation.

A second criterion is to compare the coefficient of determination R_q^2 from the subset of q predictors, with that obtained from all k predictors, R_k^2. R_k^2 is always bigger than R_q^2 if the q predictors are a subset of the k. Unfortunately, R^2 is not sensitive and can remain high even when practically important predictors are removed from the regression equation.

The third criterion is Mallows' C_p, defined as

$$C_p = \frac{SS_{error,q}}{SS_{error,k}/(n - k - 1)} - (n - 2q - 2).$$

If the subset of q predictors is equally as effective in predicting y as the full set of k predictors then $SS_{error,k}/(n - k - 1)$ is an estimate of the error variance σ^2 and $SS_{error,q}$ is an estimate of $(n - q - 1)$ times the same error variance, so C_p is roughly equal to $q + 1$, where $q + 1 = p'$, the number of constants in the selected multiple regression equation. If C_p is much greater than $q + 1$ then this indicates that $SS_{error,q}$ is much greater than $(n - q - 1)\sigma^2$ and that important variables have been omitted from the regression equation. One approach is to try several subsets of a list of potential predictors and plot the values of C_p against $q + 1$, choosing a subset that gives a C_p close to the line $C_p = q + 1$. A sudden jump in this plot as q decreases indicates that too many variables have been omitted from the regression equation. The theoretical average of C_p is $q + 1$, if all important variables are included in the equation. C_p can be less than $q + 1$ in value though it is much greater if important variables are left out of the equation. Choice of the subset with lowest C_p may lead to an unnecessarily complicated equation for practical purposes.

6.2 Automatic selection procedures

Various procedures have been suggested for searching through a set of potential predictor equations to decide which should be included in the final regression equation. One is to try all possible regressions, but with k predictors there are 2^k of these, and it may be impractical to examine such a large number of regressions ($2^{10} = 1024$). A second, and workable, method is to decide how many predictors should be used and find the subset with the specified number of predictors that is best in the sense of smallest error sum of squares. Algorithms are available in computer packages using this criterion, and in conjunction with plots of Mallows' C_p the method can be very helpful in deciding the predictors to include.

Other methods are based on an approach in which the number of predictors is changed by one at each step. In forward selection, an initial selection is made of the best predictor, then the second predictor which is best in conjunction with the first is included, then a third and so on. A disadvantage is that variables included early in the analysis may be ineffective in larger sets because of interrelationships with other predictors, but no mechanism is included for the omission of a variable once it is included. It is a useful method where the predictor variables are powers of a single variable, and thus a polynomial equation in x is used as a predictor for y.

The reverse process to forward selection is backward elimination. Here the starting point is an equation with all variables included, and the first step is to eliminate the variable that causes the smallest increase in the error sum of squares, then the variable that again adds least to prediction and so on. A compromise is the stepwise procedure, a combination of forward and backward selection. This starts as forward selection but includes a mechanism for the possible elimination of a variable at each step. This therefore needs two criteria, an F for a variable to enter the equation and an F for a variable to be removed. This stepwise procedure is the best readily available standard automatic selection method.

6.3 Examples illustrating methods of variable selection

These methods of variable selection are illustrated using the dipper data of *Table 2*. The dependent variable is the untransformed breeding density, following the results of the analysis reported in Section 4. Of seven potential predictors, three are untransformed, namely altitude x_1, water hardness x_2, and gradient x_3 and the other four are $\log_e(1 + x)$ transforms of numbers of caddis fly x_4, stonefly x_5, mayfly x_6, and other invertebrates x_7. The first step is to calculate Mallows' C_p for a range of prediction equations and plot these values against the number of predictors plus one. The command BREG (for best regression) in *Minitab* enables a selection of these to be obtained very rapidly. The dependent variable and all the potential predictor variables are entered on the command line. The package then calculates the coefficient of

```
MTB > breg c8 c1-c3 c14-c17

Best Subsets Regression of Br. Dens

                                                 G 1 1 1 1
                                                 r o o o o
                                               W a g g g g
                                                 d
                                               H i C S M O
                                             A a e a t a I
                  Adj.                       l r n d f y n
Vars     R-sq     R-sq      C-p          s   t d t d l f v

   1     58.2     56.1     19.3    0.98492           X
   1     50.4     48.0     26.3     1.0726       X
   2     69.2     66.0     11.5    0.86708       X   X
   2     69.0     65.7     11.7    0.87081     X     X
   3     77.5     73.8      6.1    0.76136       X   X X
   3     75.3     71.2      8.1    0.79836     X X   X
   4     79.3     74.4      6.5    0.75220     X X   X X
   4     78.4     73.3      7.3    0.76804     X   X X   X
   5     83.0     77.6      5.2    0.70294     X X X X   X
   5     81.6     75.8      6.4    0.73078     X X   X X X
   6     84.0     77.7      6.3    0.70283     X X X X X X
   6     83.2     76.5      7.0    0.72104   X X X X X   X
   7     84.3     76.5      8.0    0.72086   X X X X X X X
```

Figure 17. Output from *Minitab* BREG command to find an optimum multiple regression equation to predict breeding density of dippers.

determination R^2 and Mallows' C_p for the best and next best single predictor regressions; in the sense of highest R^2, highest F-ratio, or smallest C_p. Then the best and next-best regressions are found for two predictor variables and information printed. The process continues until all predictors entered on the command line are printed. Output from the BREG command is given in *Figure 17*. Unfortunately, the information calculated in BREG with *Minitab* cannot be stored automatically, and the plot of C_p against the number of predictors plus one requires these data to be entered with the keyboard. *Figure 18* plots C_p against $q + 1$ and was drawn with a graphics package so that the variables included in the regression could be printed as the points on the plot. Notice that the left-hand margin of the *Minitab* output in *Figure 17* is the number of predictors q. If a constant β_0 is included in the model, C_p is plotted against $q + 1$. The C_p for the regression with the maximum number of potential predictors included is necessarily equal to $q + 1$, and for solutions with most predictors included C_p is usually close to $q + 1$ simply because the last few of a set of predictors is rarely of any real value in the prediction equation. The most striking thing about *Figure 18* therefore is that the three-predictor solution using x_3, x_5, and x_6 is close to optimum, but there is a big jump in C_p if only two predictors are used.

Figure 19 illustrates the stepwise procedure, which allows both addition and removal of variables. In *Minitab* this is done using the STEPWISE command. The default values for the F to enter and F to remove a predictor are both

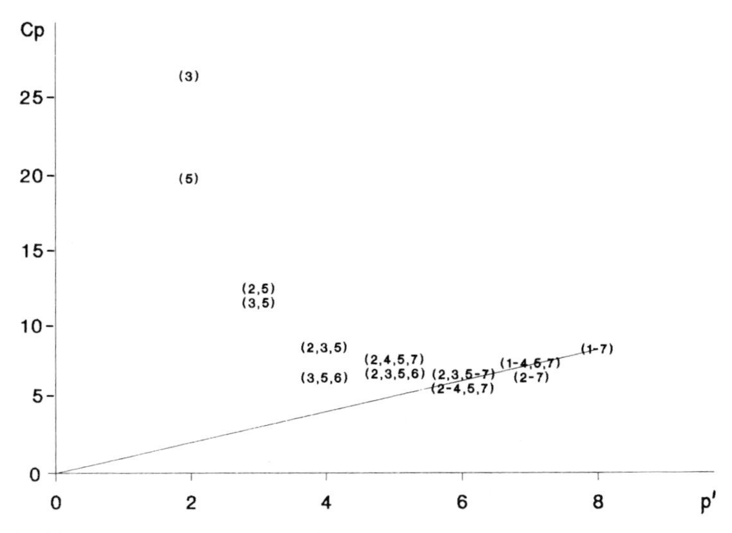

Figure 18. Mallows *Cp* plot against p' ($q + 1$) for multiple regression to predict breeding density of dippers; the straight line is at $-C_p = p'$.

equal to 4. Each column of *Figure 19* represents a step in the procedure. For each step the constant b_0, the partial regression coefficients b_j for variables in the regression, the associated Student's t statistic, the estimate of the error standard deviation s, and R^2 are printed. Notice that with the default values the steps are terminated with the three-variable solution identified with BREG. The three predictors were entered in turn, and none were removed at any step. The last line of output is a sub-command inviting the user to change the default values of the F to enter or F to remove, or to force variables in or

```
MTB > stepwise c8 c1-c3 c14-c17

 STEPWISE REGRESSION OF Br. Dens ON  7 PREDICTORS, WITH N =   22

     STEP         1         2         3
CONSTANT   -1.0076   -0.1727   -1.7747

log Stfl      1.14      0.79      0.86
T-RATIO       5.28      3.41      4.20

Gradient               0.096     0.096
T-RATIO                 2.61      2.97

log Mayf                         0.232
T-RATIO                           2.58

S            0.985     0.867     0.761
R-SQ         58.21     69.23     77.53
 MORE? (YES, NO, SUBCOMMAND, OR HELP)
SUBC> no
```

Figure 19. Output from *Minitab* STEPWISE command to find an optimum multiple regression equation to predict breeding density of dippers.

out of the regression equation. In this illustration the routine was terminated by typing the word 'no'.

Forward selection and backward elimination can be done in *Minitab* by changing the defaults. The F to remove (FREMOVE) is the criterion for removal of a predictor, if the F-ratio for removal of any predictor is less than FREMOVE, the variable with the smallest F-ratio is removed. By setting this to zero therefore, the removal of variables is made impossible. Since the output obtained with simply FREMOVE set to zero is identical to *Figure 19*, *Figure 20* was obtained by setting in addition the FENTER value very low (equal to 0.1) so as to illustrate more steps in the forward selection routine. The small increase in R^2 achieved by the inclusion of more than three predictors, together with the C_p plot of *Figure 18* indicates that the three-predictor model is probably the best that can be achieved with these data. Unfortunately the *Minitab* STEPWISE procedure does not print Mallows' C_p and as was mentioned earlier, the R^2 value can be an unreliable guide in variable selection. In this output it is the t-ratio that should be examined. A formal test can only be done by first calculating the degrees of freedom ($n - q - 1$) where q is the number of predictors in the model at that step. This t-ratio is the square root of the F-test for the inclusion of a predictor in the model. At

```
MTB > stepwise c8 c1-c3 c14-c17;
SUBC> fremove=0;
SUBC> fenter=.1.

 STEPWISE REGRESSION OF Br. Dens ON  7 PREDICTORS, WITH N =   22

    STEP          1         2         3         4         5         6         7
CONSTANT    -1.0076   -0.1727   -1.7747   -1.8706   -1.2301   -1.1121   -0.8806

log Stfl       1.14      0.79      0.86      0.88      0.79      0.59      0.60
T-RATIO        5.28      3.41      4.20      4.34      3.75      2.44      2.42

Gradient                0.096     0.096     0.084     0.087     0.074     0.080
T-RATIO                  2.61      2.97      2.50      2.66      2.26      2.24

log Mayf                          0.232     0.180     0.201     0.111     0.115
T-RATIO                            2.58      1.81      2.06      1.00      1.00

W Hard                                     0.0053    0.0087    0.0101    0.0100
T-RATIO                                      1.20      1.77      2.09      2.01

log OInv                                              -0.16     -0.25     -0.27
T-RATIO                                               -1.42     -2.01     -2.03

log Cadd                                                         0.41      0.41
T-RATIO                                                          1.52      1.49

Alt                                                                     -0.0018
T-RATIO                                                                   -0.51

S             0.985     0.867     0.761     0.752     0.731     0.703     0.721
R-SQ          58.21     69.23     77.53     79.28     81.60     84.04     84.33
 MORE? (YES, NO, SUBCOMMAND, OR HELP)
SUBC> no
```

Figure 20. Output from *Minitab* STEPWISE command used to calculate multiple regressions based on the forward selection procedure.

step 3 the *t*-ratio for the last variable introduced, $\log_e$ (1 + mayfly numbers), is 2.58 and the df are (22 − 3 − 1) = 18. The 5% critical value from *Appendix B.6* is 2.101, so this *t*-ratio is significant. The *t*-ratio for water hardness at the next step is not significant at the 5% level (nor indeed at the 10% level), so this test indicates that water hardness should not be included with the best three predictors. Notice that the *t*-ratio for $\log_e$ (1 + mayfly numbers) has fallen to 1.81 at this step, but this is the *t*-ratio for the inclusion of this variable if water hardness is included as well, so this statistic is not relevant.

Figure 21 illustrates the process of backward elimination. In *Minitab* this is done with the STEPWISE procedure with all the predictor variables entered at the first step and the FENTER criterion set very large. With these data and the default value of REMOVE left at 4, the procedure stops at step 3 with five variables in the predictor, and the FREMOVE criterion has been reset so as to show the elimination of all variables. This output illustrates one of the defects of the backward elimination procedure. The predictor variable $\log_e$ (1 + mayfly numbers) (x_6) is eliminated at step 3 in proceeding to the five-variable solution, but this predictor is included in the best solutions with three or four variables and from steps 4 onwards the solutions from the backward

```
MTB > stepwise c8 c1-c3 c14-c17;
SUBC> enter c1-c3 c14-c17;
SUBC> fenter=10000;
SUBC> fremove=10.

 STEPWISE REGRESSION OF Br. Dens ON  7 PREDICTORS, WITH N =   22

    STEP          1         2         3         4         5         6         7
CONSTANT   -0.8806   -1.1121   -0.7244   -1.5080   -2.3755   -1.7599   -1.0076

Alt        -0.0018
T-RATIO      -0.51

W Hard      0.0100    0.0101    0.0118    0.0137    0.0087    0.0114
T-RATIO       2.01      2.09      2.61      2.83      1.91      2.57

Gradient     0.080     0.074     0.065
T-RATIO       2.24      2.26      2.07

log Cadd      0.41      0.41      0.55      0.62      0.39
T-RATIO       1.49      1.52      2.43      2.55      1.65

log Stfl      0.60      0.59      0.51      0.71      0.97      1.12      1.14
T-RATIO       2.42      2.44      2.24      3.13      4.70      5.89      5.28

log Mayf      0.11      0.11
T-RATIO       1.00      1.00

log OInv     -0.27     -0.25     -0.27     -0.28
T-RATIO      -2.03     -2.01     -2.16     -2.05

S            0.721     0.703     0.703     0.768     0.834     0.871     0.985
R-SQ         84.33     84.04     82.97     78.40     73.05     68.97     58.21
 MORE? (YES, NO, SUBCOMMAND, OR HELP)
SUBC> no
```

Figure 21. Output from *Minitab* STEPWISE command used to calculate multiple regressions based on the backward selection procedure.

```
MTB > regress c8 3 c3 c15 c16

The regression equation is
Br. Dens = - 1.77 + 0.0963 Gradient + 0.864 log Stfl + 0.232 log Mayf

Predictor        Coef        Stdev     t-ratio        p
Constant       -1.775        1.087       -1.63    0.120
Gradient      0.09630      0.03241        2.97    0.008
log Stfl       0.8639       0.2058        4.20    0.001
log Mayf      0.23240      0.09017        2.58    0.019

s = 0.7614      R-sq = 77.5%      R-sq(adj) = 73.8%

Analysis of Variance

SOURCE         DF         SS         MS         F        p
Regression      3     35.992     11.997     20.70    0.000
Error          18     10.434      0.580
Total          21     46.426

SOURCE         DF     SEQ SS
Gradient        1     23.418
log Stfl        1      8.723
log Mayf        1      3.851

Unusual Observations
Obs.Gradient  Br. Dens        Fit Stdev.Fit  Residual    St.Resid
 15     17.4     4.700      6.374     0.312    -1.674      -2.41R

R denotes an obs. with a large st. resid.
```

Figure 22. Multiple regression to predict breeding density of dippers with the best three predictors identified in *Figures 17, 18,* and *19.* Output from *Minitab* REGRESS command.

elimination procedure are sub-optimal. Forward selection often has the same defect, a variable included early leads to sub-optimal solutions with more predictors at subsequent steps. The stepwise procedure to some extent ameliorates this problem, but even with this method optimal solutions are not guaranteed. For that reason a combination of BREG and STEPWISE should be used, with careful scrutiny of Mallows' C_p.

The full regression analysis for the best three-variable regression is given in *Figure 22*. This cannot be compared directly with the analysis in *Figure 6* since in the latter case the dependent variable is the logarithm of breeding density. However, in the three-variable model identified by the selection procedures all variables included are statistically significant. This equation may therefore form the basis of a useful investigation, though I do not suggest that the three-variable solution is optimal. One defect is that a plot of breeding density against $\log_e$ (1 + stonefly numbers) shows curvature, and the square of the latter is actually a better predictor in the statistical sense. Section 4.3 made clear that the search for optimal transformations is difficult. However, the solution proffered here is simple and fairly effective. It highlights some of the important influences on dipper breeding density. It is, however, highly tailored to this particular data set and may not be representative of other populations of dippers.

Protocol 4. Selection of variables in multiple regression

1. Identify an optimal subset of variables using a procedure that calculates the regression statistics for the best regression with a specified number of predictors.
2. Plot Mallows' C_p against $q + 1$ for a range of subsets of q predictors and look for one whose C_p is close to $q + 1$. Ignore those subsets with most predictors included unless other subsets have a C_p much greater than $q + 1$.
3. Confirm that the optimal subset is best using a stepwise procedure that both adds and removes variables to find a solution.
4. Calculate the full regression analysis for the optimal subset and follow *Protocol 1*.

7. Dummy variables in multiple regression

Qualitative factors can be included in regression models by arbitrarily ascribing numerical values to the classifications to obtain dummy or indicator variables. In a regression study on animals, for example, the sex of each animal could be incorporated in the study using a dummy variable that takes the value 1 for females and 0 for males. Dummy variables are also used to enable unbalanced factorial experiments to be analysed. The analysis of factorial experiments is described in Chapter 2, with Section 6 devoted to unbalanced experiments. The essentials of the method are that multiple regression is performed using dummy variables. A dummy variable is introduced for each level of each factor. One variable takes the value 1 for observations at level 1 of factor A and 0 for observations at other levels, a second dummy variable takes the value 1 only for observations at level 2 of factor A and so on. A complication arises in that the resulting dummy variables are collinear with the constant so in fact only $(a - 1)$ of these dummy variables are needed, with a the number of levels of factor A.

If there is a second factor, B, in the experiment this can be incorporated into the model using regression by $(b - 1)$ further dummy variables, constructed for the levels of B in a similar way to the $(a - 1)$ dummy variables for A. Dummy variables for interactions are the products of those for the factors included in the interaction. The so-called general linear model commands in packages such as *Minitab* and *SAS* calculate the necessary dummy variables automatically, so a detailed description of their construction is superfluous here. Rawlings (10, Chapter 8) contains more details of this approach to the analysis of variance. Other applications of dummy variables are mentioned by Chatterjee and Price (1).

In this chapter the use of dummy variables will be illustrated with the data given in *Table 3*. These data are the mortality rates and the logarithm of the

```
The regression equation is
M = - 0.123 + 0.133 x1 + 0.0209 x2

Predictor        Coef         Stdev      t-ratio        p
Constant     -0.12349       0.02262        -5.46    0.000
x1            0.13295       0.02270         5.86    0.000
x2           0.020947      0.003200         6.55    0.000

s = 0.005022     R-sq = 87.5%     R-sq(adj) = 84.9%

Analysis of Variance

SOURCE         DF           SS           MS          F         p
Regression      2   0.00175798   0.00087899      34.85     0.000
Error          10   0.00025219   0.00002522
Total          12   0.00201017

SOURCE         DF       SEQ SS
x1              1   0.00067755
x2              1   0.00108043

Unusual Observations
Obs.       x1         M       Fit  Stdev.Fit   Residual    St.Resid
 13      0.00   0.05147   0.04201    0.00344    0.00946       2.58R

R denotes an obs. with a large st. resid.
```

Figure 23. Multiple regression equation to predict mortality of O-group plaice using dummy variables, given in *Table 3* and described in the text, based on the natural logarithm of the maximum density.

maximum density for O-group plaice. Each row of data relates to a particular year class. The scatter plot of the data given in *Figure 1* suggests that an equation that remains constant up to a threshold value for the logarithm of maximum density equal to about 6.26 and thereafter increases linearly would be a sensible model for mortality. In fact there is some justification for the use of such an equation. The lower densities, zone 2 of *Table 3*, correspond to surveys made in the Dutch Wadden Sea. Zone 1 consists of bays in Swedish waters. It is possible that there is a relationship between the variables for the Swedish data, but not for the Dutch. The form of equation required, with y the mortality rate and x the logarithm of maximum density, is

$$y = \beta_{01} + \varepsilon \qquad \text{for } x < 6.26;$$
$$y = \beta_{02} + \beta_{12}x + \varepsilon \qquad \text{for } x \geqslant 6.26.$$

This can be achieved with the two predictor variables given as the fourth (x1) and fifth (x2) columns of *Table 3*, with the model

$$y = \beta_0 + \beta_1 x_1 + \beta_2 x_2 + \varepsilon.$$

Variable x_1 (x1, *Table 3*) is simply a dummy variable constructed according to the rules in the first paragraph of this section, whilst x_2 (x2, *Table 3*) is constructed as zeros for zone 2, to represent the constant, mean value assumed in this zone, and the values of log D_{max} for zone 1, to represent the sloping line assumed here. The effect of these dummy variables is that for the Dutch data

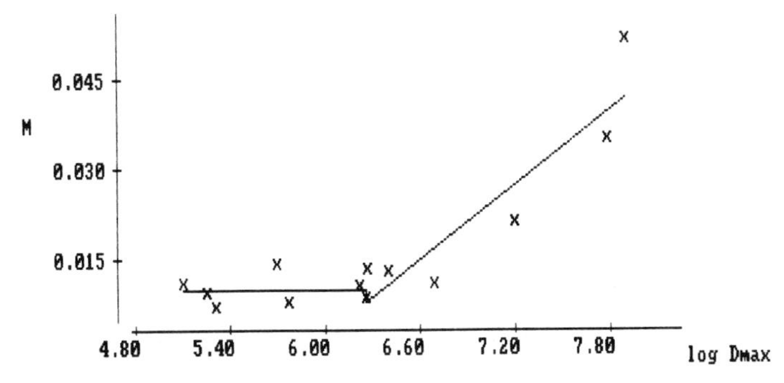

Figure 24. Scatter plot of mortality against $\log_e$ maximum density for O-group plaice together with fitted equation obtained from dummy variables.

$y = \beta_0 + \beta_1 + \varepsilon$ and for the Swedish data $y = \beta_0 + \beta_2 x + \varepsilon$ and this is equivalent to the model given above, with $\beta_{01} = \beta_0 + \beta_1$, $\beta_{02} = \beta_0$, and $\beta_{12} = \beta_2$.

Figure 23 gives the multiple regression analysis for these data, using *Minitab*. For the Dutch data the multiple regression equation gives as a prediction $y = -0.123\,49 + 0.132\,95 = 0.009\,46$ and this is equal to the mean of the y values of the Dutch data. For the Swedish data the multiple regression equation gives as a prediction $y = -0.123\,49 + 0.020\,947x$.

This is simply the regression equation of y on x for the Swedish data alone. The advantage of this dummy variable method of fitting separate equations to the two parts of the data are that a comparison can be made with the simpler model in which y and x are assumed to be related by a single straight line. Similarly, comparison could be made with some assumed curve (see Chapter 3, Section 5). *Figure 24* is a plot of the multiple regression equation given in *Figure 23*.

Further examples of the use of dummy variables are given by Draper and Smith (11), where other references on fitting segmented straight lines are given.

References

1. Chatterjee, S. and Price, B. (1977). *Regression analysis by example*. John Wiley, New York.
2. Gunst, R. F. and Mason, R. L. (1980). *Regression analysis and its application. A data-oriented approach*. Marcel Dekker, New York.
3. Atkinson, A. C. (1985). *Plots, transformations and regression. An introduction to graphical methods of diagnostic regression analysis*. Oxford University Press, Oxford.
4. Cook, R. D. and Weisberg, S. (1982). *Residuals and influence in regression*. Chapman & Hall, New York.

5. Miller, R. G. (1986). *Beyond ANOVA: Basics of applied statistics*. John Wiley, New York.
6. Kendall, M. G. and Stuart, A. (1973). *The advanced theory of statistics; Volume 2: Inference and relationship*. Griffin, London.
7. Hoaglin, D. C., Mosteller, F., and Tukey, J. W. (1985). *Exploring data tables, trends and shapes*. John Wiley, New York.
8. McCullagh, P. and Nelder, J. A. (1989). *Generalized linear models* (2nd edn). Chapman & Hall, London.
9. Kendall, M. G. and Stuart, A. (1976). *The advanced theory of statistics; Volume 3: Design and analysis, and time series*. Griffin, London.
10. Rawlings, J. O. (1988). *Applied regression analysis. A research tool*. Wadsworth and Brookside, Pacific Grove, California.
11. Draper, N. R. and Smith, H. (1981). *Applied regression analysis* (2nd edn). John Wiley, New York.

5

Ordination

P. F. RANDERSON

1. Why do we need multivariate analysis?

1.1 Multivariate data—objects and characteristics

Individuals comprising a population, or at least a sample taken from it, may be described quantitatively and compared by measurements of common characters or variables. Thus a variable is any quantity that takes different values for different individuals or for the same individual at different times, that is a quantity which can take any one of a specified set of values. A variable may be continuous, such as

- height
- density
- plant cover
- abundance

or discontinuous, such as

- integer counts
- rank orders
- binary (e.g. sex or presence/absence, which take either of two states)

By extension, a variate, or random variable, is any quantity that can take any one of a specified set of values with a specified relative frequency or probability. A variate is therefore characterized by a distribution of values, and could be transformed to an alternative distribution. Data for multivariate analysis may be selected randomly from a population, but is more often an arbitrary set of 'available' data.

Statistical tests such as analysis of variance (see Chapters 1 and 2) or the χ^2 test seek to demonstrate differences between groups of individuals in the values of a single measured variate. Where the distribution of values can be assumed to be, or can be transformed to become, approximately normal, a measure of probability that groups are really different to each other can be given. Such analyses are univariate. Where measurements of a pair of characters are made on a set of individuals, any relationship between the two variates can be detected with bivariate tests such as correlation and regression (see Chapter 3).

The biologist is often faced with multivariate data, where each individual is characterized by several measured variates. For example, to identify a bacterial culture we need to measure various aspects of its morphology, performance, and activity to relate it adequately to others. In ecology, sites are characterized by the presence of many species or by several measured environmental factors. As we may wish to compare many sites, there is often a large matrix of data comprising species-in-site, environmental-factors-in-site, and other measurements. Species measures may be qualitative by recording presence or absence at a site, or quantitative by estimating abundance. For animals, counts of numbers (estimating density) are appropriate, whereas for plants, estimates of biomass or percentage ground cover may be preferred. Similar data matrices with columns of individuals or cases versus rows of attributes or variates arise in other disciplines (*Table 1*). Using the ecological example, each individual, such as a sampling unit, station, or quadrat, has its variates, such as species or environmental factors (*Figure 1*).

1.2 The roles of multivariate analysis—classification and ordination

Multivariate analysis has the following aims (1):

- searching for pattern or structure in a set of data
- describing or summarizing the data efficiently to reduce the data matrix to a more manageable form
- searching for possible causal relationships between the distribution of the biota and that of environmental factors

Unlike most statistical analysis, where the approach is deductive, based on experiment, multivariate analysis uses an inductive, non-experimental approach to generate rather than to test hypotheses. In this respect, two approaches to multivariate analysis, classification (see Chapter 6) and ordination, are complementary, as they search the data for patterns of different form. In contrast, multiple regression (see Chapter 4) assumes that a variate can be predicted from a set of other variates, and seeks the best mathematical relationship between them.

In classification, each individual, either a site or species, is assigned to one of several classes or groups on the basis of the relative similarity of its attributes to its fellows. In ordination, each individual, either a site or species, is placed on one or more constructed axes so that its geometrical position relative to its fellows reflects its similarity to them. Hence classification imposes discontinuities on the data by assigning individuals to discrete groups, whereas ordination detects continuous variation in the distribution of

Table 1. The data matrix—individuals × attributes; some examples

Ecology
- samples by species
- sites by environmental parameters
- species by niches
- species by behavioural patterns

Taxonomy
- specimens by characteristics

Genetics
- varieties by genetic traits

Agronomy
- soils by characteristics

Paleontology & Geology
- samples by species
- samples by geochemical characteristics

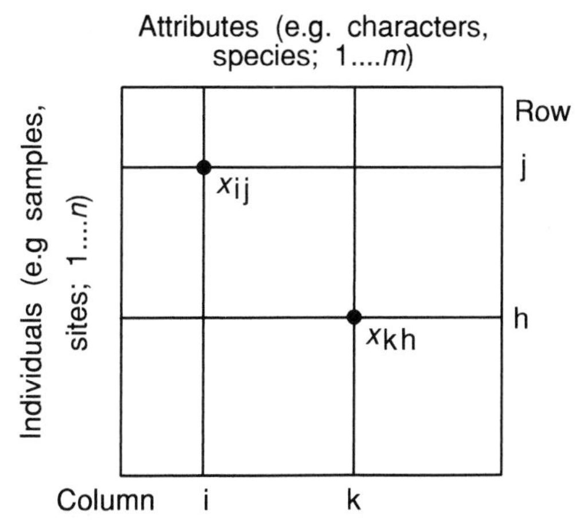

Figure 1. Raw data table structure, with columns (j, h) as attributes and rows (i, k) comprising individuals. Each cell of the table (e.g. x_{ij} or x_{kh}) contains a data value, zero, or missing value.

attributes between individuals. Ordination represents objects as points in a low-dimensional order which provides a summary of the data.

Which approach is the more appropriate depends partly on the data in question, but also on the investigator's view of the nature of variation in his or her data. The investigator might ask whether there are natural groups with clear separation, as in many taxonomic problems, or in ecological surveys of widely differing environments. Alternatively, are there extreme individuals separated by a range of intermediate forms, as in transitional environments or hybrid species? In the latter case, it may still be desirable to impose breaks along a gradient of transitional forms for convenience, or to summarize objectively and efficiently.

1.3 Looking for pattern—'new axes for old'

Data can be summarized because of two aspects of variation in a set of data (1):

- noise, or random variation; in contrast to
- redundancy, or the coordinated response among attributes—the opposite of noise

These ideas may be illustrated with reference to a bivariate situation in which individuals are characterized by two attributes.

Consider a sample of postal envelopes on which the two variates 'length' and 'width' have been measured. We have an $n \times 2$ matrix of data which can be displayed geometrically in a two-dimensional variate space (*Figure 2a*). Each individual then appears as a point on the plane, referenced by two coordinates plotted as an (x, y) pair. We can inspect the figure to search for pattern. All the points on the plot lie on or below the principal diagonal, for square or rectangular envelopes respectively. The larger the envelope, the further away from the origin it lies. We could define a trend among the data points corresponding to the trend of size, orientated at an angle, as shown in *Figure 2b*. Independently of size, we could define a trend corresponding to envelope shape, orientated at right angles, with the more oblong envelopes below and squarer ones above, for any given size (*Figure 2b*). The shape dimension is illustrated by outliers with odd shapes (long and thin envelopes), in contrast to the majority of 'normal-shaped' envelopes. We could also note that the points are aggregated into three main groups (large, medium, and small) with a few intermediates and some outliers (e.g. longer envelopes). Should we consider these 'groups' to be discrete entities, or are they nodes along a continuum? Is there a major, and opposing minor, orientation to this continuum corresponding to the 'size' and 'shape' trends noted above?

We could now construct a new coordinate system to support the set of data points (*Figure 3a*), aligned along our trend lines of 'size' and 'shape', to replace the original measured variates of 'length' and 'width'. This new pair of axes, positioned in this case subjectively by eye, retains all the information provided by the original data: the axes merely provide a new reference system which has been rotated through an angle α, and has a new arbitrary origin with respect to the old (*Figure 3a*). Of the two new axes, the longer one represents size and accounts for a larger proportion of the total variability in the data compared to the other representing shape, which appears as the shorter line.

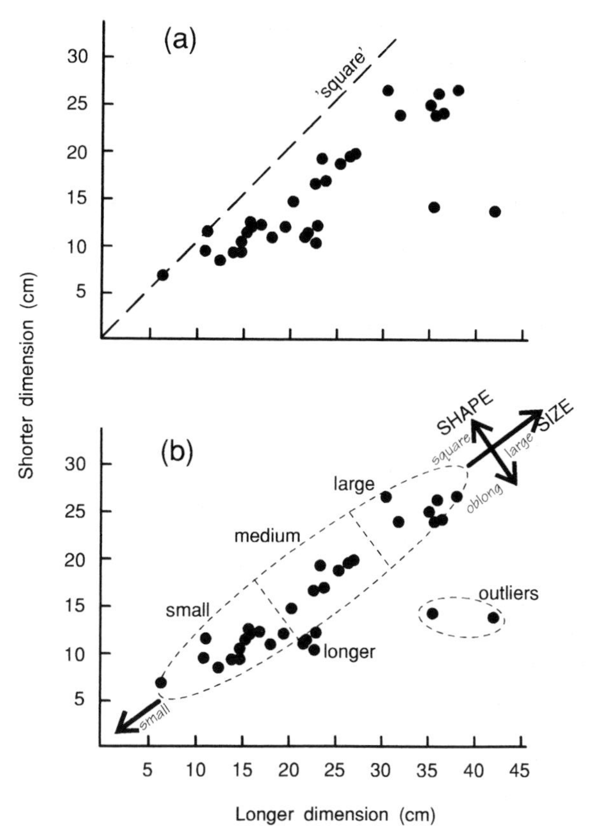

Figure 2. (a) Length and width values of a sample of 34 postal envelopes. (b) Visually defined trend lines superimposed on the points. Ellipses enclose arbitrary 'groups' of envelopes defined by size and shape.

We could, however, summarize the pattern of the data using only one of the new axes, that related to size. By ignoring shape, we would simplify our data set from a two-dimensional to a one-dimensional problem, although losing some information in the process (*Figure 3b*). By choosing the longer size axis in preference to the shape axis, we obtain the better summary. Equally, we could summarize by grouping the envelopes into three main groups (small, medium, and large) with sub-groups (thin or broad) in each case (*Figure 2b*). The first approach ordinates the data along trend lines which are more readily interpretable as general characteristics of the population, whereas the latter classifies them into conveniently identifiable groups.

In a similar way, we can illustrate a bivariate data set which describes the top speeds and engine capacities of motor cars (taken from *Appendix 5.1*) as an (x, y) coordinate plot (*Figure 4*). We can identify a trend in these data corresponding to increasing size of car, again orientated diagonally with

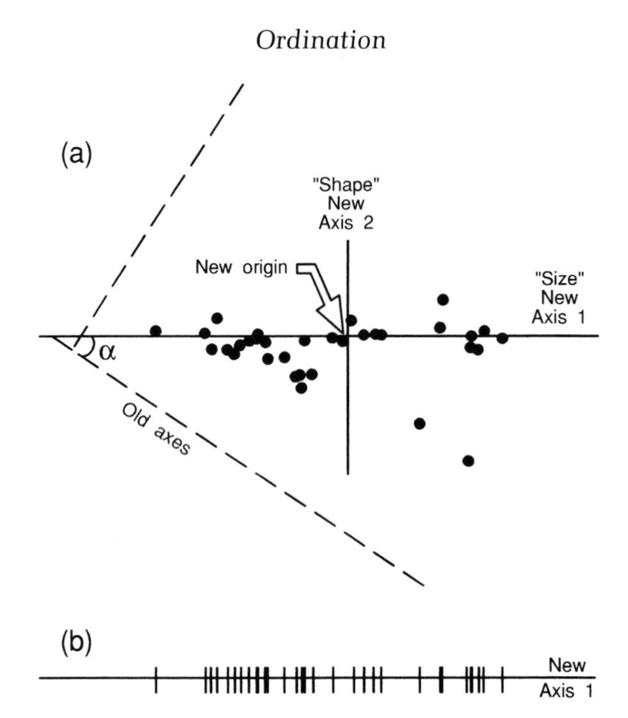

Figure 3. (a) Postal envelopes as in *Figure 2a*, positioned on a new pair of visually rotated axes conforming to the 'size' and 'shape' trends of *Figure 2b*. (b) Envelopes positioned in one dimension along new axis 1.

respect to the original coordinates. Using our knowledge of the cars in the sample, we can interpret the trend as ranging from compact, cheap family cars to large, expensive luxury models. Diverging from this orientation we could recognize a trend in 'sportiness', faster cars for any given size such as the sports cars and GTs positioned above corresponding standard models on the plot. Again, we have ordinated these data by arbitrarily rotating the coordinate axes to produce a new pair of axes which represent interpretable general characteristics of motor cars.

With only two initial dimensions, such graphical manipulation is easy to perform to match a visually defined end point. With multivariate data, the situation is more complex. A tri-variate data set (also from *Appendix 5.1*), such as we would have if horsepower were included with the above data on cars, may be illustrated on two-dimensional paper (*Figure 5*) as a solid figure on which ordination axes can be subjectively imposed with respect to the shape of the cloud of points comprising the data. Intuitively, we would consider the major dimension of our three new coordinates to run through the length of the sausage-shaped cloud of points, because this dimension carries the largest divergence of points away from its centre, that is the largest variability. Subsequent coordinates defining the width and depth of the sausage have less variation about the centroid of the cloud.

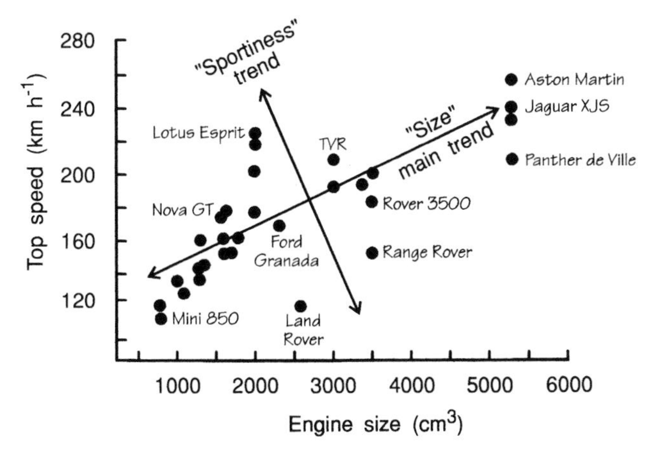

Figure 4. Engine size (cm^3) and top speed (km/h) values of 27 models of motor car (from *Appendix 5.1*) with visually defined trend lines representing 'size of car' and 'sportiness' superimposed on the points.

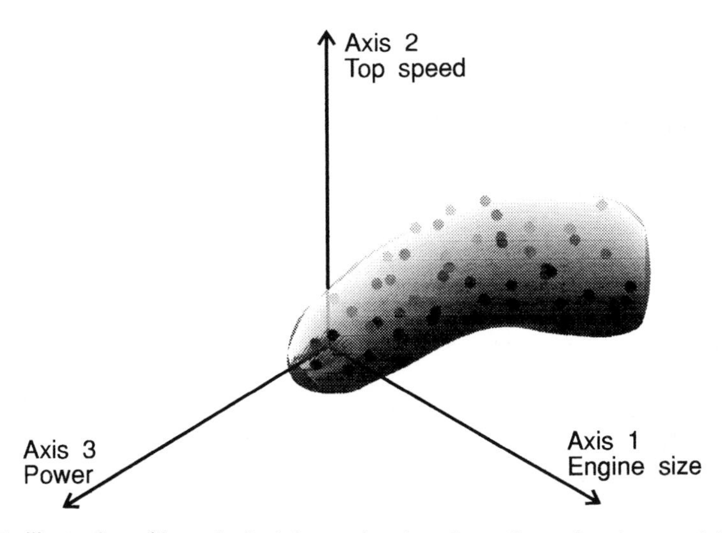

Figure 5. Illustration of hypothetical data points in a three-dimensional space defined by three axes (such as measures of top speed, engine size, and power in the cars; *Appendix 5.1*), and bounded within a sausage-shaped envelope.

In principle, the process of ordination, by constructing one or more new axes which pass through a cloud of points, is the same whatever the number of dimensions supporting the cloud, although we cannot draw an n-dimensional 'hypersausage' on paper. Instead of visual rotation of the original coordinates, it is necessary to calculate optimal positions for the new axes by objective, statistical methods. Although various methods exist, they each seek to minimize the variation left over after each ordination axis is fitted through the cloud of points. This process is similar to regression (see Chapters 3 and 4), and with a bivariate ordination the first axis will be close to the regression line.

1.4 Data 'spaces'—measuring the similarity/distance between individuals

In the above examples of envelopes and cars we have used a pair of attributes as geometric coordinates to position the individuals in so-called attribute space, or A-space, which defines the locations of n individuals, which may be sites or samples, on m axes representing attributes, which may be species or characters. With many attributes comprising the columns of the data matrix, each row provides a set of values or a vector locating a point for each individual with respect to the origin (see *Figure 1* of Chapter 6). Conversely we could also represent the data in individual space or I-space, which defines the locations of m points, now the attributes, on n axes, now the individuals, each column of the data matrix again comprising a 'position vector'.

One possible measure of resemblance between individuals is simply the direct linear distance between them in A-space, the Pythagorean or Euclidean distance. In two dimensions this is easily measured graphically or calculated by Pythagorean triangles (*Figure 6*, and *Figure 2* of Chapter 6):

$$D_{jh} = \sqrt{(x_{ij} - x_{ih})^2 + (x_{kj} - x_{kh})^2},$$

whereas in m dimensions an extension of the same formula can be used (*Table 2*).

There are many options for the kind of mathematical index or resemblance function relating the individuals, which may take the form of either similarity

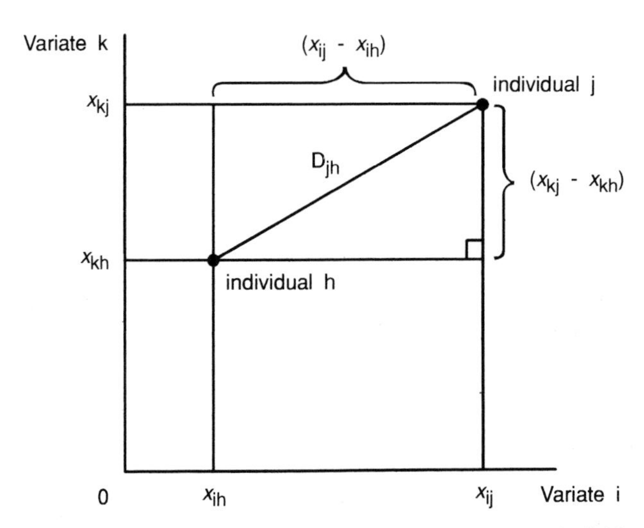

Figure 6. Geometric representation of Euclidean distances between individuals j and h in bivariate 'A-space' defined by variates i and k.

Table 2. Examples of resemblance coefficients and data transformations[a]

Sorensen (Czekanowski) coefficient (non-Euclidean)
Either Q- or R-mode (C_{jh} or C_{ik}).
$C_{jh} = 2W/(A + B)$, where:

- A = sum of attribute scores for case j
- B = sum of attribute scores for case h
- W = sum of lesser scores of attributes common to both cases j and h

$$\text{i.e. } C_{jh} = 2 \sum_{i=1}^{m} \min(x_{ij}, x_{ih}) \Big/ \left(\sum_{i=1}^{m} x_{ij} + \sum_{i=1}^{m} x_{ih} \right)$$

Euclidean distance (Pythagorean distance)
Q-mode (interstand distance D_{jh}) or R-mode (D_{ik}):

$$D_{jh} = \sqrt{\sum_{i=1}^{m} (x_{ij} - x_{ih})^2}$$

Product-moment (Euclidean) similarity
Coefficients correlation coefficient (Pearson correlation)
R-mode:

$$r_{ik} = \text{covariance}_{ik} / \sqrt{(\text{variance}_i)(\text{variance}_k)}$$

Implicit transformations:

- Centred by attribute mean $(x_{ij} - \bar{x}_{i.})$
- Standardized by attribute standard deviation $(x_{ij}/s_{i.})$

Q-mode:

$$r_{jh} = \text{covariance}_{jh} / \sqrt{(\text{variance}_j)(\text{variance}_h)}$$

Implicit transformations:

- Centred by individual mean $(x_{ij} - x_{.j})$
- Standardized by individual standard deviation $(x_{ij}/s_{.j})$

Covariance
R-mode (Dispersion)

$$S_{ik} = \sum_{i=1}^{n} (x_{ij} - \bar{x}_{i.})(x_{kj} - \bar{x}_{k.})$$

Implicit transformation:

- Centred by attribute mean $(x_{ij} - \bar{x}_{i.})$

Q-mode

$$S_{jh} = \sum_{i=1}^{m} (x_{ij} - \bar{x}_{.j})(x_{ih} - \bar{x}_{.h})$$

Implicit transformation:

- Centred by individual mean $(x_{ij} - \bar{x}_{.j})$

Note: the Q-mode coefficient which provides the same transformation as dispersion above is the weighted similarity coefficient (WSC):

$$W_{jh} = \sum_{i=1}^{m} (x_{ij} - \bar{x}_{i.})(x_{ih} - \bar{x}_{k.})$$

Implicit transformation:

- Centred by attribute mean $(x_{ij} - \bar{x}_{i.})$

[a] Subscripts j,h denote individuals, subscripts i,k denote attributes, a dot in a subscript indicates a row or column statistic (e.g. $\bar{x}_{i.}$ is the attribute mean), resemblance between any pair of attributes i,k is R-mode, and resemblance between any pair of individuals j,h is Q-mode

(closeness) or dissimilarity (distance) between each pair (see also Chapter 6). Perhaps the most commonly used is the product-moment or Euclidean similarity coefficient, derived as the sum of squares and cross products between either the individuals SS_Q or the attributes SS_R of a matrix of data values, or some function of them.

Euclidean coefficients have a simple geometrical interpretation in Euclidean space (*Figure 7*). They possess the important property of metric inequality, whereby the distance between any two individuals *j* and *h* is less than or equal to the sum of their distances from a third individual *l*:

$$D_{jh} \leqslant D_{jl} + D_{hl}.$$

Non-Euclidean distance measures may violate this property, so that the three inter-point distances cannot be represented in Euclidean space (*Figure 7*). A complementary relationship exists between Euclidean similarity and distance in a given space:

$$D_{jh}^2 = S_{jj} + S_{hh} - 2S_{jh}.$$

Where the resemblance function is calculated between all possible pairs of attributes, such as species or environmental factors, the index is termed an

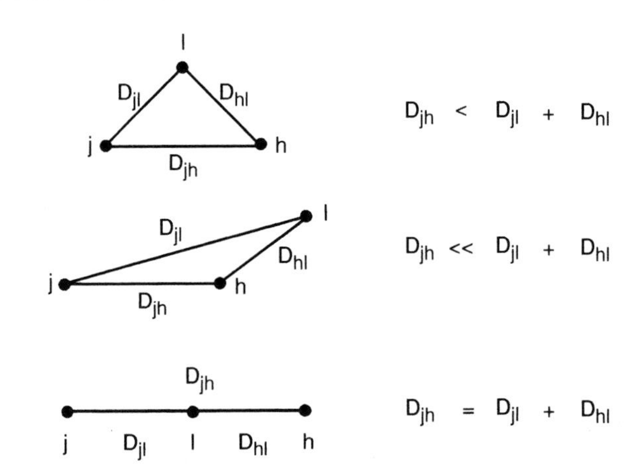

Figure 7. Geometric representation of inter-point distances.

R-statistic and the analysis is *R*-mode or an *R*-approach. A between-individuals index, such as between-sites, would be a *Q*-statistic and the analysis *Q*-mode or a *Q*-approach. Euclidean distance illustrated in *Figure 6* is an *R*-statistic, being represented geometrically as inter-point distances in *A*-space. Such indices of resemblance, *R* or *Q*, which form the basis for ordinating the individuals, can be displayed as a symmetric matrix in which the principal diagonal expresses the self-comparisons which are zeros for a distance measure, and the upper and lower triangles are mirrored (*Figure 8*).

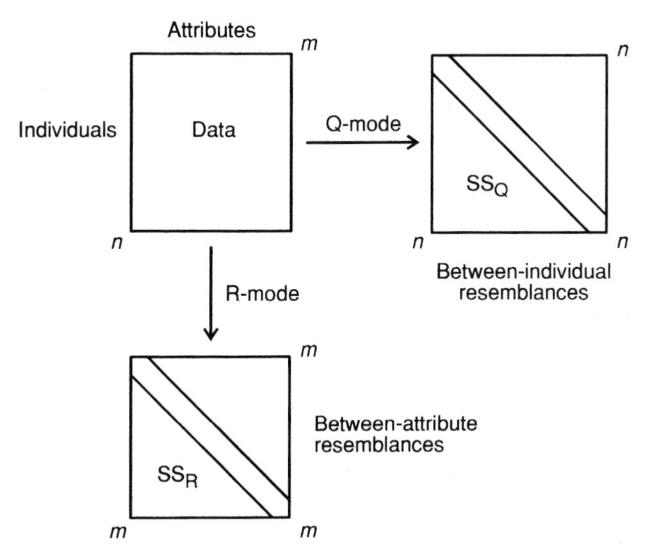

Figure 8. Deriving the alternative resemblance matrices SS_Q (between individuals) and SS_R (between attributes) from the data matrix. Self comparisons (zeros) occur on the principal diagonal and the upper and lower triangles are mirrored.

1.5 Transformations and measures of similarity

A variety of SS_Q and SS_R (*Figure 8*) may be obtained by different transformations of the data, such as centring, standardization, reduction to rank, or log, but in all cases their common Euclidean properties are maintained. This group of similarity coefficients includes several commonly used measures, such as correlation coefficient and covariance (*Table 2*), and each implicitly performs a transformation of the data prior to calculating the SS matrix (see Seciton 2.6). Computer packages commonly offer the option of one or two standard coefficients and the implied transformation is obscured. Section 2.8 considers the suitability of different coefficients in relation to the types of data to be analysed.

1.6 Geometric models in ordination—dissimilarity 'spaces'

Measures of distance between individuals, such as sites, samples, or quadrats, can be represented geometrically as a set of points in a dissimilarity space, so-called DI-space, where the axes are the measures of dissimilarity of individuals from each other (1). DI-space contains only information about the individuals and has the same numbers of axes n as points. Correspondingly, distances between attributes, such as species or characters, can become a set of points in a dissimilarity space, so-called DA-space, where the axes are dissimilarities between attributes. DA-space contains only information about the individuals and has the same number of axes m as points. The distribution of points in these n- or m-dimensional spaces is typically not random, as the points are concentrated in certain regions and along certain directions, due to patterns in species distribution. Hence the 'trick' of ordination is to project the points on to a lower-dimensional sub-space. If the points were randomly distributed, projection would not be helpful because no one configuration of axes would be superior to another in detecting pattern at the expense of noise. However, if a pattern does exist in the distribution of the points, then the data can be effectively summarized in a few new dimensions. Detecting pattern is then a matter of detecting non-randomness within the resemblance matrix, computing new coordinate positions for the points as efficiently as possible, and displaying this pattern graphically to aid interpretation.

These geometrical concepts are now put into practice using a fundamental ordination method.

2. Ordination methods

2.1 Principal components analysis

A method of ordination which has been widely used in ecology, taxonomy, and other fields, following its initial application in psychology, is that of principal components analysis (PCA), in which axes or components are successively extracted from a matrix of similarities (either SS_R or SS_Q), typically correlations or covariances between the variates. PCA is a particular form of the more general principal coordinates analysis (PCO) which can utilize either a similarity or a distance matrix, such as Euclidean distance illustrated above.

PCA was considered to be an improvement over a previous method of axis construction which made use of reference individuals to define the extremes or poles of the ordination axes; hence its name polar ordination (1). This method was based on the non-Euclidean similarity coefficient of Sorensen (*Table 2*). The axes produced would often be influenced by extreme or outlier individuals which shared little in common with the majority, whereas in PCA all individuals contribute equally to the components, avoiding dominance by outliers. Another advantage was that simultaneous ordinations for both individuals and attributes, such as sites and species, were obtained by a single analysis. PCA has found wide application in biology and is readily available as part of many computer packages such as *Minitab, SPSS/PC+* and *GENSTAT*.

2.2 Defining axis positions

We can illustrate the steps in performing and interpreting PCA using a set of five characters (the attributes) describing a non-random sample of 32 types of motor car (the individuals) (*Appendix 5.1*), as in *Protocol 1*.

Protocol 1. Steps in ordination by principal components analysis on *Minitab* using the cars data (*Appendix 5.1*)

1. Enter data into Minitab columns from the data file with the command

```
READ 'A:CARS.DAT' C1–C5
```

or from the keyboard using the data editor; the data are on drive A:.

2. Use the *Minitab* PCA command with sub-commands:

- to restrict eigenvectors and scores calculated to components
- to store eigenvectors—called 'coefficients' by *Minitab*—in three new columns
- to store principal component scores in three new columns

```
PCA C1–C5;
NCOMP 3;
COEF C11–C13;
SCOR C21–C23.
```

This will use the correlation coefficient, both centring and standardizing the variables, in an *R*-mode analysis. Note that the additional sub-command

```
COVAR;
```

would use covariance, centring but not standardizing the variables.

3. Examine the eigenvalues and the proportion of the total variance each one accounts for. Does this indicate a relatively homogeneous data set, or one with a strong single trend or discontinuity?

4. Plot the eigenvectors in all possible pairs. This is conveniently done using the *Minitab* letterplot (LPLOT) command, whereby variables 1-m will be given the first m letters of the alphabet. You will need to set up a labelling column first (C10; $m = 5$).

```
SET C10
1:5
LPLOT C12 C11 C10
LPLOT C13 C11 C10
LPLOT C13 C12 C10
```

Protocol 1. *Continued*

5. Do the same for the scores, where the labelling column is C20 (n = 32).

```
SET C20
1:32
LPLOT C22 C21 C20
LPLOT C23 C21 C20
LPLOT C23 C22 C20
```

6. Interpret the plots, identifying each point and superimposing any additional information available which may help to explain the spatial pattern.

Mathematically, PCA involves eigenanalysis of a symmetric matrix of similarities (*Figure 9*), in this case the correlation coefficients between the five characters (*Table 3*), to produce a series of eigenvalues and their corresponding eigenvectors (*Table 4*). Noting that the original variables are highly intercorrelated—top speed positively with engine size; acceleration time negatively with engine size— it is no surprise to find that the proportion of the total

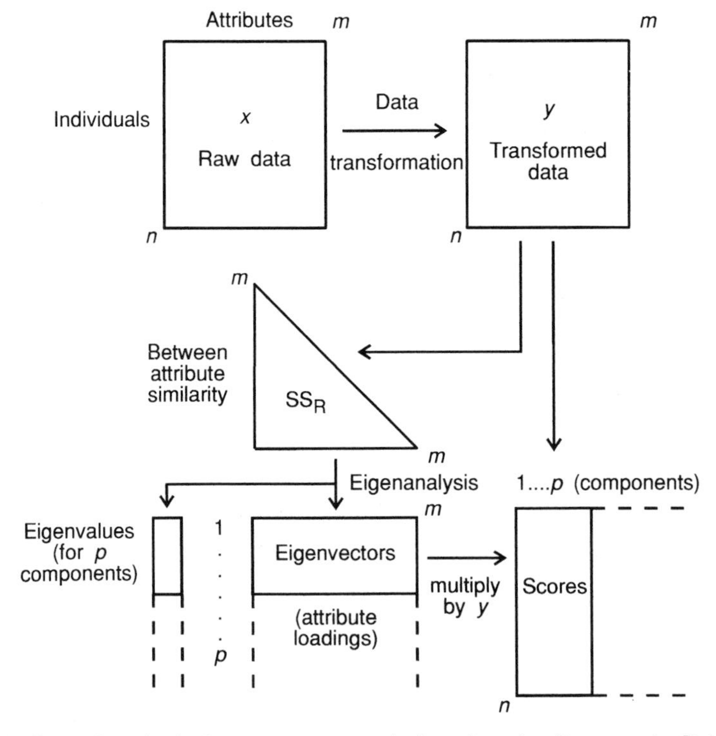

Figure 9. Steps in principal components analysis using the R-approach. Data transformation may be implicit within the chosen index of resemblance, such as correlation coefficient (Section 1.5).

Table 3. Correlation coefficients between the five variates of the cars data (*Appendix 5.1*)[a]

	Top speed	Power	Acceleration time	Engine size
Power	0.833			
Acceleration time	−0.891	−0.653		
Engine size	0.659	0.922	−0.517	
Length	0.575	0.748	−0.457	0.777

[a] Figures from the *Minitab* CORRELATE command

variance accounted for by successive components rapidly declines; that is the variability is efficiently summarized (92%) in the first two components (*Table 4*).

The components amount to a set of independent packets of variance, the first few of which frequently account for the majority of the total variation of the data, the remainder being insignificant. Thus by replacing the original m variates of the raw data by the first few p components which have relatively large eigenvalues (*Table 4a*), we effectively summarize the data and, we hope, display any inherent pattern it contains. In total, there are as many eigenvalues and eigenvectors as there were original variates. Typically, com-

Table 4. Eigenanalysis of correlations of the cars data[a]

(a) Eigenvalues and variability

Statistic	**PC1**[b]	**PC2**	**PC3**	**PC4**	**PC5**
Eigenvalue	3.8294	0.7662	0.2729	0.1055	0.0259
Proportion of variability	0.766	0.153	0.055	0.021	0.005
Cumulative proportion of variability	0.766	0.919	0.974	0.995	1.000

(b) Eigenvectors

	Attribute loadings for		
Variable	**PC1**	**PC2**	**PC3**
Top speed	−0.463	0.422	−0.035
Power	−0.489	−0.146	−0.409
Acceleration time	0.409	−0.636	−0.241
Engine size	−0.456	−0.398	−0.436
Length	−0.415	−0.488	0.763

[a] Figures calculated by the *Minitab* PCA command (*Protocol 1*, step 2)
[b] Principal components 1–5 are abbreviated as PC1 ... PC5 in the headings

puter programs calculate only the first few of these, the remainder being of little mathematical or interpretable value.

Interpretation of the components is then aided by plotting the data points using the component values as graphical coordinates. Whereas the eigenvectors provide coordinates, often termed loadings, for the attributes of the data matrix (*Table 4b*), coordinates for the individuals on the components, termed scores, are also calculated by PCA (*Figure 9*) and can be plotted independently. With suitable numerical scaling, the two sets of points can be superimposed as a biplot (2).

Plotting the eigenvectors of the first 2 components illustrates the relationships between them (*Figure 10a*). Thus the first component could be interpreted as representing the overall size of the cars, with four variables, all closely related to size, grouped at the negative end of the axis. The second, by selecting out acceleration time as the most negative variable, could represent the 'sportiness' factor at any given level of power, as in the bivariate illustration (*Figure 4*). Plotting the individual cars using their component scores reinforces this interpretation (*Figure 10b*). The cars are oriented in a band

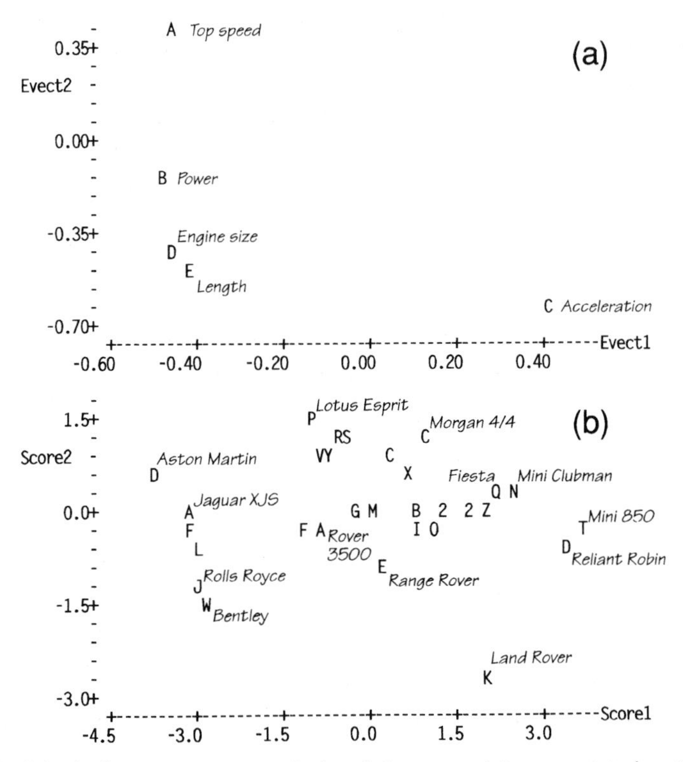

Figure 10. Principal components analysis of the cars data: annotated output from *Minitab*. (a) plot of eigenvectors for components 1 and 2, (b) plot of scores for components 1 and 2. Letter labels to identify each individual car are given in *Appendix 5.1*.

along the first component ranging from small family saloons to large, powerful limousines, whereas the second component separates sports cars and GTs of all sizes from standard models. Extreme in this respect is the Land Rover with its relatively slow acceleration.

In summary, PCA is an ordination technique for projecting a multidimensional cloud of points on to a space of fewer dimensions, using rigid rotation to derive successive orthogonal axes, which maximize the variation accounted for (1).

2.3 But what *are* the components?—a washing line analogy

Formally, the principal components (PCs) are mathematical constructs calculated as linear combinations of the original variates. The first component contains the maximum possible variance, the second contains the maximum possible of the remaining variance, with the constraint that it is orthogonal to (meaning uncorrelated with) the first, and so on. Each eigenvalue shows the variance of its corresponding eigenvector (*Table 4*). This gives the non-mathematician little 'feel' for eigenvectors or their scores, but a simple example may help to clarify.

Consider a washing machine containing several items of clothing of various lengths, widths, and weights (*Appendix 5.2*). The washing process, during which the items become thoroughly mixed is, for our purposes, analogous to calculating correlations, eigenvalues, eigenvectors, and scores for the clothes. After washing, each item is brought from the tub showing a score which indicates the position it should occupy relative to all the others along the washing line. Peg the clothes in their respective positions on the line and examine the pattern they make (*Figure 11*) along this one-dimensional ordination axis. There is a strong relationship between size and position, with small socks and a handkerchief at one end of the washing line, ranging to a bath towel and sheets at the other. This interpretation is reinforced by plotting a numerical value of size, the area, calculated as the product of length and width for each item, against its axis position (*Figure 11b*).

The clothes can also be pegged on a separate, shorter, washing line using a second set of scores (*Figure 12a*). In this case there is an apparent relationship with 'density' of the clothes as measured by the ratio of weight to area, thick or heavy materials like towelling contrasting with light nylon and thin cotton (*Figure 12b*). Similarly, a third, shorter washing line, independent of the other two, arranges the clothes by their shape, long narrow items like stockings being contrasted with the square table cloth, shorts, and handkerchief (*Figure 13*).

Each of the three washing lines, which are the first three PCs of the correlation matrix for the three variables, can be interpreted as a different facet of the items analysed, here labelled as size, density, and shape. The

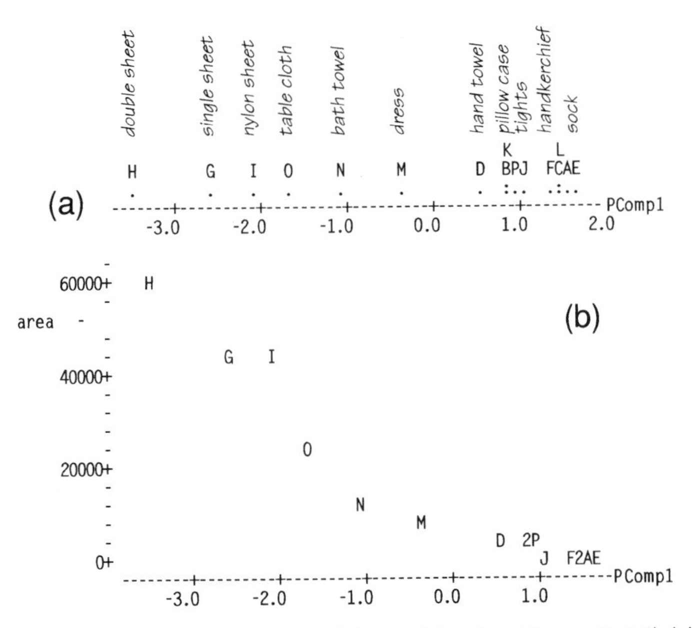

Figure 11. Principal components analysis of the washing data (*Appendix 5.2*). (a) Labelled *Minitab* DOTPLOT of scores representing 'washing line' 1 (component 1); (b) *Minitab* plot of component 1 against 'area' of items calculated as length × width. Letter labels as in *Appendix 5.2*.

increasing scatter of the explanatory plots (*Figures 11b, 12b,* and *13b*) of the scores from PC1 to PC3 represents well the decreasing variability explained by these components.

2.4 PCA of ecological data

2.4.1 Environmental data

The same type of analysis is illustrated by data for 11 environmental factors measured at 204 sites located in salt marsh and mud flats fringing the Wash, Lincolnshire, UK. The correlation matrix and eigenanalysis are shown in *Appendix 5.3, Table 5*, and *Figure 14*. Inspection of the eigenvalues for the analysis with eleven variables reveals that the last is essentially zero within rounding errors, indicating that at least one of the variables is redundant. As the last three variables are sediment fraction percentages, together adding to 100, one of them is superfluous. Data of this kind exhibit collinearity, a property which is particularly important in relation to multiple regression (see Chapter 4; Section 5). In this example, the soil data possess a strong pattern in which sediment particle size varies consistently with position up and down the intertidal zone, and this pattern was apparent whether or not % clay, one of the collinear group of variables, was included. The component values

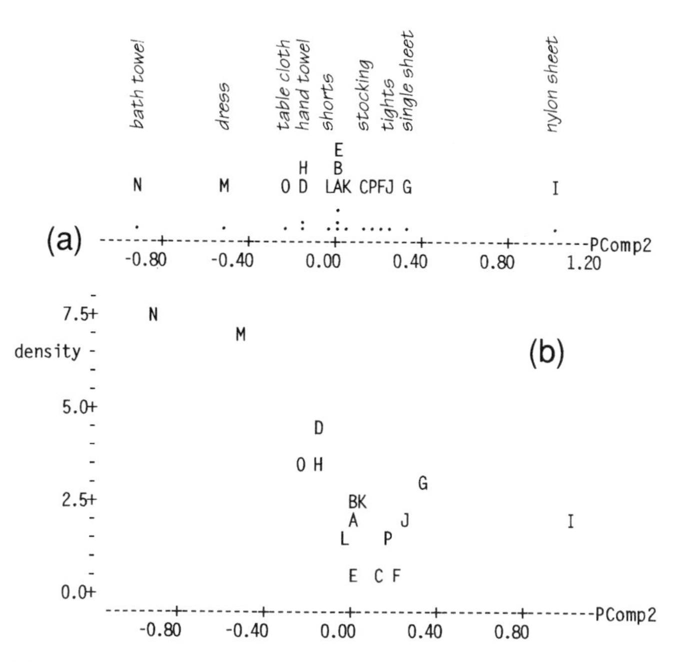

Figure 12. (a) 'Washing line' 2 (component 2); (b) plot of component 2 against 'density' of items calculated as weight/width (details as *Figure 11*).

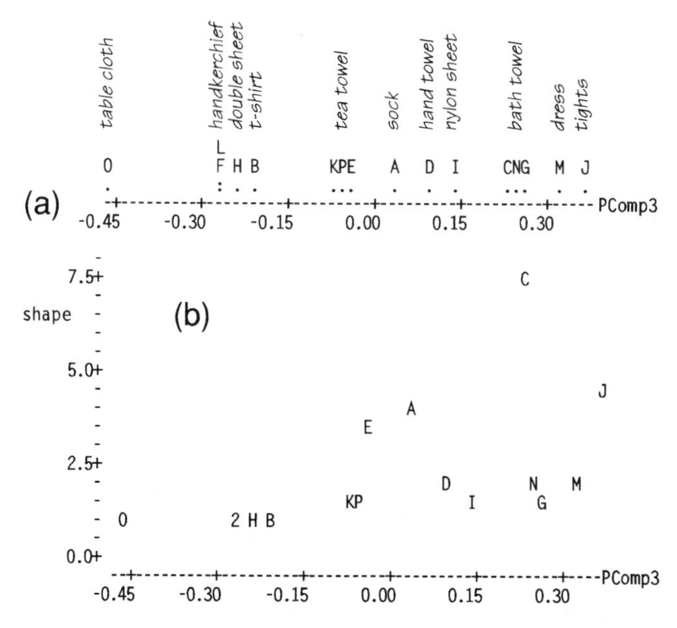

Figure 13. (a) 'Washing line' 3 (component 3); (b) plot of component 3 against 'shape' of items calculated as length/width (details as *Figure 11*).

Table 5. Eigenanalysis results of the correlation matrix for (a) 11 environmental factors and (b) 10 (excluding % clay), of the Wash mud flat samples (*Appendix 5.3*). Eigenvectors for components 1 and 2 only are shown. Lettered rows refer to *Figure 14*

	(a) 11 variables			(b) 10 variables		
Component	**Eigenvalue**	**Variation explained (%)**	**Cumulative variation explained (%)**	**Eigenvalue**	**Variation explained (%)**	**Cumulative variation explained (%)**
1	7.26759	66.0690	66.069	6.47457	64.7457	64.746
2	1.48184	13.4713	79.540	1.43306	14.3306	79.076
3	0.92325	8.3932	87.934	0.89360	8.9360	88.012
4	0.43738	3.9762	91.910	0.42039	4.2039	92.216
5	0.34492	3.1357	95.045	0.34140	3.4140	95.630
6	0.25600	2.3273	97.373	0.20852	2.0852	97.715
7	0.10771	0.9792	98.352	0.10766	1.0766	98.792
8	0.08897	0.8088	99.161	0.07001	0.7001	99.492
9	0.06867	0.6243	99.785	0.03045	0.3045	99.797
10	0.02337	0.2125	99.997	0.02035	0.2035	100.000
11	0.00028	0.0025	100.000			

		Attribute loading for eigenvector			**Attribute loading for eigenvector**	
Letter code	**Row**	**1**	**2**	**Row**	**1**	**2**
A	1	−0.344789	0.177730	1	−0.369668	0.147105
B	2	−0.324957	−0.025229	2	−0.344920	−0.051408
C	3	−0.351731	0.036760	3	−0.373924	0.006396
D	4	0.038664	−0.681587	4	0.055462	−0.666455
E	5	−0.322134	0.235748	5	−0.344058	0.222735
F	6	−0.223666	−0.299423	6	−0.237438	−0.356436
G	7	−0.319795	0.301694	7	−0.346860	0.267291
H	8	−0.335523	−0.181799	8	−0.359821	−0.009203
I	9	−0.342540	0.003775	9	−0.210612	−0.515043
J	10	−0.202485	−0.465836	10	0.364125	0.134383
K	11	0.351197	0.124677			

differed only slightly between the analyses with and without % clay included (*Table 5*).

2.4.2 Species data

Species-in-sites data may be analysed in a similar way, although with species data the covariance matrix is often preferred (see Section 2.6). Quadrat data for vegetation of an upland heath and grassland in mid-Wales (*Appendix 5.4*) were analysed with PCA using covariance. *Figure 15a* shows that a majority of the less adundant species cluster around the origin, whereas those with high values of cover and distinctive distributions occur towards the poles of

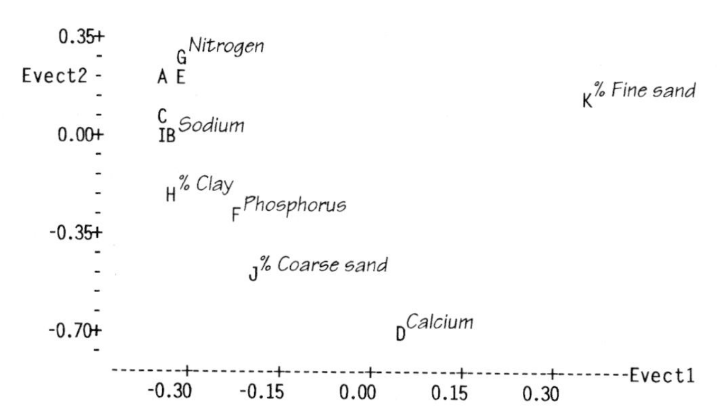

Figure 14. Principal components analysis of the Wash mudflat samples (*Appendix 5.3*). Annotated *Minitab* plot of eigenvectors 1 and 2 derived from correlation coefficients. Letters A–K indicate 11 soil factors.

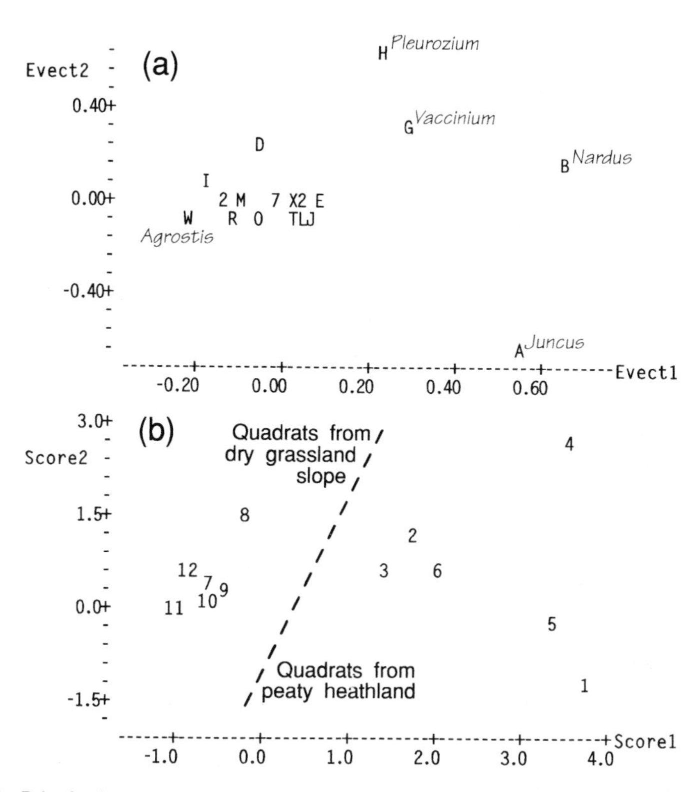

Figure 15. Principal components analysis of the Chwefru upland species data (*Appendix 5.4*). Annotated *Minitab* plots of components 1 and 2 derived from between-species covariances: (a) for 26 species (eigenvectors), (b) for 12 quadrats (scores).

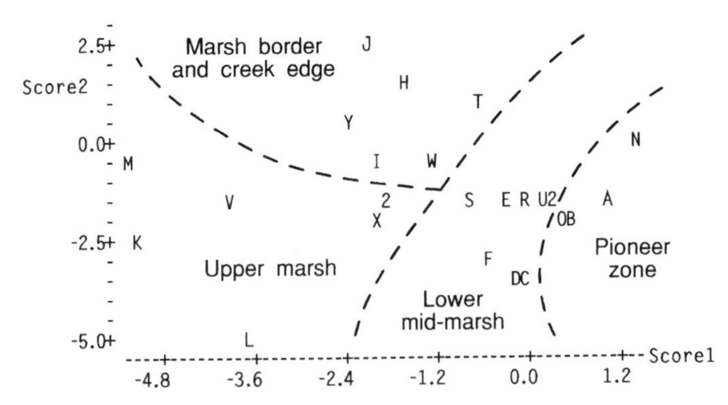

Figure 16. Principal components analysis of the Norfolk saltmarsh data (*Appendix 5.5*). Annotated *Minitab* plot of quadrat scores for components 1 and 2 derived from between-species covariances.

the two axes. Consequently, along the first PC the quadrats fall into two groups which conform to ecologially distinct habitats (*Figure 15b*). Species composition of the upland heath group varies more than in the dry grassland group, with particular dominant species affecting the position of different quadrats on component 2.

PCA of species abundance data from two transects across a Norfolk salt marsh (*Figure 16*) shows a more even distribution along the first two PCs. A landward–seaward environmental gradient on the salt marsh is reflected in the alignment of quadrats on the first component as a result of the gradual change in species along this ecocline. The second PC distinguishes creek edge quadrats, dominated by a dwarf shrub species, from the rest of the upper marsh area.

2.5 Heterogeneity of data—accounting for the variation

In the examples of PCA given in Sections 2.2, 2.3, and 2.4, relatively large proportions of the total variance of the data were extracted in the first two eigenvalues, indicating a strong trend or discontinuity in the data (*Tables 4* and 5, *Figure 17*). In some cases, however, particularly with large data sets, the first pair of PCs may account for as little as 5% of the total variance and yet be quite informative. In other cases, where the data are extremely disjunct, 90% of the variance may be accounted for, yet the result may be impossible to interpret (1). The success of PCA, as with other ordination techniques, depends on its utility for interpretation: mere percentage variation accounted for is not a reliable indicator of quality of results.

2.6 Data transformation—to standardize or not to standardize?

Minitab offers the choice of whether or not to standardize the data column by column by opting for one of two similarity coefficients. Had the correlation

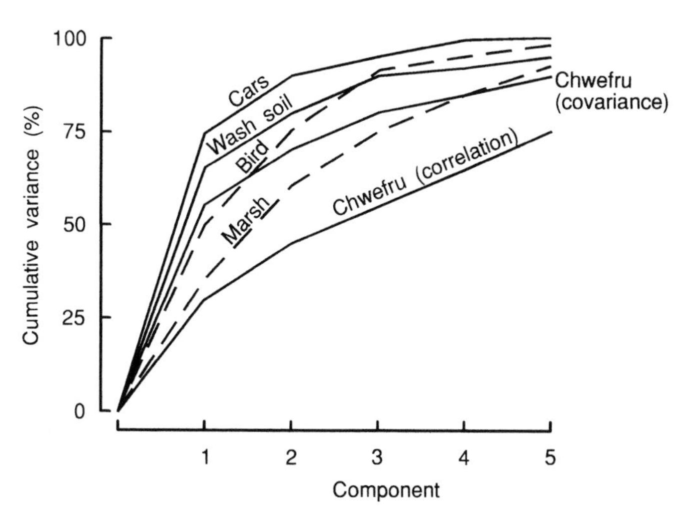

Figure 17. Cumulative proportions of total variance accounted for by successive components in analyses referred to in Section 2.

coefficient been used in the above example of species/quadrat data, the effect would have been to uprate the importance of the less abundant, infrequent species relative to that of the dominants. Whereas some ecologists would argue that rare species provide useful information as ecologial indicators and as such may help in the analysis to define plant 'communities', it is often assumed that abundance of a species at a site, being a measure of its performance under given conditions, is a better ecological indicator to differentiate sites. The covariance between species compares them without rescaling their relative abundances—in effect, the more abundant species will have the greatest influence on the analysis, whereas the rare and infrequent species will have little effect (3, 4).

Comparing the two analyses for the upland heath data (*Figures 15a, b* and *18a, b*) shows, in both cases, a contrast on the first component between two areas which comprise distinct ecological sub-habitats. The species are more evenly spread on the ordination plot when their relative abundances are evened out by the correlation coefficient, and the first few eigenvalues also account for smaller proportions of the variation (*Figure 17*).

Whereas the choice of a standardizing or non-standardizing coefficient is largely a matter of preference for species data where all variates are measured on a common scale (percentage cover values or counts of numbers), in the previous examples of cars and soil factors the choice is critical to interpretation. In these cases, each variate is measured with its own distinct units on a scale which may differ numerically from others. In our example, car engine capacities range from 850 to 5000 cm^3 whereas acceleration times vary between 6 and 30 sec. Similarly, % sand values are potentially between 0 and

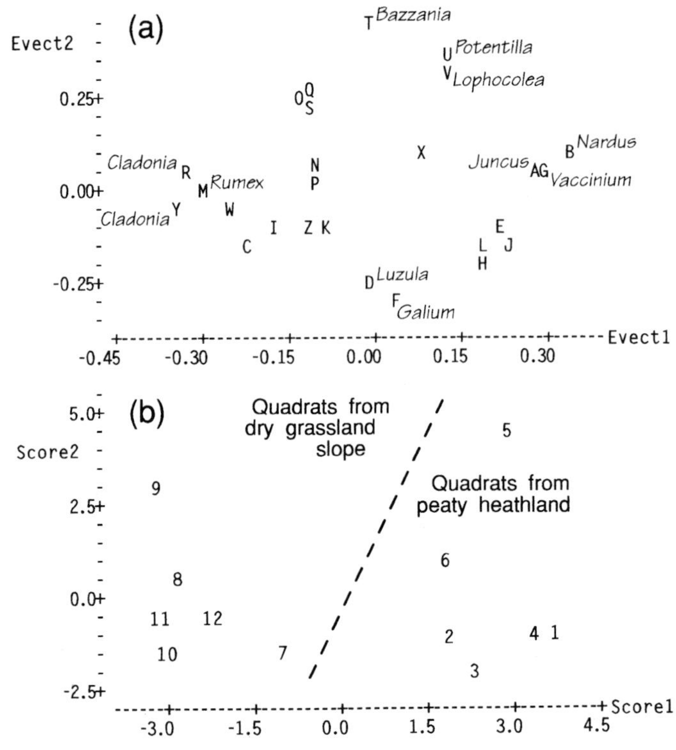

Figure 18. Principal components analysis of the Chwefru upland species data (*Appendix 5.4*). Annotated *Minitab* plot of components 1 and 2 derived from between-species correlations: (a) for species and (b) for quadrats.

100, whereas the pH range is from about 7 to 8. It is therefore necessary to standardize the scaling of all the variates, which is precisely the transformation provided by the correlation coefficient.

To illustrate the importance of this effect, the results of analysing the soils data with a covariance matrix are shown in *Figure 19*. The analysis is dominated by a single variable, calcium, which in the raw data is numerically largest. With such a distorted pattern interpretation is meaningless.

2.7 Two sides of the coin—the *Q/R* duality

PCA can be carried out in either of two modes by calculating either the *R*-similarity coefficient SS_R between attributes, or the *Q*-similarity coefficient SS_Q between individuals. This means that an identical solution is obtained whether you project the *m*-dimensional A-space or the *n*-dimensional I-space on to their respective *p*-dimensional component sub-spaces. In the *R*-mode it is the eigenvectors which position the attributes and the scores of the individuals on the new components. Reciprocally, in the *Q*-mode it is the other

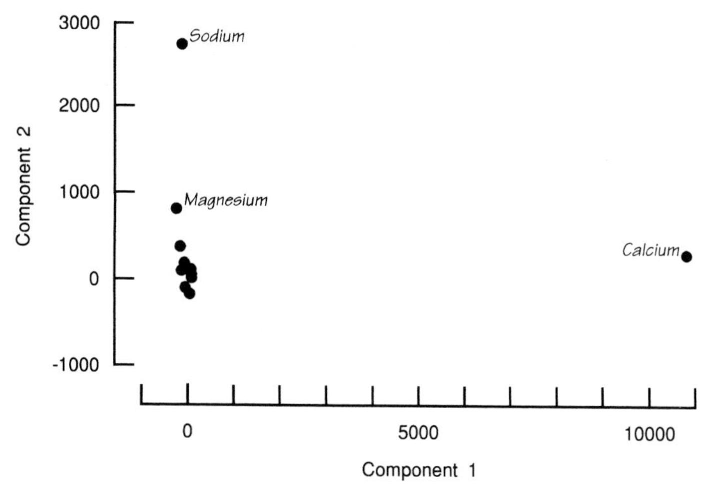

Figure 19. Principal components analysis of the Wash mudflat samples (*Appendix 5.3*). Annotated plot of eigenvectors 1 and 2 derived from covariances.

way round (*Figure 20*). The two analyses are dual to each other, but only if the same data transformation is performed prior to calculating the SS matrix.

For example, in *R*-mode, between-variates correlation coefficients would standardize the data with respect to attributes which are the row means and standard deviations of the data matrix (*Table 2*). In *Q*-mode, between-individual similarity coefficients would still have to transform by row mean and standard deviation to preserve the duality. Such a similarity coefficient would *not* be the between-individuals correlation coefficient. This creates a practical problem with respect to performing PCA on computer packages, such as *Minitab*, which provide standard coefficients (see Section 2.8). The

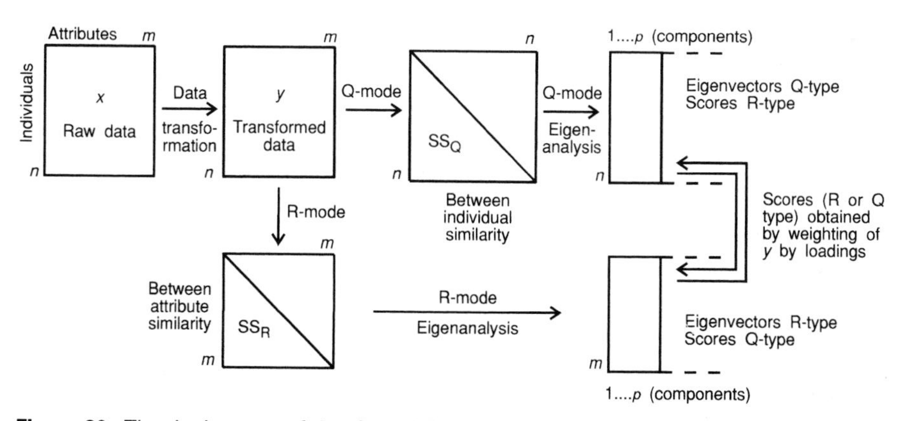

Figure 20. The dual nature of the *Q*- and *R*-mode principal components solutions.

property of duality provides a symmetric and consistent link between the two faces of a Euclidean model (A-space and I-space) and allows PCA to provide a reference structure compatible with both spaces, so that both sets of points can be superimposed and interpreted jointly (1).

Two alternative conventions exist for scaling component axes. Eigenvectors and component scores can either be scaled so that the sum of the squares of the values of the vector is equal to its eigenvalue, or in the normalized form, equal to 1. Results are often presented so that both loadings and scores are set to the relevant eigenvalue, but the duality property between the *Q*- and *R*-analyses is unaffected.

2.8 *Q*- or *R*-mode—a practical problem

In each example given above we have performed *R*-mode PCAs. We created a computer data file suitable for *Minitab*, as for most other packages, in which the variates were columns and individuals were the rows. The *Minitab* PCA command then computed the between-column correlations or covariances. Many data sets, however, have a larger number of variates than individuals, especially in ecology, where many species may be recorded in relatively few quadrats (see upland heath data, section 2.4). In such a case, if we had entered the quadrats as columns and the species as rows, we would compute the smaller *Q*-matrix of quadrat-by-quadrat similarities which would transform with respect to quadrats rather than species. Such a *Q*-mode analysis would not be dual to the normal *R*-mode (*Table 2*) and we must question whether our transformation is appropriate for our particular data set (*Table 6*). This difficulty has been discussed in the ecological literature (5, 6). Alternative coefficients have been devised for *Q*-mode analysis such as the 'weighted similarity coefficient' (WSC, *Table 2*) but these are not readily available on standard packages such as *Minitab*.

Possible solutions include:

- transpose rows and columns in the *Minitab* worksheet so that you can perform the appropriate *R*-analysis (see *Protocol 2*)
- use an alternative computer package such as *CANOCO* (see Section 3.2) which allows explicit transformations either by species or by quadrats
- accept the assumptions implicit in transforming your data by quadrat not species (see *Table 6*)

Protocol 2. Organizing data and selecting an appropriate PCA method[a]

1. If the data are measured characteristics of organisms or samples or environmental factors, proceed with step 2; if species-in-samples or species-in-quadrats community data are to be analysed, go to step 3.
2. Prepare a data file or read data directly into *Minitab* with samples as rows and attributes as columns (see *Protocol 1*, step 1). Proceed with PCA on

Minitab as in *Protocol 1*, step 2, using correlation coefficient—do not include the COVAR sub-command.

3. If a computer file is already prepared, are the species in columns and quadrats in rows? If so, proceed with step 4. If you need to swap rows/columns, go to step 8.

4. Prepare a data file, or read directly into *Minitab*, with quadrats as rows and species as columns (see *Protocol 1*, step 1).

5. Refer to *Table 6* to decide whether you prefer a quantity-oriented approach and proceed with step 6, or a phytosociological approach in which case go to step 7.

6. Proceed with PCA in *Minitab* as in *Protocol 1*, step 2, including the COVAR sub-command to use the covariance between species.

7. Proceed with PCA in *Minitab* as in *Protocol 1*, step 2, using correlation coefficient—do not include the COVAR sub-command.

8. Transpose rows and columns of the worksheet. *Minitab* on the microcomputer allows a maximum of 99 columns: more are permited on mainframe implementations.

```
LET K1 = 20              #(e.g. for 20 quadrats in columns)
COPY C1-CK1 to M1        #(copy data into a matrix)
TRANSPOSE M1 to M2       #(transpose rows/columns)
LET K2=30                #(e.g. for 30 species)
COPY M2 to C1-CK2        #(copy back to columns)
ERASE M1 M2
```

Proceed with step 5 above.

[a] If you have species data with corresponding environmental factors, canonical ordination using *CANOCO* (*Appendix 4*) would be appropriate in addition to PCA (see Section 3.2). *CANOCO* also offers reciprocal averaging and de-trended correspondence analysis.

It is possible to obtain only as many components as the smaller of the numbers of rows and columns of the data matrix. Hence if the number of columns m exceeds the number of rows n in the *Minitab* worksheet, then only n PCs can be calculated, the remaining p-n being zero. In practice, usually only the first three or four components are of interest for interpretation. For example, analysis of the upland heath data, with 12 quadrats, produced 11 non-zero eigenvalues, the remaining 15 being zero.

2.9 Limitations of PCA for species community analyses

Whereas PCA has the advantage of being relatively objective and is free of subjective weights or axis end points, it suffers from two assumptions which limit its applicability in the field of species community analysis and which arise from a mismatch between the community model of species in their

Table 6. Choice of data transformation—ecological implications for species-in-sites community data (3)

Centring	**Standardization**
• subtract mean of row or column $(x_{ij} - x_{i.})$ or $(x_{ij} - x_{.j})$ • changes the origin from zero to the average	• divide by standard deviation of row or column $(x_{ij}/s_{i.})$ or $(x_{ij}/s_{.j})$ • rescales each row or column • necessary when variates are measured in different units, such as environmental factors • not necessary for biotic measures such as biomas, % cover, or density
By species • moves reference point to an 'average site' which has average species composition. Sites are compared to this average. Species are compared to a uniform distribution across sites and to mutual independence • differences between sites rather than absolute composition is important, as is variance of species	*By species* • places all species at same level of importance regardless of relative abundance—uprates the rarer ones • consistent with phytosociological approach defining faithful/characteristic species (9), but analysis is sensitive to deviant, atypical sites
By site (quadrat) • moves reference point to 'average species' which has constant proportion $1/m$ of all species in site • species distribution profile is compared to this. Sites are important if composition departs from equal proportion of all species • not a useful assumption	*By site (quadrat)* • only necessary if sites are of different sizes—equalizes importance of rich, diverse sites and poor, uniform sites
	Non-standardized • weighting in favour of abundant species and rich stands—quantity oriented approach • highlights floristic diversity • avoids dominance by rare members • suitable approach in production ecology

environment and the underlying model of PCA (1). PCA assumes that species abundances change linearly along environmental gradients. Typically, however, species show changes in abundance which have a Gaussian or normal-shaped distribution with respect to environmental factors. This non-linearity often results in a valid first PCA axis but a second which does not convey meaningful or independent information, being a quadratic distortion of the first. This appears as an arched configuration on the plot of axis 1 versus axis 2. This problem is particularly acute when the data sample spans a wide ecological range, in which the extreme individuals may have little or nothing in common as regards presence of species. Although successive axes must be orthogonal, meaning uncorrelated with each other, this does not preclude an arch-shaped relationship, since the positive correlations on one side of the arch are balanced by the negative correlations on the other, so that overall no correlation exists between the axes. The arch or Guttman effect persists to many dimensions, the third axis being a cubic distortion of the first, the fourth a quartic, and so on. As a consequence of this, potentially interesting ecological gradients may not be represented in the first few PC axes and hence may be 'lost' to view. This is illustrated by analysis of densities of breeding birds along a successional gradient (*Figure 21* and *Appendix 5.6*).

PCA also assumes that data values of the variates are normally distributed. Whereas this may be approximately true for some environmental measures, species data are inherently non-normal, having a minimum limit of zero abundance and being constrained, in the case of percentage data, to a maximum of 100. With data of sample counts of invertebrates or estimates of bacterial numbers it is common to transform to logs before analysis to improve the approximation to normality, whereas percentage data may be subjected to arcsine transformation (see Chapter 1, Section 4.1.3). This non-linearity, together with the often non-random collection of data in the field, limits the validity of PCA axes for hypothesis testing (7). Hence species ordination has become a technique mainly for data description and hypothesis generation, making use of independently collected data of subjectively chosen environmental parameters (see Section 3.1).

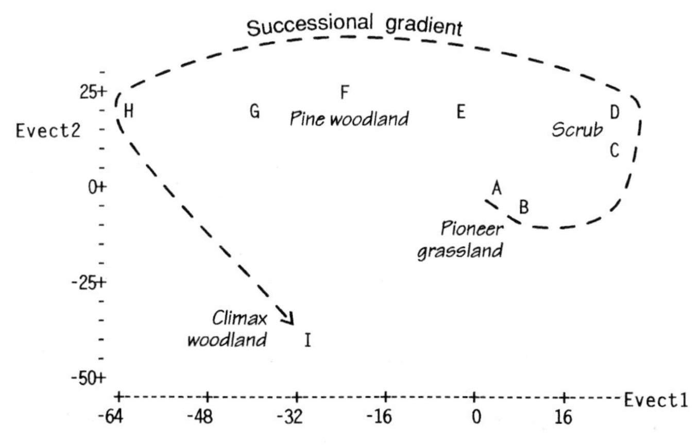

Figure 21. Principal components analysis of the birds data (*Appendix 5.6*). Annotated *Minitab* plot of eigenvectors 1 and 2 derived from between-species covariances.

2.10 Reciprocal averaging

Reciprocal averaging (RA), also called correspondence analysis (8), is an ordination technique based on eigenanalysis, but the solution is achieved directly from the data values rather than from a derived similarity coefficient. The species ordination scores calculated on RA axes are averages of the stand ordinations scores and, reciprocally, the stand scores are averages of the species scores; hence the name reciprocal averaging. Computationally, RA is very efficient, especially for large data sets, using an iterative technique to converge from an initial arbitrary position towards a stable RA axis, deriving both samples and species axes simultaneously. Subsequent axes are then derived in the same way, allowing for previously extracted axes. The set of RA axes so extracted have, as with PCA, decreasing eigenvalues representing their decreasing importance. RA achieves a compromise between the species- and site-oriented emphasis (*Table 6*). Hence, unlike PCA, the RA scores reflect particularly well the changes in community composition along a coenocline or community gradient with Gaussian species responses and moderate species turnover or β-diversity (9). For most community data sets, RA has been shown to be superior to PCA, with both simulated and field data (8, 10).

2.11 Detrended correspondence analysis

RA axes still show the arch problem, although in a less severe form than with PCA, where the ends of the arch may be re-curved or involuted (*Figure 21*). A further fault of RA is that the first-axis ends are compressed relative to the axis middle, so that a given distance of separation in the ordination does not match a consistent difference between samples, or species. As a consequence of the compromise between species- and site-emphasis mentioned above, RA may also suffer from the presence of species which are both rare and occur in samples with low total abundance, as with standardized PCA (see Section 2.6), because such species are treated as being extremely distinctive. This problem can be cured by eliminating rare species from a data set before analysis.

Detrended correspondence analysis (DCA) (11, 12), based on RA, was devised to overcome the problems mentioned above, which are common to most ordination techniques, including polar ordination, PCA, PCO, RA, non-metric multidimensional scaling, factor analysis, and canonical correlation analysis. Detrending, which is applied at each iteration of the calculation of RA scores, amounts to removing all spurious correlation between successive pairs of axes, eliminating arch effects. Axes are also rescaled to avoid end-compression, so that the degree of species turnover at the outer ends is equivalent to that at the centre. *Figure 22* compares analyses of species abundance data from a moth trap with a strongly seasonal pattern using PCA, RA, and DCA. The clear circular patterns with RA and DCA reflect the strongly seasonal changes in species abundance. This was not apparent with PCA, due to excessive grouping near the origin.

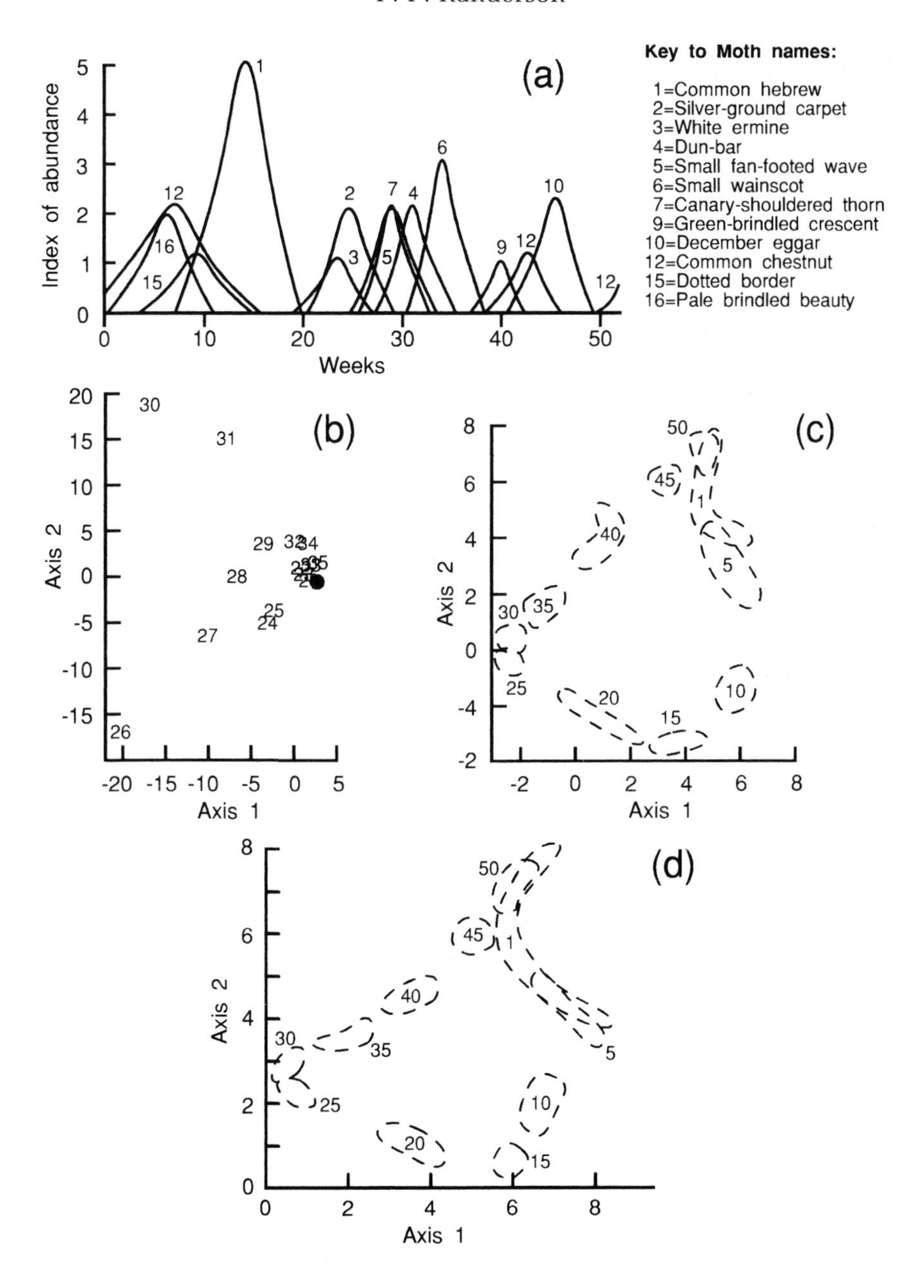

Figure 22. Analyses of moth trap catches in mid-Wales, UK. These data recorded 259 species in nightly catches over a six year period; they were analysed as weekly totals. The plots show (a) temporal changes in abundance of selected species over one year and the first two axes for (b) principal component analysis, (c) reciprocal averaging and (d) detrended correspondence analysis. In (b)–(d) the week numbers or envelopes bounding the six annual points are shown.

Both RA and DCA are provided in the Fortran package *DECORANA* (8), designed for use on the mainframe computer but now superseded by the microcomputer package *CANOCO* (see Section 3.2 below).

2.12 Relating the ordination trends to classification

As an aid to interpreting the results of ordination, it is often helpful to superimpose the groups obtained by classifying species-in-sites data (Chapter 6) on ordination axis plots. Primary classification divisions usually relate to separation of individuals on the first or second PC, whereas lower order divisions are apparent on third or fourth axes (*Figure 23*).

3. Relating species distributions with environmental factors

3.1 Explaining the trends in ordination axes

Since an aim of ordination is to attempt to explain trends in data in terms of possible causal factors, it is usual to superimpose environmental measurements upon the species-defined ordination plots and to look for trends or

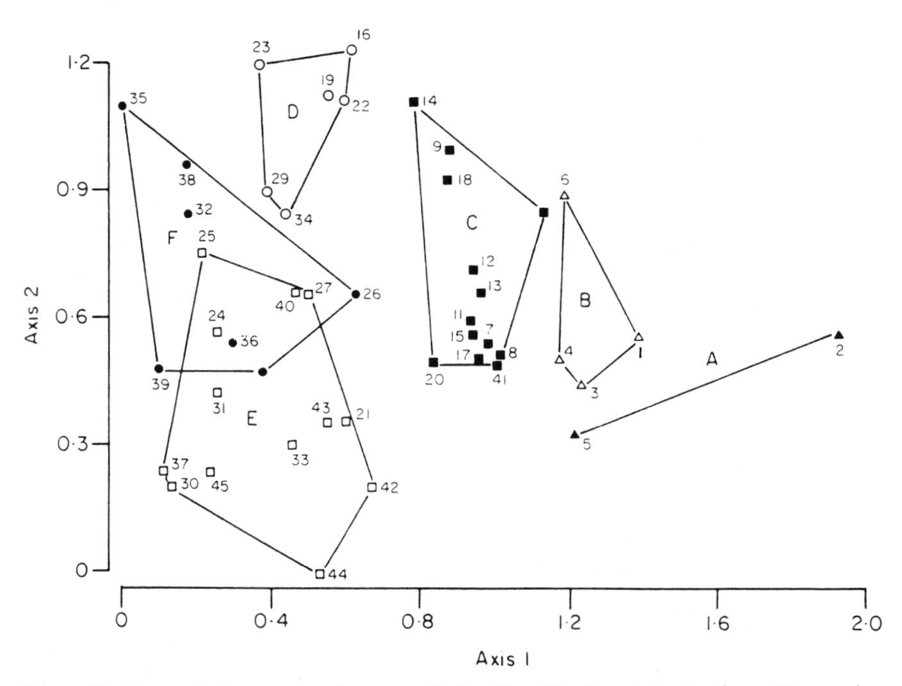

Figure 23. Detrended correspondence analysis of benthic invertebrates from 45 samples in the River Wye catchment, Wales, UK. (13); plot of the first two axes, indicating sample groups obtained by cluster analysis (see Chapter 6); primary division separates groups A, B for C–F.

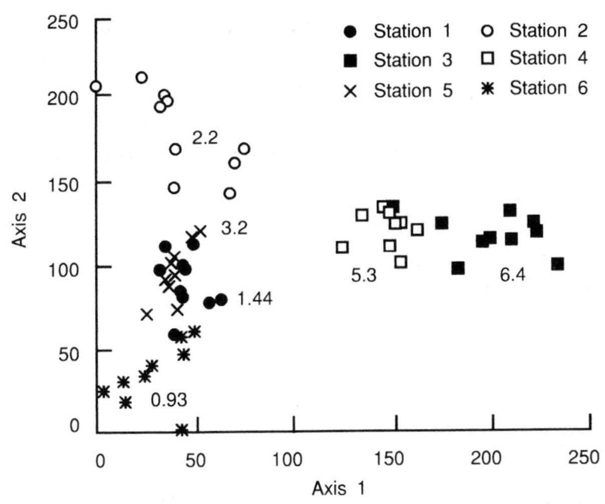

Figure 24. Detrended correspondence analysis of Algerian phytoplankton data (14) in which abundances of 227 species were determined seasonally in water samples at six river stations. Plot of 57 samples on the first two axes; mean values of salinity are superimposed.

delimit contours (*Figure 24*). In this case axis 1 reflects the different species composition at the more saline stations 3 and 4, whereas water velocity differentiates station 2 from 6, separated on axis 2. Axis 3 (not shown) differentiated station 1 from 5. Seasonal variation in species abundance is not apparent relative to these between-station differences.

Relating PC values with particular environmental factors is largely a subjective process, although correlation (see Chapter 3) and linear regression (see Chapters 3 and 4) may be instructive (*Table 7* and *Figure 11b*). Its success is limited by the environmental data available, which in turn depends on selecting appropriate factors to measure.

In the same way, we may also superimpose species occurrence data or species-defined groups on plots arising from PCA of environmental data (*Figure 25* and *Appendix 5.7*).

3.2 Canonical methods—constrained ordination and partial ordination (15–17)

Instead of regressing final values for species-defined axes on environmental factors, such regressions can be performed at each stage of the iterations in correspondence analysis which derive the axes. Hence these so-called canonical axes become constrained to be linear combinations of particular environmental factors. This amounts to inserting a regression model into the species ordination so that the ordination now has an in-built environmental basis.

Table 7. Correlations between site scores on *DECORANA* axes 1 and 2 and environmental variables (17)[a]

Variable	Axis 1	Axis 2
Slope (log)	NS	(−)***
Altitude (log)	(+)***	(−)***
Stream link magnitude (log)	NS	(+)***
Discharge category	NS	(+)***
Substratum category	NS	NS
Mean depth (log)	NS	(+)***
Distance from source (log)	NS	(+)***
Mean conductivity (log)	(−)***	NS
Mean total hardness (log)	(−)***	NS
Mean pH	(−)***	NS
Minimum pH	(−)***	NS
Mean nitrate (log)	(−)***	NS
Mean orthophosphate (square root)	NS	NS

[a] NS not significant
** $P < 0.01$
*** $P < 0.001$
(+) or (−) indicates the sign of the correlation coefficient, if significant

An alternative approach is to use regression to eliminate the effect of particular environmental variables on species community data by treating them as covariables. After several such environmental effects have been 'partialled out' by regression, the remaining variation in the community data is subjected to partial ordination to identify any remaining trends.

Both of these techniques, as well as traditional PCA, RA, and DCA, are available in the microcomputer package *CANOCO*—Canonical Community Ordination (18). *CANOCO* also provides an improved algorithm for RA, an improved method of detrending in DCA, and a 'Monte Carlo' or probability test for significance of the relationship between species-ordination trends and environmental factors. Like the *DECORANA* package, it allows data input in the more convenient Cornell compressed data entry format (*Appendix 5.8*). Provided with the package is *CANOPLOT* which allows the axis values for species and sites arising from each selected analysis to be plotted with a choice of scaling. Alternatively, axis values could be read into *Minitab* and plotted as in *Protocol 1*, steps 4 and 5.

3.3 Relating species groups to environmental factors—an objective method

Multiple discriminant analysis (MDA) relates species-defined classification groups with environmental measurements at a common set of sites. A series

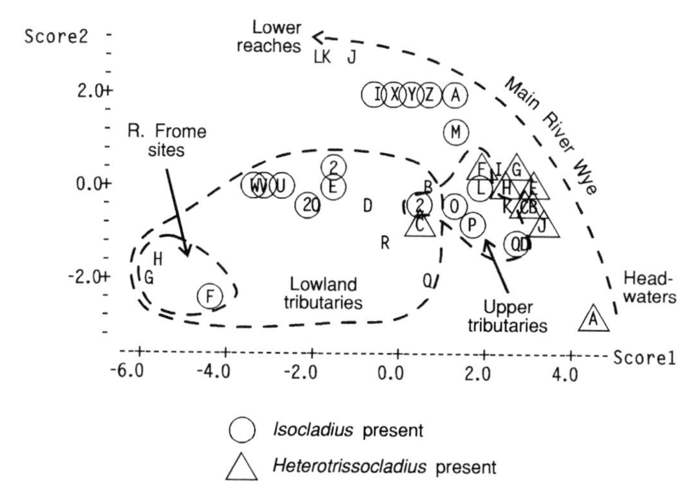

Figure 25. Principal components analysis of the River Wye physico-chemical factors (*Appendix 5.7*). Annotated *Minitab* plot of the distribution of 43 sampling sites on the first two components. Superimposed at each site is the presence of two species of midge with contrasting ecological preferences.

of discriminant functions (DF) are calculated which amount to ordination axes on which each variable can be positioned. As in PCA, the first DF has the largest eigenvalue and accounts for the largest proportion of the total variance. Positions for 'average members' or centroids of each classification group on the DFs are calculated. MDA then attempts to predict the membership of each site to its classification group from the environmentally determined DFs. How successful this is indicates the closeness of the relationship between the species composition and environmental character of a site. MDA can be performed on both *Minitab* and *SPSS/PC+* using their respective DISCRIMINANT commands.

3.4 A note on factor analysis

Another technique superficially similar to PCA, which has been extensively used especially in the field of psychology, is factor analysis (FA). Like PCA, it involves eigenanalysis of the correlation or covariance matrix but it differs mathematically from PCA in several respects. In PCA, *all* the variance is attributed to components, even though only the first few may be displayed, whereas in FA only some of the variance is attributed to the factors—which are then *not* linear combinations of the original variates. As a result there is no unique solution in FA. By 'rotating' the factors there is a multiplicity of possible solutions and selecting one which suits the user is highly subjective. It is intended that this will aid interpretation of the individual factors in terms of explanatory variables. For example, a set of examination marks for students would be replaced by factors of intelligence or mathematical or artistic ability. Whereas PCA explains the variances, FA explains the variances and covariances together.

With PCA the unique solution obtained has the benefit of explaining the maximum variance, although individual species-derived PCs may not neatly align with particular environmental variables. This objective of interpretation is perhaps better achieved using the canonical constrained ordination approaches referred to in Section 3.2.

References

1. Gauch, H. G. (1982). *Multivariate analysis in community ecology*. Cambridge University Press, Cambridge.
2. Gabriel, K. R. (1981). In *Interpreting multivariate data* (ed. V. Barnett), pp. 147–73. John Wiley, Chichester.
3. Noy-Meir, I. (1973). *J. Ecol.* **61,** 329–41.
4. Noy-Meir, I., Walker, D., and Williams, W. T. (1975). *J. Ecol.* **63,** 779–800.
5. Orloci, L. (1967). *Syst. Zool.* **16,** 208–12.
6. Ivimey-Cook, R. B., Proctor, M. F. C., and Wigston, D. L. (1969). *J. Ecol.* **57,** 673–5.
7. Strong, D. R. (1980). *Synthese* **43,** 271–85.
8. Hill, M. O. (1974). *J. Roy. Stat. Soc. Ser. C* **23,** 340–54.
9. Persson, S. (1981). *Vegetatio* **43,** 103–22.
10. Noy-Meir, I., Walker, D., and Williams, W. T. (1975). *J. Ecol.* **63,** 779–800.
11. Hill, M. O. (1979). *DECORANA: a FORTRAN program for detrended correspondence analysis and reciprocal averaging*. Cornell University, Ithaca, NY.
12. Hill, M. O. and Gauch, H. G. (1980). *Vegetatio* **42,** 47–58.
13. Ormerod, S. J. and Edwards, R. W. (1987). *Freshwat. Biol.* **17,** 533–46.
14. Al-Asadi, M. S. (1991). *The effect of ecological factors on algae in six Algerian river sites*. Ph.D. Thesis, University of Wales, UK.
15. Gittins, R. (1985). *Canonical analysis. A review with applications in ecology*. Springer, Berlin.
16. Ter Braak, C. J. F. (1986). *Vegetatio* **69,** 69–77.
17. Ter Braak, C. J. F. (1987). In *Data analysis in community and landscape ecology* (ed. R. H. G. Jongman, C. F. J. Ter Braak, and O. F. R. Van Tongeren). Pudoc, Wageningen.
18. Ter Braak, C. J. F. (1988). *CANOCO: a FORTRAN program for canonical community ordination by [partial] [detrended] [canonical] correspondence analysis, principal components analysis and redundancy analysis (version 2.1)*. Technical Report: LWA-88-02, Jan. 88. Agricultural Mathematics Group, Wageningen.
19. Odum, E. P. (1971). *Fundamentals of ecology*, 3rd edn. Saunders, Phildadelphia.
20. Learner, M. A. (1983). *The distribution of chironomidae (Diptera) in the River Wye system based on collections of pupal exuviae*. Internal Report, UWIST, Cardiff, UK.

Appendix 5.1. Contents of the file CARS.DAT[a]

A	238	213	7.8	5343	487	Jaguar XJS
B	153	54	15.6	1748	399	Leyland Maxi
C	172	64	10.5	1599	366	Morgan 4/4
D	258	261	5.7	5340	465	Aston Martin V8
E	155	97	15.8	3528	447	Range Rover
F	235	213	8.1	5343	495	Jaguar XJ5.3
G	188	101	13.3	2994	443	Reliant Scimitar GTE
H	145	44	16.2	1256	394	Vauxhall Chevette
I	158	61	15.6	1798	445	Leyland Princess
J	190	209	9.0	6750	516	Rolls Royce Camargue
K	116	63	30.0	2625	465	Land Rover 109
L	209	198	7.5	5343	518	Panther de Ville
M	167	81	11.5	2293	463	Ford Granada 2.3L
N	129	34	17.6	1098	340	Mini Clubman Estate
O	153	54	15.5	1593	433	Ford Cortina 1.6L
P	222	119	6.0	1973	419	Lotus Esprit
Q	135	34	16.1	957	361	Ford Fiesta Ghia
R	201	113	6.8	3523	371	Morgan Plus 8
S	210	79	7.5	2994	391	TVR (sports)
T	113	25	25.2	848	305	Leyland Mini 850
U	156	51	15.6	1294	424	Chrysler Alpine GL
V	213	119	7.8	1973	446	Lotus Eclat
W	185	194	10.2	6750	517	Bentley Corniche
X	174	40	11.0	1600	420	Vauxhall Nova GT
Y	201	119	7.9	1973	446	Lotus Elite
Z	134	40	16.5	1275	385	Austin Allegro 1300
A	184	116	10.3	3500	470	Rover 3500
B	163	56	14.3	1584	445	Vauxhall Cavalier 1.6GL
C	177	78	9.9	1998	406	Triumph TR7
D	117	30	24.4	848	333	Reliant Robin
E	143	43	15.9	1297	398	Ford Escort 1.3L
F	188	120	11.0	3442	495	Daimler Sovereign 3.4

[a] The file is organized as 32 rows relating to different models of motor car; data extracted from Automobile Association statistics. Rows are lettered A ... Z, A ... F for reference to *Figure 10b*. The five numerical columns give data for top speed (km/h), power output (kW), acceleration time for 0–100 km/h (sec), engine size (cm^3), and length (cm) for each model, followed by text indicating the make and model name. The first text field (A ... Z, A ... F) is not in the file and the second text field is ignored by *Minitab* when the READ command is used in free format (*Protocol 1*)

Appendix 5.2. Contents of the file WASHING.DAT[a]

A	40	10	20	sock
B	60	50	115	t-shirt
C	60	8	3	stocking
D	90	45	210	hand towel
E	30	9	5	sock
F	40	40	15	handkerchief
G	260	176	550	single sheet
H	260	224	780	double sheet
I	250	180	325	nylon
J	94	23	40	tights
K	70	45	120	pillow case
L	30	30	50	shorts
M	133	60	410	dress
N	150	80	600	bath towel
O	160	160	540	table cloth
P	70	45	75	tea towel

[a]The file is organized as 16 rows relating to differrent items of clothing. Rows are lettered A ... P for reference to Figures 11, 12, and 13. The three numerical columns give data for length (cm), width (cm), and weight (g), for each item followed by text describing the item. The first text field (A ... P) is not in the file and the second text field is ignored by *Minitab* when the READ command is used in free format

Appendix 5.3. Contents of the file WASHSOIL.COR[a]

1.000	0.771	0.856	−0.241	0.824	0.490	0.951	0.760	0.857	0.401	−0.829
0.771	1.000	0.901	0.018	0.835	0.478	0.664	0.764	0.741	0.410	−0.778
0.856	0.901	1.000	−0.128	0.855	0.543	0.805	0.823	0.824	0.489	−0.854
−0.241	0.018	−0.128	1.000	−0.218	0.012	−0.405	0.115	−0.039	0.162	−0.054
0.824	0.835	0.855	−0.218	1.000	0.331	0.782	0.734	0.785	0.219	−0.771
0.490	0.478	0.543	0.012	0.331	1.000	0.447	0.520	0.450	0.613	−0.526
0.951	0.664	0.805	−0.405	0.782	0.447	1.000	0.644	0.785	0.339	−0.730
0.760	0.764	0.823	0.115	0.734	0.520	0.644	1.000	0.872	0.534	−0.974
0.857	0.741	0.824	−0.039	0.785	0.450	0.785	0.872	1.000	0.425	−0.957
0.401	0.410	0.489	0.162	0.219	0.613	0.339	0.534	0.425	1.000	−0.544
−0.829	−0.778	−0.854	−0.054	−0.771	−0.526	−0.730	−0.974	−0.957	−0.544	1.000

[a] The file comprises the full matrix of correlation coefficients between 11 factors in soil samples at 204 locations in the mud flats and salt marshes fringing the Wash, UK. The file is organized as 11 columns and 11 rows, each cell containing a correlation between each of the 11 variables, as follows: % loss on ignition, sodium, potassium, calcium, magnesium, phosphorus, nitrogen, % clay, % silt, % coarse sand, and % fine sand. Raw data are not given. PCA of a correlation matrix may be performed in *Minitab* using the commands:

```
READ 'A:WASHSOIL.COR' C1–C11    # (read correls. into cols.)
COPY C1–C11 M1                  # (create a matrix structure)
EIGEN M1 C13 M2                 # (eigenanalysis –
                                # (eigenvalues into C13;
                                # (eigenvectors into M2)
COPY M2 C21–C31                 # (copy M2 to columns
                                # (for plotting)
```

Appendix 5.4. Contents of the file CHWEFRU.DAT[a]

```
4.0  2.0  0.5  0.0  0.5  1.0  0.5  1.0  0.5  0.5  0.5  0.5  0.0  0.0  0.0  0.0  0.0  0.0  0.0  0.0
0.0  0.0  0.0  0.0  0.0  0.0
0.5  2.0  1.0  1.0  0.0  1.0  0.5  1.0  0.5  0.5  0.0  0.0  0.0  0.0  0.0  0.0  0.0  0.0  0.0  0.0
0.0  0.0  0.0  0.0  0.0  0.0
1.0  1.0  0.5  0.5  0.0  2.0  0.5  1.0  0.5  0.5  0.5  0.5  0.0  0.0  0.0  0.0  0.0  0.0  0.0  0.0
0.0  0.0  0.0  0.0  0.0  0.0
1.0  3.0  0.5  0.5  0.5  1.0  2.0  3.0  0.5  0.0  1.0  0.0  0.0  0.0  0.0  0.0  0.0  0.0  0.0  0.0
0.0  0.0  0.0  0.0  0.0  0.0
2.0  3.0  0.5  0.0  0.0  0.5  1.0  0.5  0.0  0.0  0.5  0.0  0.0  0.0  0.5  0.0  0.0  0.0  0.0  0.5
0.5  0.5  0.0  0.0  0.0  0.0
1.0  2.0  0.5  0.0  0.0  0.5  1.0  1.0  0.5  0.5  0.5  0.0  0.0  0.0  1.0  0.0  0.0  0.0  0.0  0.0
0.0  0.0  0.5  0.5  0.0  0.0
0.0  0.0  1.0  1.0  0.0  1.0  0.0  2.0  1.0  0.0  0.5  0.0  0.5  0.0  0.0  0.0  0.0  0.0  0.0  0.0
0.0  0.0  0.5  0.0  0.5  0.0
0.0  0.0  0.5  0.0  0.0  0.5  0.0  0.5  1.0  0.0  0.5  0.0  0.5  0.5  0.5  0.5  0.0  0.5  0.0  0.0
0.0  0.0  0.5  0.0  0.5  0.0
0.0  0.0  1.0  0.0  0.0  0.5  0.0  0.5  1.0  0.0  0.5  0.0  0.5  0.0  0.5  0.0  0.5  0.5  0.5  0.5
0.0  0.0  0.5  0.0  0.5  0.0
0.0  0.0  2.0  0.0  0.0  2.0  0.0  0.5  0.0  0.0  1.0  0.0  0.5  0.0  0.5  0.0  0.0  0.5  0.0  0.0
0.0  0.0  0.5  0.0  0.5  0.5
0.0  0.0  1.0  0.5  0.0  1.0  0.0  0.0  1.0  0.0  1.0  0.0  0.5  0.0  0.5  0.0  0.0  0.5  0.0  0.0
0.0  0.0  2.0  0.0  0.5  0.0
0.0  0.0  1.0  1.0  0.0  0.5  0.0  0.5  2.0  0.0  0.5  0.0  0.0  0.0  0.5  0.0  0.0  0.5  0.0  0.0
0.0  0.0  1.0  0.0  0.5  0.0
```

[a] The file is organized as 24 rows comprising species abundance values in 12 quadrats, two rows per quadrat, collected from 2 areas of the Chwefru upland, mid-Wales, UK. In each pair of rows are values of plant cover estimated in 50 × 50 cm quadrats on an arbitrary scale (0.5, 1, 2, 3, 4, 5) for 26 species, as follows: *Juncus squarrosus*; *Nardus stricta*; *Festuca ovina*; *Luzula campestris*; *Carex* sp.; *Galium saxatile*; *Vaccinium myrtilus*; *Pleurozium schreberi*; *Dicranum scoparium*; *Rhytidiadelphus squarrosus*; *Polytrichum juniperinum*; *Mnium undulatum*; *Rumex acetosella*; *Poa annua*; *Hypnum cupressiforme*; *Bryum* sp.; *Cladonia floerkiana*; *Cladonia pyxidata*; *Ulex* sp.; *Bazzania* sp.; *Potentilla erecta*; *Lophocolea bidentata*; *Agrostis tenuis*; *Calluna vulgaris*; *Cladonia impexa*; *Pseudoscleropodium purum*.

The first six quadrats (rows 1–12) were placed randomly on a heathland plateau area with waterlogged, peaty soil, and the remaining six quadrats (rows 13–24) on a steeply sloping hillside with dry, acidic mineral soil.

This data set can be entered into *Minitab* with a formatted READ command from drive A: as follows:

```
READ 'A:CHWEFRU' C1–C26;
FORMAT (20F4.0/6F4.0).
```

Appendix 5.5. Contents of the file MARSH.DAT[a]

.5	0.	0.	0.	2.	0.	0.	1.	0.	0.	3.	1.	0.
.5	0.	0.	0.	2.	0.	0.	2.	0.	0.	.5	2.	0.
2.	0.	.5	0.	4.	0.	0.	1.	0.	.5	.5	2.	0.
2.	0.	1.	0.	4.	0.	0.	1.	0.	.5	.5	1.	0.
2.	2.	0.	0.	3.	0.	0.	0.	0.	.5	.5	1.	0.
3.	1.	1.	0.	4.	0.	0.	0.	0.	.5	.5	.5	.5
2.	0.	.5	2.	2.	0.	1.	1.	0.	1.	.5	.5	0.
1.	3.	0.	2.	1.	1.	.5	1.	0.	.5	0.	0.	0.
1.	1.	1.	2.	2.	1.	1.	1.	.5	1.	0.	.5	0.
1.	5.	.5	2.	.5	0.	.5	.5	0.	1.	0.	0.	0.
3.	0.	1.	2.	2.	0.	.5	1.	1.	5.	1.	.5	0.
3.	0.	.5	0.	4.	0.	1.	.5	0.	4.	0.	1.	3.
2.	.5	.5	4.	1.	1.	.5	1.	0.	4.	.5	.5	0.
0.	0.	0.	0.	.5	0.	0.	0.	0.	0.	5.	0.	0.
1.	0.	0.	0.	2.	0.	0.	1.	0.	0.	.5	2.	0.
1.	0.	.5	0.	2.	0.	0.	.5	0.	0.	.5	1.	0.
1.	1.	0.	0.	2.	0.	.5	.5	0.	0.	.5	2.	0.
2.	.5	.5	0.	2.	0.	0.	.5	0.	0.	.5	.5	0.
1.	1.	1.	0.	2.	0.	.5	.5	0.	1.	.5	.5	.5
1.	3.	.5	.5	.5	0.	.5	.5	0.	.5	1.	0.	0.
1.	0.	0.	0.	2.	0.	0.	1.	0.	0.	.5	0.	0.
1.	0.	.5	1.	1.	0.	1.	.5	0.	4.	0.	0.	.5
1.	.5	1.	.5	1.	0.	.5	1.	0.	1.	0.	0.	0.
1.	0.	1.	.5	2.	0.	.5	.5	.5	2.	0.	.5	1.
1.	.5	.5	3.	5	0.	.5	.5	0.	1.	0.	0.	0.
2.	0.	1.	0.	1.	0.	.5	.5	.5	2.	.5	.5	0.

[a] The file is organized as 26 rows comprising species abundance values in 26 quadrats collected from a salt marsh community at Blakeney Point, Norfolk, UK. Each row gives values of plant cover estimated on an arbitrary scale (0.5, 1, 2, 3, 4, 5) for 13 species, as follows: *Aster tripolium*; *Halimione portulacoides*; *Limonium vulgare*; *Puccinellia maritima*; *Salicornia herbacea*; *Salicornia perennis*; *Spartina anglica*; *Suaeda maritima*; *Triglochin maritima*; *Bostrychia scorpioides*; *Enteromorpha* sp.; *Fucus volubilis*; *Pelvetia canaliculata*.

The quadrats were spaced at 20 m intervals in two seaward–landward transects (rows 1–13 and 14–26 respectively)

Appendix 5.6. Contents of the file BIRD.DAT[a]

10.	5.	0.	0.	0.	0.	0.	0.	0.	0.	0.	0.	0.	0.	0.	0.	0.	0.	0.	0.
0.	0.	0.	0.	0.	0.	0.	0.	0.	0.										
30.	10.	0.	0.	0.	0.	0.	0.	0.	0.	0.	0.	0.	0.	0.	0.	0.	0.	0.	0.
0.	0.	0.	0.	0.	0.	0.	0.	0.	0.										
25.	0.	35.	15.	5.	5.	5.	0.	0.	0.	0.	0.	0.	0.	0.	0.	0.	0.	0.	0.
0.	15.	0.	0.	0.	0.	0.	0.	0.	0.										
0.	2.	48.	18.	16.	4.	8.	8.	6.	8.	0.	0.	0.	0.	0.	0.	0.	0.	0.	0.
0.	0.	0.	0.	0.	0.	0.	0.	0.	0.										
0.	0.	25.	0.	0.	9.	13.	6.	6.	0.	16.	6.	0.	0.	0.	0.	0.	0.	0.	0.
0.	0.	0.	0.	0.	0.	0.	0.	0.	0.										
0.	0.	8.	0.	0.	10.	10.	4.	0.	4.	34.	13.	4.	2.	2.	0.	0.	0.	0.	0.
0.	0.	0.	0.	0.	0.	0.	0.	0.	0.										
0.	0.	3.	0.	0.	14.	15.	0.	0.	5.	43.	13.	5.	5.	13.	2.	10.	9.	6.	3.
3.	3.	1.	1.	1.	1.	0.	0.	0.	0.										
0.	0.	0.	0.	0.	20.	15.	0.	0.	0.	55.	15.	20.	5.	0.	5.	1.	10.	10.	5.
30.	10.	3.	2.	10.	5.	1.	0.	0.	0.										
0.	0.	0.	0.	0.	23.	0.	0.	0.	0.	0.	10.	10.	5.	13.	0.	3.	10.	15.	7.
11.	43.	5.	5.	6.	23.	9.	8.	5.	5.										

[a] The file is organized as 18 rows giving the distribution of passerine birds at nine stations, two rows per station, along a successional gradient in the Piedmont region, Georgia, USA (19). In each pair of rows are densities of 30 species of breeding birds, as follows: Grasshopper sparrow; Meadowlark; Field sparrow; Yellowthroat; Yellow-breasted chat; Cardinal; Towhee; Bachman's sparrow; Prairie warbler; White-eyed vireo; Pine warbler; Summer tanager; Carolina wren; Carolina Chickadee; Blue-gray gnatcatcher; Brown-headed nuthatch; Wood pewee; Hummingbird; Tufted titmouse; Yellow-throated vireo; Hooded warbler; Red-eyed vireo; Hairy woodpecker; Downy woodpecker; Crested flycatcher; Wood thrush; Yellow-billed cuckoo; Black and white warbler; Kentucky warbler; Acadian flycatcher.

The nine stations were located as follows: A, 1–2 year, forb stage; B, 2–3 year grass; C, 15 year grass-shrub; D, 20 year grass shrub; E, 25 year young pine forest; F, 35 year pine forest; G, 60 year pine forest; H, 100 year old pine forest; I, 150–200 year Oak–Hickory climax forest.

This data set can be entered into *Minitab* with a formatted READ command from drive A: as follows:

```
READ 'A:BIRD' C1–C30;
FORMAT (20F4.0/10F4.0).
```

Appendix 5.7. Contents of the file WYENV.DAT[a]

320.	36.	3.	0.30	6.2	45.	0.20	1.5	2.	0.06	16.93
272.	64.	3.	0.32	6.4	53.	0.42	2.2	3.	0.10	4.06
244.	86.	3.	0.33	6.6	61.	0.50	3.4	5.	0.07	3.72
270.	31.	2.	0.31	7.3	75.	0.46	6.1	19.	.1352	8.02
223.	121.	1.	0.34	6.7	67.	0.58	3.9	5.	0.09	3.96
210.	141.	3.	0.60	6.3	50.	0.43	5.2	6.	0.16	3.14
180.	271.	2.	0.34	6.7	64.	0.57	6.2	9.	0.05	4.48
208.	130.	2.	0.36	7.1	74.	0.68	5.2	10.	0.07	3.91
150.	288.	3.	0.37	6.4	59.	0.49	3.6	4.	0.11	2.56
254.	25.	4.	0.31	6.3	44.	0.22	2.9	8.	0.05	5.86
198.	45.	4.	0.32	6.8	57.	0.37	6.1	8.	0.04	4.48
174.	138.	3.	0.33	7.3	88.	0.56	5.5	18.	0.13	3.21
126.	658.	3.	0.39	7.1	101.	0.81	14.5	20.	0.13	2.27
160.	196.	3.	0.34	7.8	183.	1.35	25.9	45.	0.16	3.54
219.	112.	4.	0.33	7.5	163.	1.20	11.9	40.	0.05	2.07
262.	44.	3.	0.32	7.5	160.	0.53	30.7	40.	0.01	4.69
318.	22.	3.	0.31	7.4	134.	0.45	10.7	31.	0.01	7.09
194.	21.	3.	0.37	7.8	296.	2.87	39.4	103.	0.11	5.86
132.	52.	4.	0.55	7.9	300.	3.04	64.1	103.	0.13	2.12
97.	96.	3.	0.67	8.0	328.	3.25	50.5	118.	0.08	4.23
68.	219.	3.	0.64	7.9	401.	4.00	34.3	144.	0.17	0.90
55.	251.	4.	0.63	8.0	432.	4.19	23.3	158.	0.24	0.65
48.	267.	4.	0.62	8.0	457.	4.37	22.7	178.	0.23	0.65
63.	940.	4.	0.45	7.5	166.	1.23	11.5	48.	0.08	0.50
76.	873.	3.	0.43	7.4	150.	1.15	21.2	40.	0.06	0.59
88.	846.	3.	0.42	7.3	132.	0.98	22.8	32.	0.06	1.20
91.	753.	1.	0.41	7.3	109.	0.82	22.0	24.	0.05	1.20
138.	37.	3.	0.37	7.6	196.	1.37	12.3	59.	0.10	2.50
170.	31.	3.	0.40	7.8	203.	2.55	22.9	63.	0.06	6.10
132.	48.	3.	0.58	7.8	269.	3.08	16.5	92.	0.16	4.84
83.	61.	4.	0.60	7.9	315.	3.62	10.5	113.	0.11	2.72
107.	32.	3.	0.43	7.9	604.	5.85	33.5	224.	0.80	2.24
72.	45.	5.	0.56	8.1	647.	5.95	67.0	239.	0.51	1.97
50.	74.	5.	0.52	8.1	658.	5.98	63.3	242.	0.43	1.65
46.	969.	3.	0.47	7.6	192.	1.58	23.2	52.	0.12	0.40
46.	1336.	2.	0.52	7.7	226.	2.31	32.5	72.	0.14	0.40
32.	1354.	4.	0.55	7.8	256.	2.39	30.9	80.	0.12	0.46
15.	1442.	4.	0.57	7.9	266.	2.47	31.2	85.	0.11	0.46
46.	335.	3.	0.53	8.0	390.	1.96	14.4	167.	0.11	1.61
63.	291.	3.	0.54	8.0	391.	2.00	10.9	168.	0.12	2.44
76.	44.	3.	0.45	7.9	466.	3.14	16.1	210.	0.11	2.22
124.	76.	1.	0.43	7.8	335.	1.15	10.5	147.	0.09	6.10
229.	41.	3.	0.55	8.0	278.	1.13	8.6	121.	0.09	12.19

[a] The file is organized as 43 rows comprising 11 physico-chemical variables at stations on the main river and tributaries of the River Wye, Wales, UK (20). In each row, the 11 columns are:

A Altitude (m O.D.)
B Stream link magnitude
C Stream bed code (1 bedrock, 2 boulders, 3 cobbles, 4 pebbles, 5 gravel)
D Base flow index (low values = 'flashy' flows, high values = steady, even flows)
E pH
F Conductivity (μS/cm)
G Total nitrogen (mg/l)
H Suspended solids (mg/l)
I Alkalinity (mg $CaCO_3$/l)
J Orthophosphate (mg P/l)
K Slope (m/km)

Appendix 5.8. Contents of the file CHWEFRU.CAN[a]

```
ABI04'83 50*50CM QUADRAT. Chwefru UPLAND HEATH : STEEP GRASS SLOPE. 26spp;12qu's
(I2,9(I3,F4.0))
          09
01 01 4.0 02 2.0 03 0.5 05 0.5 06 1.0 07 0.5 08 1.0 09 0.5 10 0.5
01 11 0.5 12 0.5
02 01 0.5 02 2.0 03 1.0 04 1.0 06 1.0 07 0.5 08 1.0 09 0.5 10 0.5
03 01 1.0 02 1.0 03 0.5 04 0.5 06 2.0 07 0.5 08 1.0 09 0.5 10 0.5
03 11 0.5 12 0.5
04 01 1.0 02 3.0 03 0.5 04 0.5 05 0.5 06 1.0 07 2.0 08 3.0 09 0.5
04 11 1.0
05 01 2.0 02 3.0 03 0.5 06 0.5 07 1.0 08 0.5 11 0.5 15 0.5 20 0.5
05 21 0.5 22 0.5
06 01 1.0 02 2.0 03 0.5 06 0.5 07 1.0 08 1.0 09 0.5 10 0.5 11 0.5
06 15 1.0 23 0.5 24 0.5
07 03 1.0 04 1.0 06 1.0 08 2.0 09 1.0 11 0.5 13 0.5 23 0.5 25 0.5
08 03 0.5 06 0.5 08 0.5 09 1.0 11 0.5 13 0.5 14 0.5 15 0.5 16 0.5
08 18 0.5 23 0.5 25 0.5
08 03 1.0 06 0.5 08 0.5 09 1.0 11 0.5 13 0.5 15 0.5 17 0.5 18 0.5
09 19 0.5 20 0.5 23 0.5 25 0.5
10 03 2.0 06 2.0 08 0.5 11 1.0 13 0.5 15 0.5 18 0.5 23 0.5 25 0.5
```

```
10  26  0.5
11  03  1.0  04  0.5  06  1.0  09  1.0  11  1.0  13  0.5  15  0.5  18  0.5  23  2.0
11  25  0.5
12  03  1.0  04  1.0  06  0.5  08  0.5  09  2.0  11  0.5  15  0.5  18  0.5  23  1.0
12  25  0.5
00
JUNCSQUANARDSTRIFESTOVINLAZUSPECCARESPECGALISAXAVACCSPECPLEUSPECDICRSPECRHYTSPEC
POLIJUNIMNIUUNDURUMEACITPOA   ANNUHIPNSPECBRIUSPECCLADFLOECLADPYXIULEXSPECBIZZSPEC
POTESPECLOFABIDEAGROTENUCALLSPECCLADIMPEPSEUSPEC
TOP1      TOP2      TOP3      TOP4      TOP5      TOP6      SLO1      SLO2      SLO3      SLO4
SLO5      SLO6
```

[a] The file, comprising the same species data as *Appendix 5.3*, is organized as 31 rows according to the format for input to *CANOCO* (*Appendix A*), as follows:

- row 1: title describing the data (≤80 characters)
- row 2: Fortran-type fixed field format for reading data from row 4 onwards. This format provides for a single two-character integer (quadrat number) followed by up to nine data 'couplets' each comprising a species number and its cover value
- row 3: maximum number of data couplets (here nine) to be read per row
- rows 4–25: values for species cover in 12 quadrats. Following the quadrat number, the quantity of each species present is given after the species number as a couplet. Up to nine couplets are specified per row, with continuation rows if more species are present in a quadrat
- row 26: value zero for quadrat number indicates end of species data
- rows 27–29: abbreviated names for species 1–26 (10 per row), coded as four characters for the genus followed by four characters for the species in each case, for example JUNCSQUA: *Juncus squarrosus* (see *Appendix 5.3* for list of species)
- rows 30–31: Alpha-numeric labels for quadrats 1–12 (10 per row); eight characters for each quadrat.

6

Classification

P. D. BRIDGE

1. Introduction

The use of statistical and numerical methods to derive and investigate classifications is well established within systematics, and such methods are generally referred to by the collective term 'numerical taxonomy'. Numerical taxonomy has in turn been defined by Sneath and Sokal (1) as 'the grouping by numerical methods of taxonomic units into taxa on the basis of their character states'. The history and philosophy of numerical taxonomy has already been well documented by a number of authors (e.g. 1–4), and although numerical taxonomy did not become widely used until the relatively recent introduction of computers, the basic principles involved can be traced back to the nineteenth century and earlier (1).

In practice, numerical taxonomy generally involves calculating resemblances between different individuals, often referred to as operational taxonomic units (OTUs). Resemblances are calculated as either similarities or differences within sets of characters or properties of the OTUs and these OTUs are then ordered and grouped into ranks or classes on the basis of the resemblance measures. A number of methods, which are collectively termed cluster analysis, may be used to place similar OTUs together into groups or clusters, and these groups are in turn represented graphically, most often as dendrograms or clustered similarity matrices. Additional analysis can then be undertaken on the dendrogram to assess the distinctness and validity of clusters, and constant characters for later use in diagnostic schemes can be determined.

The above procedure usually involves a clustering method which is essentially hierarchic, as opposed to other multivariate methods such as principle component analysis and other ordinations (see Chapter 5) which yield non-hierarchic arrangements. Although biological classifications are usually considered to be hierarchic, ordination techniques have been used in numerical taxonomic studies, particularly in cases where it has been suspected that individuals represented a continuous spectrum of variation, rather than a number of distinct groups. Ordination techniques, such as principal component and principle coordinate analysis have been extensively used in ecological and other studies, and the application of these methods in systematics has been reviewed elsewhere (e.g. 1, 5–7).

Numerical taxonomy and cluster analysis have been used widely in biological systematics during the last 30 years. The types of characters used have varied considerably between different studies, and have included simple morphological features (e.g. 8), physiological and biochemical properties (e.g. 9), and molecular data such as isoenzyme patterns and DNA and protein sequences (e.g. 10, 11).

Protocol 1. Steps in deriving a classification from resemblances and cluster analysis

1. Collect data on individuals, i.e. laboratory tests, observations, or literature.
2. Code data into a form suitable for producing an n (individuals or OTUs) by t (attributes or characters) table.[a] This step is most commonly undertaken when entering data into a computer package, although some packages allow for limited transformation of data.
3. Select resemblance coefficient to calculate a similarity or difference matrix. The choice of coefficient can be particularly important and care must be taken to ensure that the coefficient selected is relevant for the characters used, i.e. qualitative, quantitative, etc.
4. Calculate resemblance values between all possible pairs of individuals. For assigning storage space during computations it is important to remember that there are $n\,(n + 1)/2$ values for all possible pair comparisons if each individual is compared with itself, and $n(n - 1)/2$ values if individuals are not compared with themselves.
5. Select cluster analysis method, most commonly single or average linkage (see Section 3).
6. Compute clustered similarity or difference values.
7. Represent clustered individuals graphically, most commonly as dendrograms and clustered matrices.
8. Assess clustering (a) empirically and (b) from cophenetic values (see Section 4).
9. Consider individual clusters by listing constant and variable characters and by significance tests for clusters (see Section 4.3).

[a] In numerical taxonomy literature, n has commonly been used for characters and t for OTUs, this is reversed here for consistency between chapters.

The above protocol lists the steps involved in arriving at a numerical classification from original data. Not all of the steps involved rely on computation, and in fact the most important parts of the procedure, data collection and selection of coefficient and clustering method, should only be made after careful consideration. In this chapter I will first describe some of the more common coefficients and clustering methods that have been used in classification studies and then attempt to give some details on data coding, testing classifications, and some examples of applications. The methods described here are fully detailed in three textbooks that provide comprehensive reviews of the subject, *Numerical taxonomy* by Sneath and Sokal (1), *Taxonomic analysis in biology* by Abbott *et al.* (7) and *An introduction to mathematical taxonomy* by Dunn and Everitt (12), and these texts should be consulted if further details are required. The data used for examples in this chapter are taken from a multidisciplinary study of the filamentous fungus genus *Penicillium* (13) and includes morphological, physiological, and biochemical data.

2. Measures of resemblance

To calculate resemblances between individuals it is first necessary to generate a data matrix—a table listing the different character states or attribute values for the individuals under study. In theory, any set of taxonomic attributes may be used, although care must be taken if characters are related or not exclusive (see Section 5.2). An example of a possible table for the penicillia is given in *Table 1*. These tables are often referred to as $n \times t$ tables or matrices, where n is the number of individuals and t is the number of characters.

Formulae for calculating a coefficient of resemblance between individuals can for practical purposes be divided into two groups: those for quantitative data, which give a measure of distance between individuals, and those for qualitative data, which give an estimate of similarity based on the character states (association coefficients). However, it should be noted that the groups are not strictly exclusive and some similarity coefficients can be directly related to distance measures, as will be seen in Section 2.2.

Table 1. $n \times t$ table of 10 characters for 5 different penicillia

	Characters[a]									
Organism	**1**	**2**	**3**	**4**	**5**	**6**	**7**	**8**	**9**	**10**
A *Penicillium expansum*	−	−	+	−	−	−	−	−	+	−
B *P. echinulatum*	−	−	+	−	−	+	+	−	−	−
C *P. roquefortii*	+	+	−	−	+	+	−	−	−	−
D *P. hordei*	−	−	−	+	−	−	−	−	+	−
E *P. brevicompactum*	+	−	−	−	+	−	−	+	−	+

[a] Characters: 1 = growth on nitrite, 2 = growth on acetic acid, 3 = production of basic metabolites from creatin, 4 = yellow mycelium, 5 = velvet colonies on agar, 6 = dark-green conidia, 7 = echinulate conidia, 8 = production of brevianamide, 9 = production of cyclopenol, 10 = colony on agar < 25 mm

2.1 Distance coefficients

To explain the concept of distance coefficients it is necessary first to consider the individuals to be compared as represented in a form of hyperspace called A-space (attribute space, 14). A-space has t dimensions, one for each attribute or character, and individuals may be plotted in this space according to their relative properties (*Figure 1*). Individuals can be arranged along a single axis (dimension) when a single character such as spore size is considered (*Figure 1a*). When a second character, colony size, is added then this becomes a two-dimensional plot, similar to a conventional graph (*Figure 1b*). When a third dimension is added, production of penicillin, a box graph is produced (*Figure 1c*). This principle can be continued in theory until there are t-dimensions, where t is the total number of attributes or characters, although it cannot be easily represented. Distance coefficients are those that result in a measure of the distances between individuals in A-space.

2.1.1 Euclidean distances

The most widely used measure of distance in numerical taxonomy is probably the Euclidean or taxonomic distance (1, 7). In the geometric model outlined

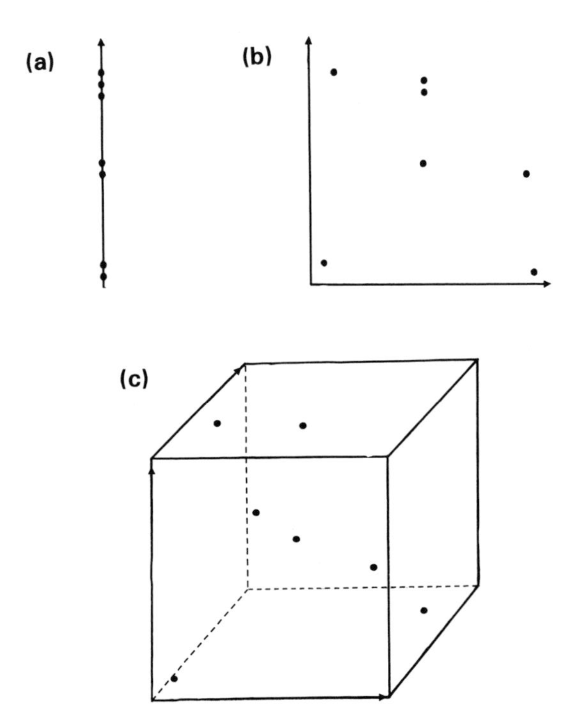

Figure 1. Arrangement of individuals in A-space: (a) one character (dimension), (b) two characters, and (c) three characters.

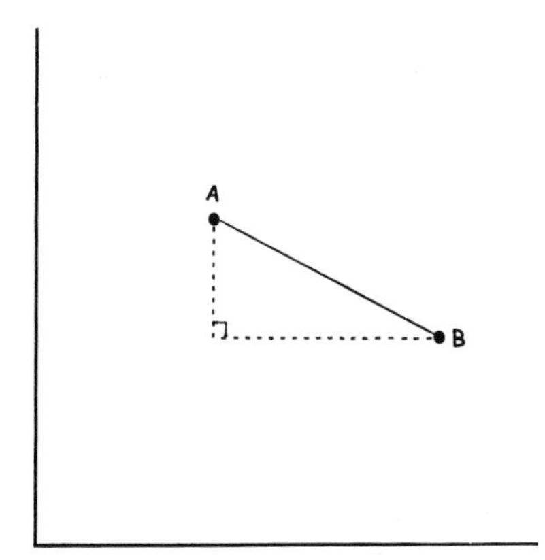

Figure 2. Euclidean (——) and Manhattan (— —) distances between two individuals in two-dimensional A-space.

above, Euclidean distance (Δ_{AB}) between the two individuals A and B is calculated by Pythagoras' theorem extended to t dimensions (see *Figure 2*):

$$\Delta_{AB} = \sqrt{(X_{iA} - X_{iB})^2 + (X_{2A} - X_{2B})^2 \cdots\cdots + (X_{tA} - X_{tB})^2},$$

where X_{iA}, X_{iB} are the states of character $i(i = 1, 2, \ldots, t)$ for the two individuals. One failing of this measure is that it increases as the number of characters increases and so an average distance (d_{AB}) is often calculated (1):

$$d_{AB} = \frac{\Delta_{AB}}{\sqrt{t}}.$$

This is the taxonomic distance. It can be calculated from the binary data for the first two individuals in *Table 1*. The first step is to calculate the differences between each character state.

Comparison	**Character** 1	2	3	4	5	6	7	8	9	10
A:B	0 − 0	0 − 0	1 − 1	0 − 0	0 − 0	0 − 1	0 − 1	0 − 0	1 − 0	0 − 0
$(X_A - X_B) =$	0	0	0	0	0	−1	−1	0	1	0
$(X_A - X_B)^2 =$	0	0	0	0	0	1	1	0	1	0

$$\Sigma\,(X_A - X_B)^2 = 3;$$

$$\Delta_{AB} = \sqrt{3};$$

$$d_{AB} = \frac{\sqrt{3}}{\sqrt{10}} = 0.5477.$$

2.1.2 City-block metrics

Another commonly used distance coefficient is the Manhattan or city-block metric (1, 7). This is the sum of the absolute values of the differences between the character states, that is, disregarding the signs of the differences, and in the geometric model is analogous to the distance between the two individuals along lines parallel to the axes (*Figure 2*):

$$D_{AB} = \sum_{i=1}^{t} | X_{iA} - X_{iB} | .$$

There are a large number of other distance coefficients that have been used in the taxonomic literature and a good review of these can be found in Sneath and Sokal (1).

2.2 Association coefficients

Calculation of association coefficients is not readily represented in A-space. Association coefficients are usually calculated from binary data and give a direct similarity measure.

2.2.1 Simple matching coefficient

The simplest similarity coefficient is the proportion of common results for the individuals tested. This is also known as the simple matching coefficient (S_{SM}), and can be defined as

$$S_{SM} = (w + z)/(w + x + y + z),$$

where w, x, y, and z are as in *Table 2*. This can be demonstrated for individuals A and B from *Table 1* where number of characters positive for both, $w = 1$, characters positive for A and negative for B, $x = 1$, characters positive for B and negative for A, $y = 2$, and characters negative for both A and B, $z = 6$. So S_{SM} for A and B $= (1 + 6)/(1 + 1 + 2 + 6) = 0.7$.

Table 2. Calculation of similarity values

		Individual B Number of characters	
Individual A		**Positive**	**Negative**
Number of characters	Positive	w	x
	Negative	y	z

Although calculated differently, the simple matching coefficient is directly related to the taxonomic distance for binary data by the expression $d = \sqrt{(1 - S_{SM})}$. For the example data, where the S_{SM} value has been calculated as 0.7, $\sqrt{(1 - S_{SM})}$ is $\sqrt{0.3} = 0.5477$, the same as the d_{AB} value calculated earlier.

2.2.2 Jaccard's coefficient

One feature of the simple matching coefficient is that it counts both positive and negative correlations as similarities. As a result, two individuals with a large number of negative responses for characters can be considered very similar. Unfortunately, a large number of negative results may be due to factors such as inappropriate character selection, or slow growth in a microbial culture. To minimize errors in this situation, Sneath and Sokal (1) have suggested the use of a similarity coefficient derived by Jaccard (S_J) which discounts matching negative characters and is expressed simply as

$$S_J = w/(w + x + y).$$

For the individuals A and B in *Table 1* this gives a similarity value of $1/(1 + 1 + 2) = 0.25$, compared with 0.7 obtained with the S_{SM}.

2.3 Other coefficients

2.3.1 Gower's coefficient

Both of the above association coefficients have been used widely in numerical taxonomic studies with binary data. However, many studies result in data that is not binary, or more commonly, is a mixture of binary qualitative data and multistate quantitative data. For this type of study Gower's general similarity coefficient (S_G) as given in Sneath and Sokal (1) is often used. This assigns a score of between 0 and 1 to a character based on its range, and a weight of 1 or 0 depending on whether the comparison is considered valid. In most cases the weight is set at 1, but can be set to 0 where data are unknown or missing or where negative matches are to be excluded. The character score for the ith character is defined as

$$S_{iAB} = 1 - (|X_{iA} - X_{iB}|/R_i),$$

where R_i is the quantitative range for character i over the population. Gower's coefficient is then expressed as

$$S_G = \frac{\sum_{i=1}^{t} (w_{iAB}\, s_{iAB})}{\sum_{i=1}^{t} w_{iAB}}$$

where w_{iAB} is the weight assigned to the comparison of character i. If all comparisons (including matching negative results) are made in a complete data set then $w_{AB} = 1$ in each case and the formula simplifies to

$$S_G = \frac{\left(\sum_{i=1}^{t} s_{iAB}\right)}{t}.$$

As with distance coefficients there are a large number of other similarity coefficients that can be used in numerical taxonomic studies and the reader is again referred to Sneath and Sokal (1).

2.3.2 Pattern coefficient

One further type of association coefficient that is finding increasing application in numerical taxonomy is the Pattern coefficient (D_P) (15, 16). As was mentioned earlier, in microbiology negative matches between characters may result from suboptimal culture growth under the conditions used. While this may be a fundamental difference between some cultures, suboptimal growth can also be due to a number of relatively minor environmental and experimental conditions. In these cases neither excluding nor including negative matches is entirely appropriate. The Pattern coefficient has been developed to minimize differences related to growth rate differences and is based on the apparent differences in vigour between individuals. For binary characters, vigour can be defined simply as the proportion of positive test results and the difference in vigour between two individuals is the difference in this proportion. This difference in vigour can be related to the total difference between the individuals by

$$D^2_{TAB} = D^2_{VAB} + D^2_{PAB},$$

where D_{TAB} is the total difference between individuals A and B and is given by $1 - S_{SM}$, D_{VAB} is the difference in vigour and D_{PAB} is the Pattern difference.

For the first two individuals in *Table 1*, the proportions of positive results are 0.2 and 0.3 respectively, so $D_{VAB} = 0.1$. S_{SM}, the simple matching coefficient, has already been calculated as 0.7, and so $D_{TAB} = 1 - S_{SM} = 0.3$. Thus D_{PAB} can be calculated as $D^2_{PAB} = 0.3^2 - 0.1^2$ and so in this case $D_{PAB} = \sqrt{0.08} = 0.283$. The formulation for multistate data is considerably more complicated and is described by Sackin (16). In this coefficient the vigour of the individuals is considered as the proportion of positive results and so the data should be of a type where positive values indicate greater activity. It should be noted that although derived from similarity data, the Pattern coefficient is a measure of difference and so identical individuals would have a Pattern difference of 0, while for completely different individuals the value would be 1.

2.3.3 Trace derived data

One type of data that is increasingly being used in clustering studies is machine-read data, which are often output through a conventional chart recorder, e.g. from a densitometer or an HPLC. These data can be compared by treating the continuous trace as a series of coordinates, which results in a large number of characters (time points) of varying values (trace heights). The data set can then be considered by one of the distance coefficients, although as each value represents only part of a trace, it may be more correct to use a correlation coefficient, such as r (see Section 2.4), or an angular distance coefficient such as cosine η (1). It should be remembered that when these types of coefficients are used with trace data, they are essentially comparing the 'shapes' of the traces, and so traces with the same shape but with different overall heights will show a good or perfect score. However, as the individual data values in the two traces are not identical, these measures should not strictly be considered as similarity coefficients.

2.4 Summary

As can be seen from this section, there are a large number of types and forms of resemblance measure that can be used to generate matrices for cluster analysis. In most circumstances it is unlikely that many users will encounter more than a small number of these and a summary of the general features of the most commonly used coefficients are given in *Table 3*.

Table 3. Summary of resemblance coefficients

Coefficient and symbol	Type of measure	Usual type of data used	Coefficient type
Taxonomic distance (d)	Dissimilarity	Quantitative	Distance
Manhattan distance (D)	Dissimilarity	Quantitative	Distance
Simple matching (S_{SM})	Similarity	Binary	Association[a]
Jaccard (S_J)	Similarity	Binary	Association
Gower (S_G)	Similarity	Mixed data types	Association
Pattern difference (D_P)	Dissimilarity	Binary & Quantitative	Association[b]
Correlation coefficient (r)	0 – 1[c]	Quantitative	Correlation
Cosine η ($\cos \eta$)	−1 – 1	Quantitative	Angular distance

[a] Many association coefficients can be related directly to distance measures
[b] The Pattern coefficient can more correctly be referred to as a shape coefficient
[c] Although the correlation coefficient varies between 0 and 1, and cosine η varies between −1 and 1, complete correlation does not imply that all values being compared are identical, so they are not strictly similarity measures

3. Clustering methods

Once a table of resemblances between each pair of individuals has been calculated, the next step is to order these so that individuals showing the greatest resemblance are put together. This process can be termed clustering, and the table of resemblances is often referred to as a similarity or triangular matrix. *Table 4* shows the similarity matrix derived with the S_{SM} coefficient for the example data in *Table 1*.

Many types of clustering procedure are available. However, for numerical

Table 4. Similarity matrix of S_{SM} values for the example *Penicillium* data

Individual					
A *Penicillium expansum*	X				
B *P. echinulatum*	0.7	X			
C *P. roquefortii*	0.4	0.5	X		
D *P. hordei*	0.8	0.5	0.4	X	
E *P. brevicompactum*	0.4	0.3	0.6	0.4	X
	A	B	C	D	E
			Individual		

taxonomic studies, sequential, agglomerative, hierarchic, non-overlapping methods (SAHN) are most commonly used (see 1). The two most commonly used SAHN methods are single linkage clustering, also known as the nearest neighbour technique, and unweighted averge linkage clustering, also known as unweighted pair group method analysis (UPGMA).

3.1 Single linkage clustering

In single linkage clustering, an individual is placed in a group on the basis of its highest similarity with any member of that group. This results in groups that are formed from single links between individuals. To cluster the example data in *Table 4* by single linkage, the first step would be to locate the highest similarity level. The highest value is the single value of 0.8 between individuals A and D, so this forms the first pair in the clustering (*Table 5a*). The next highest value is 0.7 between individuals A and B. Although A is already linked with D, this is the single highest similarity for individual B and so links B with A and D (*Table 5b*). At this point the first three individuals have been linked by two values; the next highest value is 0.6 between individuals C and E, and as these have not yet been linked to any others they form a new pair (*Table 5c*). The next highest value in the matrix is 0.5, which enables individuals B and C or B and D to be joined. In this case B and D are already linked and so 0.5 forms the link between the group containing C (C–E) and the group containing B (A–B–D; *Table 5d*). At this point all five individuals have been linked by the four highest values and the clustering is completed. The final clustering may be represented as the minimum spanning tree as shown in *Figure 3*, or as a dendrogram (*Figure 4a*). It should be noted that although the original similarity matrix consisted of 10 individual values, the final graphical representation is based only on the four highest. An alternative strategy is to rearrange the original table to bring similar individuals and groups together. In writing the table after clustering, the order of the OTUs in the table becomes that implied by the clustering, and so areas of high similarity are grouped together along the diagonal of the table (*Figure 4b*).

Table 5. Single linkage clustering: (a) first link, (b) second link, (c) third link, (d) final (fourth) link

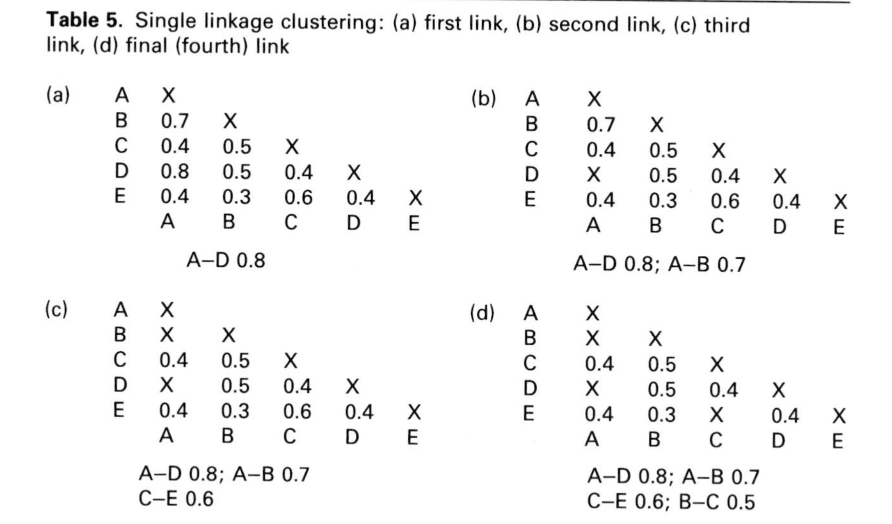

(a)

A	X				
B	0.7	X			
C	0.4	0.5	X		
D	0.8	0.5	0.4	X	
E	0.4	0.3	0.6	0.4	X
	A	B	C	D	E

A–D 0.8

(b)

A	X				
B	0.7	X			
C	0.4	0.5	X		
D	X	0.5	0.4	X	
E	0.4	0.3	0.6	0.4	X
	A	B	C	D	E

A–D 0.8; A–B 0.7

(c)

A	X				
B	X	X			
C	0.4	0.5	X		
D	X	0.5	0.4	X	
E	0.4	0.3	0.6	0.4	X
	A	B	C	D	E

A–D 0.8; A–B 0.7
C–E 0.6

(d)

A	X				
B	X	X			
C	0.4	0.5	X		
D	X	0.5	0.4	X	
E	0.4	0.3	X	0.4	X
	A	B	C	D	E

A–D 0.8; A–B 0.7
C–E 0.6; B–C 0.5

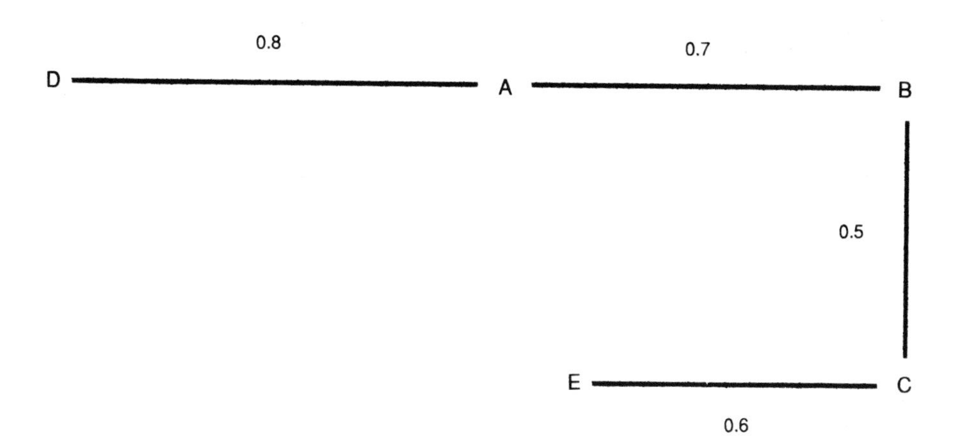

Figure 3. Representation of single linkage clustering as a minimum spanning tree.

3.2 Unweighted average linkage clustering

In unweighted average linkage clustering, individuals are grouped on the basis of their arithmetic average similarities to each other and to the groups of individuals already formed. In practice, the first step is the same as in single linkage and is to identify the highest link in the similarity matrix, which for the example data is 0.8 for individuals A and D (*Table 6a*). This forms the first

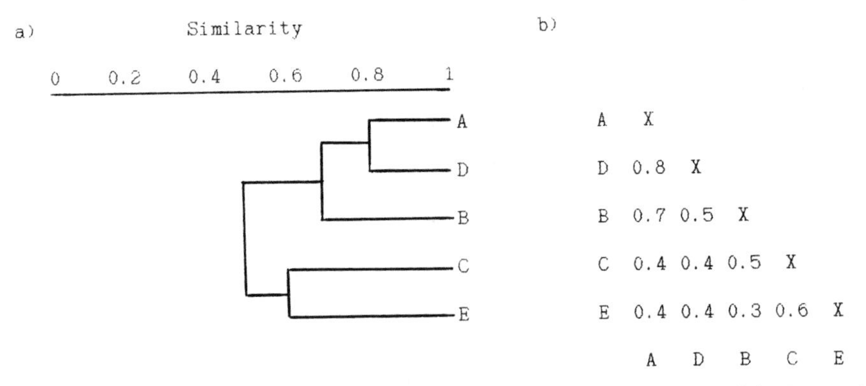

Figure 4. Representation of single linkage clustering: (a) dendrogram, (b) clustered matrix.

pair in the clustering. The pair A and D is now considered as a group and the similarity matrix should be transformed to represent this, with a single entry for the A–D pair. The values giving the new comparisons to the A–D pair are the arithmetic averages of the separate values to A and to D (*Table 6b*). In this case the value for the A–D pair to B becomes 0.6 (average similarity of A and B, 0.7 and D and B, 0.5). The next step is to find the next highest links. The value for individuals C and E remains 0.6 and the value for A–D and B is 0.6, so individuals C and E link to form a second group at 0.6 and B joins A and D to form a triplet. The similarity matrix is then transformed again to give the average values between groups and individuals, although now there are only two columns (*Table 6c*). The remaining value is the arithmetic average of the individual values between the groups ADB and CE, which in this case is 0.4. The resulting dendrogram (*Figure 5a*) is in this case topologically equivalent to the one derived from single linkage clustering

Table 6. Transformation of similarity matrix during average linkage clustering: (a) original similarity matrix, (b) similarity matrix after formation of first link, (c) similarity matrix after second and third links

(a)

A	X				
B	0.7	X			
C	0.4	0.5	X		
D	0.8	0.5	0.4	X	
E	0.4	0.3	0.6	0.4	X
	A	B	C	D	E

(b)

A + D	X			
B	0.6	X		
C	0.4	0.5	X	
E	0.4	0.3	0.6	X
	A + D	B	C	E

(c)

A + D + B	X	
C + E	0.4	X
	A + D + E	C + E

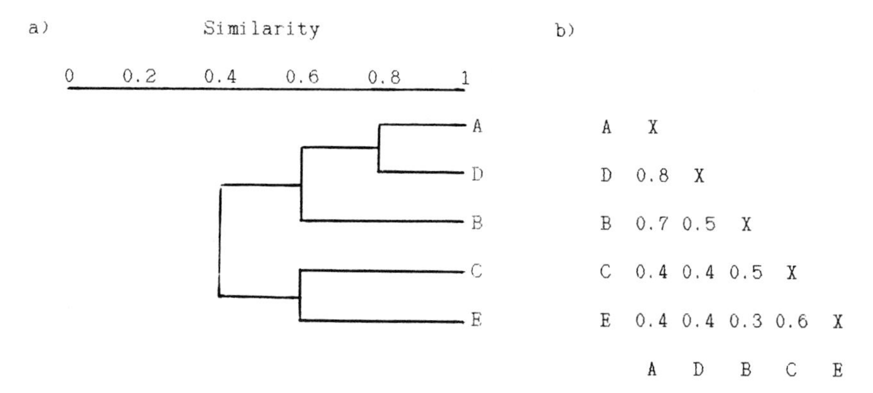

Figure 5. Representation of average linkage clustering: (a) dendrogram, (b) clustered matrix.

(*Figure 4a*), although the overall similarity levels are lower and the two groups appear less closely related. Again, this can be represented by re-arranging the similarity matrix into the new order (*Figure 5b*), although in this case the result is the same as the single linkage matrix.

3.3 Choice of clustering method

The above two examples show the two clustering strategies most widely used in taxonomic studies to produce classifications. There are, however, many other clustering strategies available, including complete linkage, centroid clustering, median clustering, Ward's method and weighted average linkage. The choice and naming of clustering methods has been the subject of debate between taxonomists and statisticians and comprehensive reviews are available in Sneath and Sokal (1) and Abbott *et al.* (7). In general, average linkage clustering has been preferred in numerical taxonomy, as it is an intermediate method lacking some of the extremes that may occur with other clustering methods, and although it has been described as 'the worst of both worlds' (see 7), as it averages both large and small differences, it continues to find favour in both traditional phenetic and modern molecular studies (e.g. 17, 18).

4. Testing classifications

The final output from a cluster analysis classification is generally a dendrogram and/or sometimes a clustered similarity or difference matrix. As has been seen in Section 3, these are representations of the overall resemblances between the individuals, based on their true similarities or differences. It is therefore desirable to obtain some measure of how well a particular dendrogram represents the original data, and how suitable the data was for hierarchical clustering.

4.1 Cophenetic correlation

The most common way to measure how well the original data match the hierarchical clustering is to compare the resemblance values from the original similarity or difference matrix with those implied from the dendrogram (cophenetic values). This process is termed 'cophenetic correlation' and although a number of different coefficients have been proposed (see 1, 7), the usual method is to calculate a product-moment correlation coefficient (r) between the two sets of values (19, 20). Obviously, a dendrogram which gave a perfect representation of the data would yield a cophenetic correlation value of 1. In practice this is never obtained, and in microbiological studies values between 0.6 and 0.95 have been reported; a value of greater than 0.8 is generally considered acceptable (20). The cophenetic correlation coefficients for the single and average linkage dendrograms of the example *Penicillium* data are given in *Table 7*. As can be seen, the cophenetic correlation coefficient for the single linkage dendrogram is 0.876, which is lower than the 0.904 obtained for the average linkage case, although both values are acceptable. This finding would be expected from a direct comparison of the dendrograms (*Figures 4* and *5*) as they are topologically identical and show the same classification. In general, amongst clustering methods that do not allow reversals, unweighted average linkage clustering gives the highest cophenetic coefficients (20, 21). Low values for the cophenetic correlation coefficient obviously show a low correlation between the dendrogram and the original

Table 7. Calculation of the cophenetic correlation coefficient for the single and average linkage dendrograms of the *Penicillium* data: (a) original similarity matrix from S_{SM} coefficient, (b) implied (cophenetic) matrix from single linkage dendrogram, (c) implied (cophenetic) matrix from the average linkage dendrogram

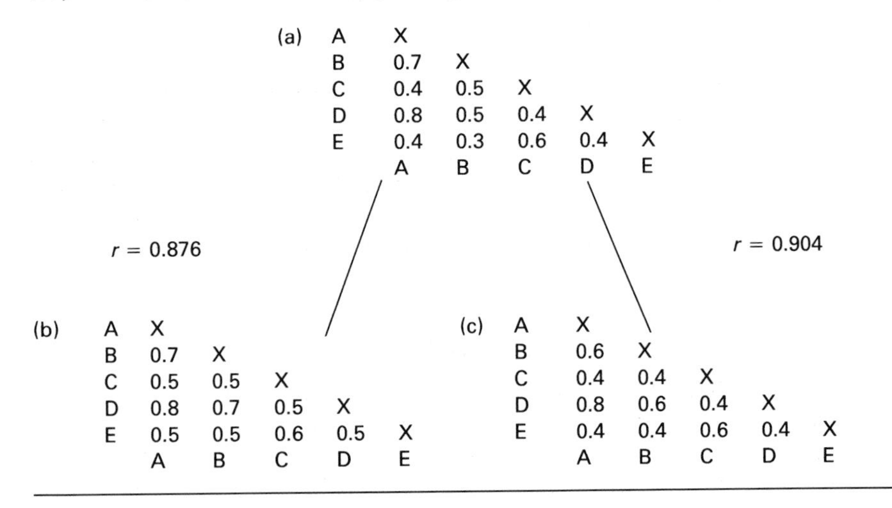

(a)

A	X				
B	0.7	X			
C	0.4	0.5	X		
D	0.8	0.5	0.4	X	
E	0.4	0.3	0.6	0.4	X
	A	B	C	D	E

$r = 0.876$ (b)

A	X				
B	0.7	X			
C	0.5	0.5	X		
D	0.8	0.7	0.5	X	
E	0.5	0.5	0.6	0.5	X
	A	B	C	D	E

$r = 0.904$ (c)

A	X				
B	0.6	X			
C	0.4	0.4	X		
D	0.8	0.6	0.4	X	
E	0.4	0.4	0.6	0.4	X
	A	B	C	D	E

similarities, so in these cases the dendrogram would not give an accurate representation of the relationships between the individuals.

4.2 Determining clusters

While the cophenetic correlation is a useful measure of the distortion within a dendrogram, it should not be taken as the only test of the final classification. It must be remembered that in a cluster analysis the purpose of clustering regimes is to put the most similar organisms together, and to continue this until all individuals are linked. Hence a very different individual included in an analysis of otherwise similar individuals will be linked to them in the dendrogram, albeit at a low similarity. A number of numerical taxonomy studies have included a small number of very dissimilar individuals within the main classification as 'markers' and these usually appear in the final dendrograms as either single branches or very loose clusters (e.g. 13). Careful examination of the individuals in these loosely formed clusters usually shows that they have few character values in common, but are similar in that they are all significantly different from the individuals in the bulk of the dendrogram. It is therefore important, once clusters have been identified, to determine the constant characters within them and to consider which characters differentiate individual clusters.

There is no single simple algorithm or rule to determine at what level in a dendrogram clusters are formed, and Milligan and Cooper (22) list some 30 methods. One common procedure is to examine the final clustering and then to designate a similarity or difference level above which individuals are considered grouped. To illustrate some of the difficulties with this, the dendrograms obtained for the *Penicillium* data (*Figures 4* and *5*) can be studied. Both clustering strategies have given acceptable cophenetic values and both dendrograms show a split into two possible clusters (A, D, and B and C and E) at a similarity of 0.6. The characteristics of these clusters are given in *Table 8a*. As can be seen, only two characters (characters 1 and 5) are differential between the clusters and between four and five of the characters are variable within a cluster. A better interpretation of the results would be to consider the dendrogram as having two clusters (A and D, and C and E) and one ungrouped individual (B). This arrangement is characterized in *Table 8b* and results in four characters that give either positive or negative responses for the clusters (characters 1, 5, 7, and 9). Intuitively, this is a better arrangement than before.

4.3 Testing distinctness of clusters

Once clusters have been identified, they may be further tested with significance tests. Reviews of significance tests for cluster analysis have been given by Sneath (23) and Perruchet (24). One of the most commonly used methods is to estimate their overlap in Euclidean space (25). This provides a means of

Table 8. Characteristics of clusters from *Penicillium* data:
(a) considering two clusters, (b) considering individual B ungrouped

		Characters									
Cluster	**Individuals**	1	2	3	4	5	6	7	8	9	10
1	A, B, and D	–	–	v	v	–	v	v	–	v	–
2	C and E	+	v	–	–	+	v	–	v	–	v

		Characters									
Cluster	**Individuals**	1	2	3	4	5	6	7	8	9	10
1	A and D	–	–	v	v	–	–	–	–	+	–
2	C and E	+	v	–	–	+	v	–	v	–	v
	B	–	–	+	–	–	+	+	–	–	–

v = variable result for character within cluster

determining whether the overlap between any two clusters is significantly greater than a chosen figure. The method assumes that the clusters are approximately spherical within hyperspace and involves calculating the distances along the axis of these hyperspheres. This is useful for demonstrating whether clusters are well separated with little overlap or whether the clusters are in fact adjacent regions of a homogeneous swarm of individuals with little or no gap between them (26). Such tests can be extremely useful in practical studies where it is otherwise difficult to ascertain whether a group of clusters are in reality subgroups of a single taxon. An example of this can be found in Bridge *et al.* (13) where overlap criteria were used to measure the disjunction between a group of clusters that individually showed few diagnostic characters.

Other aids to determining the composition and characteristics of clusters include comparing resemblance values within groups of clustered OTUs and the measurement of typicality (see 1).

4.4 Comparing classifications

In many cases it is desirable to compare the dendrograms produced from different cluster analyses. These cases may be where different coefficients or clustering strategies have been used, or where different studies have been undertaken on similar or possibly overlapping populations. The comparison of classifications has been reviewed by Sackin (27) and Gordon (28), and there would appear to be no single recommended method. Most methods of comparing dendrograms are based on topological or cophenetic measures, although additional descriptors allowing multivariate comparisons have also been described (29).

One approach, based on cophenetic values, was used in a comparison of coding schemes by Bridge and Sackin (30). In this case the cophenetic values, that is, the resemblance values implied by the dendrogram, were compared between dendrograms derived from different data sets by means of the product-moment correlation coefficient. The values obtained were then tested for significance with a χ^2 test. The average and single linkage dendrograms obtained for the example *Penicillium* data (*Figures 4* and *5*) can be compared in this manner, and give a correlation of 0.968. This is a very high value and is in fact greater than the values for either of the dendrograms to the original data (0.876 and 0.904; see *Table 7*). This is not surprising as the two dendrograms are topologically equivalent, and the high value supports this.

Protocol 2. Assessing a classification from a cluster analysis

1. Consider dendrograms from cluster analysis, particularly noting differences (if any) between single and average linkage dendrograms.
2. Calculate cophenetic correlations for individual dendrograms.
3. If significant topological differences between dendrograms, calculate cophenetic correlation between dendrograms.
4. Consider characteristics of clusters by identifying constant and varying characters.
5. Consider membership of clusters, both individually and in relation to each other.
6. Consider range of resemblance values included in cluster.
7. Calculate significance tests for clusters.

Protocol 2 lists the steps that should be taken in assessing dendrograms from a cluster analysis. This is a comprehensive protocol, but should be followed to arrive at a reliable interpretation of the dendrograms.

5. Character coding and weighting

One of the basic principles of numerical taxonomy is that '*a priori*, every character is of equal weight in creating natural taxa' (1). Although non-weighted statistical methods are used to produce classifications, a certain degree of character or attribute weighting may result from the methods of character coding and the inclusion of dependent linked characters.

5.1 Character coding

The coding of characters before undertaking a cluster analysis is perhaps one of the most important parts of the study. Characters can be coded as binary (e.g. +/− results), quantitative (e.g. measurement data) or multistate qualitative (e.g. a single character scale for pigmentation or shape). In most cases the best form of the character will be self-evident but conversion between the different forms is possible. One example of this is measurement data. These are quantitative, and single measurements such as spore length may be treated as single characters. However, it is also possible to partition measurements data to give size classes that can then be coded as a number of binary characters, such as small spores, medium spores, and large spores. Although this process can introduce character linking (see Section 5.2), it is a common procedure in classifications based on association coefficients.

Another consideration in coding characters is whether the characters are truly quantitative or qualitative, and this in turn is important in the selection of the resemblance coefficient. As an example of this, let us consider pigment production by some micro-organisms, where yellow, orange, or brown pigments are produced by different individuals. If these pigments are different chemical compounds then they can be coded in a binary scheme as three independent characters. If, however, the colour difference is due only to different concentrations of the same compound, it may be more correct to code this as a single quantitative character.

A further factor to consider in character coding schemes is whether the observed property is in fact an active or non-active state, as resemblance coefficients such as the Pattern coefficient assume that positive results are related to greater vigour and activity. This becomes significant with characters such as sensitivity to antibiotics in bacteria. Here the observed feature may be an individual's sensitivity to a particular compound, although the actual character could be better termed resistance, as resistance implies a greater vigour.

A final feature of coding schemes is that they should allow accurate comparisons to be made—for example, in a comparison of plants it would not be entirely correct to score an individual plant as negative for a large number of characters relating to flower structure if that plant had not produced a flower. Most coefficients can be implemented with a facility for a 'missing' or 'no comparison' result (1), which in practice is the best course of action in such cases. As a result it is important to allow for this situation in the numerical algorithm used.

5.2 Linked characters

Most of the coefficients used in classification studies require the assumption that the characters selected are exclusive and independent. In some character sets non-independent characters can be easily identified. For example, in carbon source utilization data for micro-organisms the ability to utilize a disaccharide such as sucrose is linked to the ability to utilize its monosaccharide components glucose and fructose. However, in practice it is often difficult to recognize linked characters before the classification is completed.

Character linking can also come about from coding schemes. For example, the conversion of a single quantitative measurement into a series of binary size classes results in linked characters, as a positive result in one class automatically precludes positive results for the others. This is also true of characters relating to other qualitative characters, such as shapes and colours. One solution to this is to adopt an 'all present' system whereby single characters are split into a number of secondary characters, combinations of these being used to describe the original feature. For example, the green spores of *Penicillium* may be coded from a set of colour characters such as green, yellow, blue, and dark and so combinations of these characters can be used to describe blue–green, dark–green etc. Schemes such as this and the use of primary and secondary characters have been reported in numerical classifications, and examples can be found in Proctor and Kendrick (31) and Mugnai *et al.* (32).

In practice, most classifications contain a small number of linked characters. Linked characters can theoretically affect the weighting of particular features and this has been investigated in some taxonomic schemes (33). Recently, the effect of character coding and linkage has been investigated in two numerical classifications (30). In this study, a proportion of the characters were recoded to give a maximum and a minimum number and dendrograms were computed from each data set; although some minor differences were apparent, none of these was considered significant. If the final classification produced from a cluster analysis is a true reflection of the relationships between individuals it will, in the majority of cases, be sufficiently stable and robust not to be significantly affected by these changes.

6. Some applications of cluster analysis in classification

6.1 Systematics

There have been many studies which have used cluster analysis for both phenetic and cladistic classification in biological systematics. As early as 1973, Sneath and Sokal (1) provided a list of more than 500 numerical taxonomy studies, of both living and fossil organisms, from mammals to viruses, of which more than half involved some form of cluster analysis. It is likely that a similar exercise today would give more than double that number.

Cluster analysis methods have been employed at all levels of traditional biological systematics, and so have been used in studies that have grouped individual organisms into species and subspecies (13), individuals and species into genera (34), and genera into families (18). In many cases classifications derived from cluster analyses of traditional phenotypic characters have been supported by similar ordinations (17) and subsequent studies, such as DNA homologies and chemosystematic characters. One example of this can be seen clearly in the taxonomy of fission yeasts, originally described as the single genus *Schizosaccharomyces*. A cluster analysis of physiological and biochemical characters of some 60 strains of fission yeast, based on Gower's coefficient with average linkage clustering, gave three distinct clusters (35). Genetic, chemical, and nucleic acid studies within *Schizosaccharomyces* have supported the separation of the genus into three groups (36, 37) and the fission yeasts have now been formally described as three separate genera *Schizosaccharomyces, Octosporomyces,* and *Hasegawaea* (37).

6.2 Cladistics

Up to now I have described cluster analysis classifications where individuals are grouped together solely on the basis of their resemblance, calculated from a number of characters or attributes. These are phenetic classifications, as the attributes studied are essentially phenotypic. One can imagine that such dendrograms might represent evolutionary or phylogenetic lines, but to try to reconstruct such lineages it is important to choose methods that embody appropriate assumptions, such as constant evolutionary rates and maximum parsimony. The usual phenetic techniques so far described do not do this. An alternative approach is cladistics, where an attempt is made to reconstruct phylogeny. A wide variety of phenotypic and genotypic characters have been used in cladistic analyses, and cladistic analyses are often undertaken on characters derived from macromolecular data, such as protein or nucleic acid sequences. Many of the coefficients and clustering procedures used in cladistic analyses are included in Felsenstein (38). In cladistic studies the resulting tree diagrams are often referred to as cladograms, and are often presented with divergence, time, or evolutionary distance axes. The arms of the cladogram can be taken as representing different evolutionary lineages or events.

There are a large number of published reviews and texts dealing specifically with cladistics and cladistic methods and these should be consulted for further details (1, 7, 39, 40).

6.3 Population and ecological studies

Another area in biology where cluster analysis has been successfully implemented is the study of populations and ecology. These studies have involved the clustering of organisms into groups from particular hosts or environments, such as the types of vegetation within an ecological niche (41) and clusters of a fungal species associated with different insect hosts (32). An example of this type of analysis will be given for the data in *Table 2*, of Chapter 4, which lists the characteristics of 22 breeding sites for dippers. Although there are only eight characters for each site, these data can be clustered by site to give the dendrogram shown in *Figure 6*, where breeding sites with similar characteristics can be seen. In this case, with Gower's coefficient and average linkage clustering the breeding site data give one large cluster of 10 sites, one of three

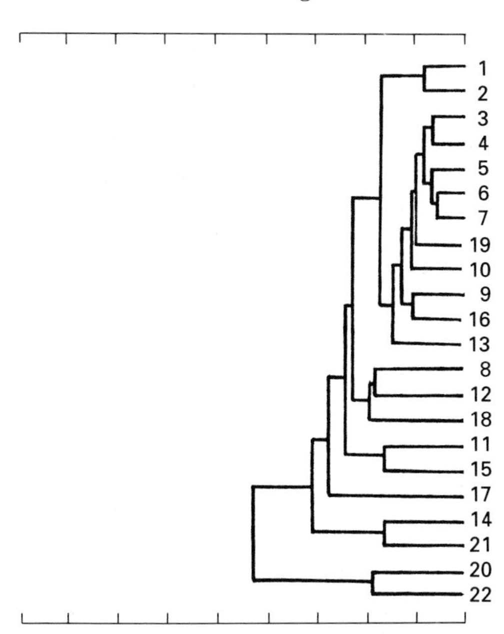

Figure 6. Average linkage dendrogram for breeding sites of dippers.

and four clusters of two sites, with one site, 17, remaining only loosely linked. Examination of the original data with reference to the dendrogram can show characters that are clustered together; for example, the pair of sites 1 and 2 differ from the next group of 10 in having a larger river gradient and smaller numbers of caddisfly and mayfly larvae. In addition, the last pair in the dendrogram, sites 20 and 22, are the sites at highest altitude.

There are many other examples of cluster analysis in biology other than the traditional and molecular systematics area and some examples of these can be found in Sneath and Sokal (1) and Legendre (5). It is also worth remembering that cluster analysis techniques are used widely outside traditional biology, in disciplines such as social sciences and animal behaviour (e.g. 42).

7. Computation

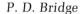

The formulae and calculations given in this chapter are all relatively straightforward mathematically, and all the calculations for the small demonstration data were performed with pencil and paper and the aid of a simple calculator. Indeed some complete numerical taxonomies have been undertaken with a calculator rather than a computer (e.g. 43). The major requirement for computers in these types of analysis is not the complexity of the equations, but the sheer number of calculations necessary. When considering a set of n

individuals, there are $n(n - 1)/2$ pairwise comparisons. As a result, to work with the demonstration data of five individuals, 10 (= 5 × 4/2) similarity or distance values need to be calculated, each based on the 10 characters. If the demonstration data consisted of 10 individuals then 45 (= 10 × 9/2) values are required. To undertake a full scale classification involving some 100 characters for 200 individuals would therefore require the calculation of 19 900 values, each calculated from 100 character values. Similarly, in the clustering described here, there is one fewer link in the dendrogram than there are individuals to be clustered, so a large study of 200 individuals would require the calculation of 199 links. While this may not be too enormous a task for single linkage clustering, the associated transformations of the data matrix with average linkage and the subsequent cophenetic correlations based on sets of 19 900 values require computer assistance.

Computing requirements for cluster analysis are mainly space-related, and any computer used should have sufficient space to store and manipulate the very large matrices and arrays that are produced. The introduction of micro-computers with hard disks has made this much less of a problem than it was. For most workers, computing speed is of secondary importance as large cluster analyses are usually the end point of an already long period of research or observation.

Historically, computer packages for numerical taxonomy have been written in a variety of computer languages by the workers who required them. The vast majority of these are unpublished, although a selection are briefly described by Sackin (44). In addition to these, smaller individual programs have been

Table 9. Comparison of cluster analysis features provided by some generally available statistical packages

	Method provided[a] by			
Feature	*Systat*	*SPSS/PC+*	*CLUSTAN[b]*	*GENSTAT[b]*
Resemblance measure				
Euclidean distance	+	+	+	+
City-block metric	+*	+	−	+
Simple matching coefficient	+*	−	+	+
Jaccard's coefficient	+*	−	+	+
Gower's coefficient	−	−	?	+
Pattern coefficient	−	−	+	−
Clustering method				
Single linkage	+	+	+	+
Average linkage	+	+	+	+

[a] + = provided, − = not provided, +* = provided within the correlation subprogram; the matrix must be saved and read into the clustering module

[b] Data from Sackin (44)

published for specific procedures, such as those for cluster overlap statistics (45) and comparing trace data (46). Of the commercially available packages, those that have been used in a number of studies are *GENSTAT* (47), *SPSS* (SPSS Europe, Gorinchem, The Netherlands), and *CLUSTAN* (Clustan, Edinburgh, UK). These packages are available for mainframe computers (e.g. VAX) and some are available for smaller machines such as the IBM-compatible PCs. A brief comparison of some of the features of some commercially available packages is given in *Table 9*. Software available for phylogenetics and cladistics, such as *PHYLIP* (J. Felsenstein, University of Washington, Seattle, USA) and *PAUP* (D. Swofford, Illinois Natural History Survey, Champaign, USA) has recently been reviewed by Swofford and Olsen (40).

Acknowledgement

I am extremely grateful to M. J. Sackin, Department of Microbiology, Leicester University, for his critical reading of the manuscript and his many helpful comments and suggestions.

References

1. Sneath, P. H. A. and Sokal, R. R. (1973). *Numerical taxonomy*. W. H. Freeman, San Francisco.
2. Gilmour, J. S. L. (1951). *Nature* **168,** 400.
3. Sneath, P. H. A. and Sokal, R. R. (1962). *Nature* **193,** 855.
4. Sokal, R. R. (1985). In *Computer-assisted bacterial systematics* (ed. M. Goodfellow, D. Jones, and F. G. Priest), pp. 1–20. Academic Press, London.
5. Legendre, P. (1983). In *Numerical taxonomy* (ed. J. Felsenstein), pp. 505–23. Springer, Berlin.
6. Alderson, G. (1985). In *Computer-assisted bacterial systematics* (ed. M. Goodfellow, D. Jones, and F. G. Priest), pp. 227–64. Academic Press, London.
7. Abbott, L. A., Bisby, F. A., and Rogers, D. J. (1985). *Taxonomic analysis in biology*. Columbia University Press, New York.
8. Mueller, G. M. (1985). *Mycologia* **77,** 121.
9. Manczinger, L. and Polner, G. (1987). *Syst. Appl. Microbiol.* **9,** 214.
10. Selander, R. K., Caugant, D. A., Ochman, H., Musser, J. M., Gilmour, M. N., and Whittam, T. S. (1986). *Appl. Environ. Microbiol.* **51,** 873.
11. Sneath, P. H. A. (1989). *Syst. Appl. Microbiol.* **12,** 15.
12. Dunn, G. and Everitt, B. S. (1982). *An introduction to mathematical taxonomy*. Cambridge University Press, Cambridge.
13. Bridge, P. D., Hawksworth, D. L., Kozakiewicz, Z., Onions, A. H. S., Paterson, R. R. M., Sackin, M. J., and Sneath, P. H. A. (1989). *J. Gen. Microbiol.* **135,** 2941.
14. Williams, W. T. and Dale, M. B. (1965). *Advances in Botanical Research* **2,** 35.
15. Sneath, P. H. A. (1968). *J. Gen. Microbiol.* **54,** 1.
16. Sackin, M. J. (1981). *J. Gen. Microbiol.* **122,** 247.
17. Bridge, P. D. and Sneath, P. H. A. (1983). *J. Gen. Microbiol.* **129,** 565.

18. Blanz, P. A. and Gottschalk, M. (1986). *Syst. Appl. Microbiol.* **8,** 121.
19. Sokal, R. R. and Rohlf, F. J. (1962). *Taxon.* **11,** 33.
20. Jones, D. and Sackin, M. J. (1980). In *Microbiological classification and identification,* (ed. M. Goodfellow and R. G. Board), pp. 73–106. Academic Press, London.
21. Austin, B. and Priest, F. (1986). *Modern bacterial taxonomy.* Van Nostrand Reinhold, Wokingham.
22. Milligan, G. W. and Cooper, M. C. (1985). *Psychometrika* **50,** 159.
23. Sneath, P. H. A. (1980). In *Data analysis and informatics* (ed. E. Diday *et al.*), pp. 491–508. North-Holland, Amsterdam.
24. Perruchet, C. (1983). In *Numerical taxonomy* (ed. J. Felsenstein), pp. 199–208. Springer, Berlin.
25. Sneath, P. H. A. (1977). *Classification Society Bulletin* **4,** 2.
26. Sneath, P. H. A. (1977). *Mathemat. Geol.* **9,** 123–43.
27. Sackin, M. J. (1985). In *Computer-assisted bacterial systematics* (ed. M. Goodfellow, D. Jones, and F. G. Priest), pp. 21–36. Academic Press, London.
28. Gordon, A. D. (1987). *J. Roy. Statist. Soc. A* **150,** 119.
29. Podani, J. and Dickinson, T. A. (1984). *Can. J. Bot.* **62,** 2765.
30. Bridge, P. D. and Sackin, M. J. (1991). *Mycopathologia* **115,** 105.
31. Proctor, J. R. and Kendrick, W. B. (1963). *Nature* **167,** 716.
32. Mugnai, L., Bridge, P. D., and Evans, H. C. (1989). *Mycol. Res.* **92,** 109.
33. Kendrick, W. B. and Proctor, J. R. (1964). *Can. J. Bot.* **42,** 65.
34. Dabinett, P. E. and Wellman, A. M. (1978). *Can. J. Bot.* **56,** 2031.
35. Bridge, P. D. and May, J. W. (1984). *J. Gen. Microbiol.* **130,** 1921.
36. Sipiczki, M., Kucsera, J., Ulaszewski, S., and Zsolt, J. (1982). *J. Gen. Microbiol.* **128,** 1989.
37. Yamada, Y. and Banno, I. (1987). *J. Gen. Appl. Microbiol.* **33,** 295.
38. Felsenstein, J. (1983). *J. Roy. Statist. Soc., A* **146,** 246.
39. Felsenstein, J. (1983). In *Numerical taxonomy* (ed. J. Felsenstein), pp. 315–34. Springer, Berlin.
40. Swofford, D. L. and Olsen, G. J. (1990). In *Molecular systematics* (ed. D. M. Hillis and C. Moritz), pp. 411–501. Sinauer Associates, Sunderland, USA.
41. West, N. E. (1966). *Ecology* **47,** 975.
42. Schnell, G. D. and Woods, B. L. (1982). In *Numerical taxonomy* (ed. J. Felsenstein), pp. 562–81. Springer, Berlin.
43. Carlsson, J. (1968). *Odontologisk Revy* **19,** 137.
44. Sackin, M. J. (1987). In *Methods in microbiology,* Vol. 19 (ed. R. R. Colwell and R. Grigorova), pp. 59–94. Academic Press, London.
45. Sneath, P. H. A. (1980). *Computers and Geosciences* **6,** 267.
46. Jackman, P. J. H., Feltham, R. K. A., and Sneath, P. H. A. (1983). *Microbios Letters* **23,** 87.
47. Nelder, J. A. (1979). *GENSTAT reference manual.* Scientific and Social Service Program Library, University of Edinburgh.

7

Time series analysis

F. D. J. DUNSTAN

1. Introduction

In many biological and medical situations a variable is observed sequentially over a period of time. The resulting set of observations, ordered with respect to time, is called a time series. For example if the temperature in a certain place is measured at noon on each day for a year, the resulting set of values is a time series of length 365 (provided the year is not a leap year). Similarly, if the acidity level of a lake is measured monthly for five years, a time series of length 60 results. While, in many branches of statistics, when a set of observations is made they are assumed to be independent for subsequent analysis, one of the key features of a time series is that the observations are almost invariably dependent. The analysis of the series acknowledges this dependency in modelling the series and, in some applications, exploits this dependency to forecast future values. In the past, time series analysis has been developed largely in the areas of economics and engineering, but recently there has been a growing realization that it is a subject with important applications in biology and medicine and there is increasing interest in its use in these fields.

Before introducing any formal notation, some more examples are considered:

(a) the temperature in a hothouse is measured continuously and recorded as a trace on a graph

(b) the EEG activity of a patient is recorded by a set of sensors at a rate of 256 times per second

(c) the number of male deaths in the UK due to ischaemic heart disease is recorded every quarter

(d) the amount of urine excreted by a patient every 24 hours is recorded

(e) the annual yield of a certain crop is recorded every year

In (a) and (b) the variable being monitored could, in principle, be monitored continuously. In practice, to facilitate data storage and analysis, the value is recorded at regular intervals, as in the EEG example. The sampling interval can be made as small as required to ensure that no detail is lost. By contrast, in (d) and (e) there can only be one value recorded in each time period—a day in (d) and a year in (e). In all but (c) the variable being recorded is continuous in nature while in (c) it is discrete—the number of deaths must be integer-valued. Unless the set of possible values is very small, such as a case in which the value can only be 0 or 1 say, this makes little difference in practice. We generally assume, therefore, that the variable of interest is a continuous variable and is recorded at a discrete set of time points. It is usually convenient to assume that these time points are equally spaced. Sometimes this may be only approximately so; for example if a variable is recorded monthly, then not all months have the same length and so observations are not exactly equally spaced. In such cases, so long as the intervals between observations are approximately equal, the assumption is reasonable. If the gaps between successive observations are very irregular, then standard methods of analysis cannot be used. The problem is beyond the scope of this chapter; the analysis requires more sophisticated techniques. The interested reader is referred to Priestley (1). We shall assume, therefore, that observations are equally spaced and we will denote them simply by x_1, $x_2, \ldots, x_n$ where n is the length of the series. Thus a general value x_t refers to observation number t; this value t is not the actual time but can be converted easily into such a time. If values are recorded monthly, starting in January, then x_{20} refers to the value in August of the second year.

The examples considered above are all of single series. In some situations, several series are of interest. For example the number of each of several species of animals in a certain area might be recorded at regular intervals. Because of predator–prey relationships, these series might be linked—as the number of predators increases, the number of prey might decrease, and conversely. When EEG readings are taken, they are usually recorded from several sensors simultaneously and clearly the resulting series would be expected to depend on each other in some way. A series recording daily energy consumption will be linked to one recording the average daily temperature. Such problems will be discussed briefly in Section 8; until then a single series will be considered.

The aims of a time series analysis are not usually so clear cut as, for example, in fitting a regression model. Part of the analysis is often exploratory in nature, the object being to obtain an understanding of the process which has produced the series. Subsequently a model may be fitted to the data and this may be used, in some contexts, to obtain forecasts of future values of the series. This is clearly particularly important in economic applications, but is sometimes useful in biological ones. This lack of a single aim is reflected in the standard statistical software. In *Minitab* a single command, with a range of sub-commands, covers most situations for regression analysis. In time series, however, there are several commands which may be used to produce diagnostic tools which are used to choose the type of model which might be fitted. Another command is then used to fit a given model, but the user has to decide on the best model by some method. The situation, therefore, is that the software does not act as a black box into which the data are fed and which produces a simple answer; the user has much more work to do. The range of facilities for time series analysis is limited in many of the basic packages; some specialized ones, which are less likely to be available to the ordinary user, have a wider range. In this Chapter, *Minitab* will be used, with macros provided where needed to fill gaps in the facilities provided. Sometimes these will not be ideal, in the sense that a more efficient method is possible, but cannot be implemented easily in *Minitab*. For simplicity, however, it seems best to work with the single package, despite its limitations. The material presented here is only a brief summary of some of the methods of time series analysis. For further details there are several texts of moderate mathematical complexity, including those of Chatfield (2) and Diggle (3). Cryer (4) is quite readable and also indicates how some of the analysis can be carried out in *Minitab*, complementing some of the material here. We should also mention the famous book of Box and Jenkins (5), the first to present a unified theory. It is a good source, if rather technical.

2. Preliminary analysis

2.1 Plotting a series

The first step in examining a series is to plot it on a graph. The *Minitab* command TSPLOT is provided to do this but, unless the series is very short, it is fairly useless; each data point is represented by an integer 1, 2, 3, . . . and it is usually very difficult to interpret the plot. It is very easy to produce a clearer plot using the high resolution graphics command GPLOT with the sub-command LINES. The macro TPLOT, listed in *Appendix 7.11*, produces a simple plot in which the individual points are not plotted but are joined together by straight lines. This is the conventional approach for plotting series and generally gives a clear picture. The default setting for a *Minitab* graph chooses the *y*-axis so that the observations fully utilize the range. Note that this macro, and all others referred to in the chapter, are listed in *Appendices 7.11–7.20* and are available on a disk. Sometimes it is a little difficult to interpret a series plotted in this way—there seems to be too much variation and the result can be misleading, just as if the series is compressed into a very narrow range. For this reason a second macro SCTPLOT (see *Appendix 7.12*) has been provided which allows the user to choose the scaling and also to display a section of the series if required. The macro initially prints out the range of both the times and the series values and the user has to specify the section required.

Figure 1 shows the results of using these macros for a number of series. The series are described briefly in the figure captions and in more detail in *Appendices 7.1–7.4*. From these graphs we can see that a series may be made up of a number of components of different type. These are often referred to as trend,

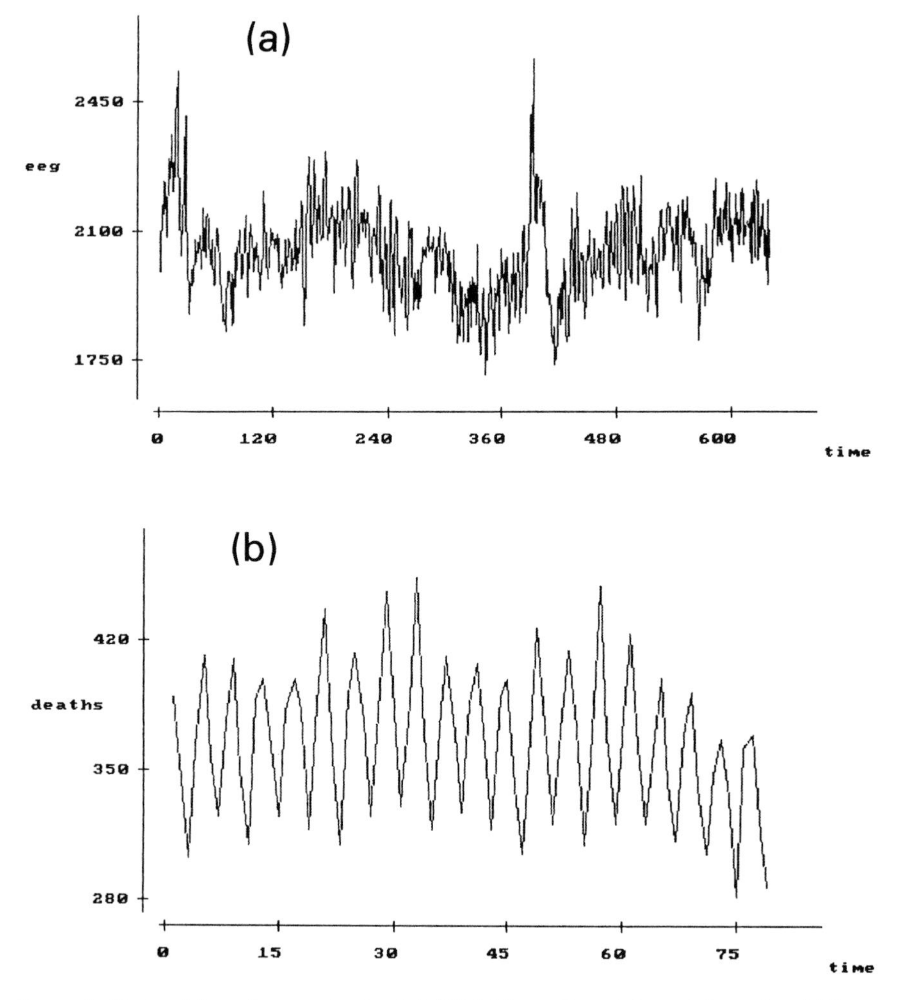

Figure 1. Plots of four time series for (a) 640 EEG readings taken at the rate of 64 per second, (b) number of deaths per quarter among males in the UK from ischaemic heart disease, (c) growth of a colony of *Paramecium aurelium* over 18 days, and (d) number (1000s) of passengers travelling on scheduled UK airline flights per month.

seasonal, and random components. The trend represents a long term movement or change in mean level. Many economic series, such as the Retail Price Index, show this clearly—that index in recent years has increased more or less steadily. The series in *Figure 1c*, the growth of the protozoal colony, clearly shows an upward trend, seemingly tailing off near the end of the series. A seasonal or periodic component occurs if the series varies in a fairly systematic periodic fashion. Many economic series again display this type of behaviour and so do many biological ones. For example, the daily average temperature

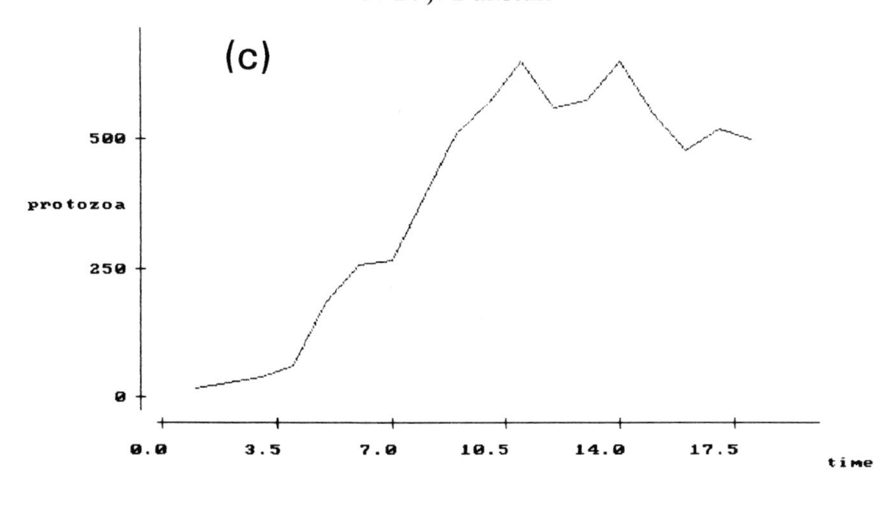

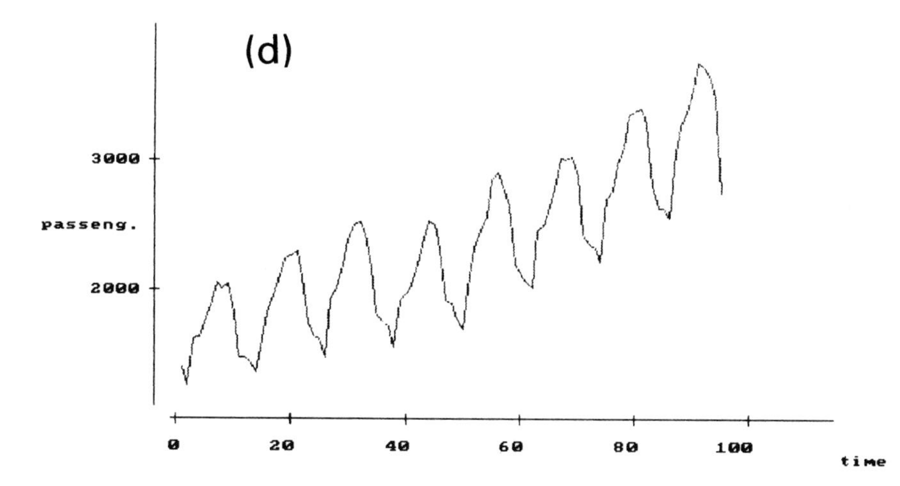

varies throughout the year in a fashion which is fairly consistent from year to year; we say that there is a periodic component with period one year. The deaths due to heart disease (*Figure 1b*), show clear periodic behaviour, again of an annual nature. In some series a periodic component can be masked by random variation and will not be apparent from a simple plot. Later we shall see how the presence or not of such a component can be investigated fairly easily by calculating certain functions from the data. Some series contain both trend and seasonal components; the series of *Figure 1d* is such a case. The overall level increases steadily from year to year but within each year there is very clear seasonal variation. In none of these examples is the seasonal component perfectly regular; there seems to be a random component, sometimes called noise, superimposed on the systematic part of the series; this is the random component referred to earlier. In many series, such as the EEG series of *Figure 1a* there is no obvious trend or seasonal component; the series seems to consist simply of this random component.

Faced with series like these, how does an analysis proceed? A standard method is to try to divide a series into these different components and to deal with each one separately. This is often easier than trying to model the whole series in a single step. Modelling is generally easiest if the series is stationary. By a stationary series we mean, loosely speaking, one which does not change systematically over time; the appearance of a graph of the series in one time period is similar to that in a different period. More formally we can define it as one whose statistical properties do not change over time. Thus a series whose mean or variability changes, or which has a seasonal component, is not stationary. Suppose we have a series which contains a trend and seasonal effect, such as in *Figure 1d*. To proceed we can try to estimate these systematic components and to remove them from the series values, leaving a random component. This can then be analysed, including an examination to see if the resulting series is in fact stationary, a model can perhaps be fitted, and then the whole series can be combined for forecasting future values, if that is an aim.

2.2 The moving average approach

2.2.1 Identifying and removing a trend

Consider first the case of a trend. One way of estimating it is by using regression methods. If the trend is approximately linear, then a linear regression against time (see Chapter 3, Section 2) will estimate the trend, while if it is possibly quadratic, or higher order, then a polynomial regression as described in Chapter 3, Section 5.1 could be used. There are certain theoretical difficulties with this approach but it can often be profitably employed and is discussed in Section 7. An alternative method is to compute a simple moving average. This is a weighted average of some series values, designed to smooth out local fluctuations to estimate the true means at the time. Suppose, for illustration, that a series displays an annual periodicity, being high in the summer and low in the winter, and that it is recorded at four-monthly intervals in March, July, and November. How do we estimate the underlying mean, as opposed to the seasonally affected mean, in July? The recorded value will overstate the position because of the seasonal effect. It seems reasonable to average over neighbouring values, but we must do so in such a way that each part of the cycle has equal weight. If not, then we will not remove the effect of the seasonal variation. To estimate the mean in a given July, therefore, it seems reasonable to average that July figure with the previous March value and the following November value. The time points for which we calculate the average are centred about the current time point and all parts of the cycle have the same weight. Thus we would calculate

$$y_t = (x_{t-1} + x_t + x_{t+1})/3.$$

The seasonal effect and local variations should have largely disappeared from the series $\{y_t\}$, which should also be much smoother.

If the data are recorded monthly, with an annual effect, then we proceed in the same sort of fashion. There is a slight complication, however. To estimate the mean now for a given July, we average values centred on July. If we are to cover all parts of the cycle equally, then we should go back six months to the preceding January and on to the following January. But then January appears twice in the calculation. To avoid this we give the two January values half the weight of the others. We thus use a formula like

$$y_t = (x_t + x_{t-1} + x_{t+1} + \ldots + x_{t-5} + x_{t+5} + \tfrac{1}{2}x_{t-6} + \tfrac{1}{2}x_{t+6})/12$$

to estimate the mean. The divisor 12 is used since effectively 12 terms are being averaged. To remove the trend from the series, we now simply subtract the smoothed value y_t from the original observation x_t. The remaining series should consist of a random component and seasonal component. This process is illustrated in *Figure 2a* where the series of deaths from heart disease of *Figure 1b* is shown, with the moving average representing the trend superimposed. The calculations were carried out by the macro SMOOTH (see *Appendix 7.13*), which requires merely the number of observations per cycle as input. The trend curve is reasonably smooth; to make it smoother we could average over a two year period, rather than a single year. If the series does not have a seasonal component in the first place, then calculation of the above moving average will not necessarily be appropriate. Any average of a reasonable number of observations centred on the current one will be fairly effective in isolating the trend. That employed in the macro SMOOTH1 (*Appendix 7.14*) is due to Henderson (see Kenny and Durbin, 6) and is slightly different in that more weight is given to the observations nearest the current time and slightly less to those more distant. The basic principle is the same, however. This smoothing process is illustrated in *Figure 3* using the series of protozoal growth from *Figure 1c*. The graph representing the trend is a fairly smooth curve and clearly reflects the overall mean behaviour.

Note that it is not possible with any method of this type to calculate these smoothed values right up to the end of the series, since the formulae use future values as well as past values. A method has to be modified if it is essential for smoothed values to extend right to the end, using values from one side only.

2.2.2 Identifying and removing seasonal effects

If there is a seasonal effect, then we an easily estimate it by using the detrended values obtained by the above process. To estimate the seasonal effect at a given part of the cycle we merely average all the detrended values from that point of the cycle. Thus, in the above example of monthly data, to estimate the effect in October we simply average all the October values for the whole series. To remove this seasonal effect we simply subtract this

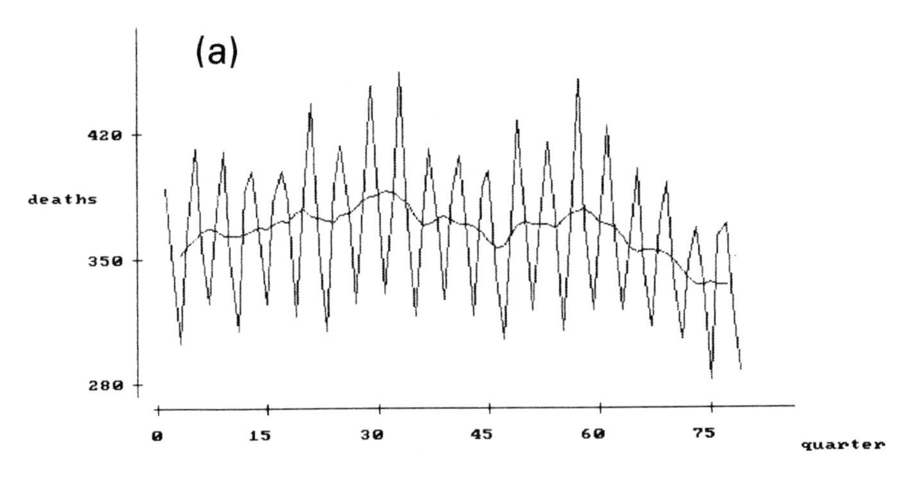

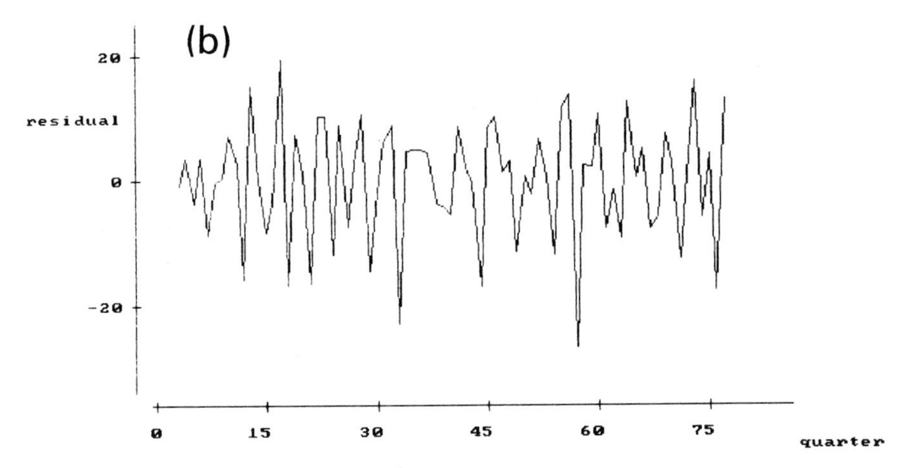

Figure 2. The series of (a) heart deaths with superimposed trend calculated by a moving average and (b) heart deaths with trend and seasonality removed by the moving average method.

average from all the October values. The result of applying this to the heart deaths data is shown in *Figure 2b*. This graph was generated by the macro SMOOTH which carries out the calculations for the whole of this smoothing process. The values remaining after this process should constitute the random part of the series. In this example the final series does not contain any obvious systematic components, although these are not always easy to spot. Later we shall describe a method which can highlight periodic variation in a very simple way. Further details of smoothing can be found in Chatfield (2) or Kendall and Stuart (7).

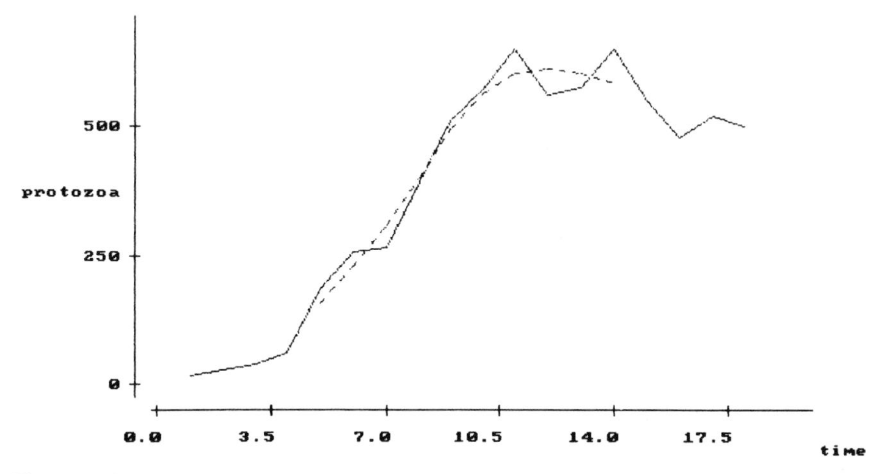

Figure 3. Protozoan growth series with trend calculated by the Henderson formula.

A problem with this moving average approach arises if we wish to project the series into the future. The seasonal effect does not cause difficulties, but it is not clear how to extrapolate the trend. Indeed, as was noted earlier, we cannot even reach the end of the series without modifying the approach. Sometimes the trend is extrapolated by eye but this is not entirely satisfactory. Although it is possible to produce methods which can extend an estimated trend, other approaches are often used to avoid this problem. One possibility already referred to is the use of polynomial regression to estimate the trend, and this readily leads to extrapolation. Another widely used method does not estimate the trend and seasonal effects directly, but removes these to try to produce a stationary series.

2.3 Differencing methods

As indicated above, the technique of differencing is used to remove non-stationary factors. The series of first differences is given by

$$y_t = x_t - x_{t-1} \text{ (sometimes written as } \nabla x_t),$$

i.e. the previous observation is subtracted from the current one. If there is a linear trend, then this should be removed by such a difference. If there is a quadratic trend then the series of first differences should be reduced to a linear trend and applying the method again, to calculate the second differences, should remove the trend. We thus find

$$\nabla^2 x_t = \nabla y_t = y_t - y_{t-1} = x_t - 2x_{t-1} + x_{t-2}.$$

The same technique can be used for removing a seasonal component. Illustrating it with the monthly series with annual periodicity, we simply take the differences between values in corresponding months. Thus from the July value of one year we subtract the July value of the previous year, and so on. We thus form the new series

$$\nabla_{12}x_t = x_t - x_{t-12}.$$

If a series contains both trend and seasonal effects then we can combine both types of differences, in either order. *Minitab* does have a command to calculate differences, namely DIFFERENCES. The command

```
DIFFERENCES k C1 C2
```

will take a series in column C1 and difference it by subtracting the first value from the $(k + 1)$th value, the second from the $(k + 2)$th, and so on, putting the results in column C2. There will, of course, be no values for observations $1,2,\ldots,k$. To remove a linear trend and annual periodic effect for monthly data we would therefore use

```
DIFFERENCES 1 C1 C2
DIFFERENCES 12 C2 C3
```

and end up with the final series in C3. If these were applied, the resulting series would have 13 missing values at the start and many *Minitab* commands would cease to work. For this reason the macro DFF (*Appendix 7.15*) has been supplied to allow the user to take a number of differences, plotting the series after each so that a decision can be made as to whether or not further differencing is required. For the series of *Figure 4a*, of monthly data with an annual period, we take a first difference followed by a twelfth difference, as we know there is an annual effect. The result is shown in *Figure 4b*. The periodic component has certainly decreased in magnitude, but has not entirely disappeared. Why is this? If we look at the graph of the original series we see that the seasonal effect seems to grow in magnitude as the overall mean increases. The trend and seasonality are combining in a multiplicative way rather than an additive way. To overcome this we have to transform the data by taking logarithms; this converts the multiplicative effect into an additive one. The transformed series is plotted in *Figure 4c,* while *Figure 4d* shows the result of taking the first and twelfth differences; the periodic variation has been removed more effectively. Other transformations are sometimes employed, but their use is really beyond the scope of this chapter.

As we shall see later, even if a series has been differenced it is still possible to forecast future values by reversing the differencing process, and this is an advantage over the moving average method.

3. Autocorrelation

Suppose that, by one of these methods, the systematic variation has been removed so that what remains is a random series. How can we explore this to gain an insight into its behaviour? The first stage is usually an examination of the dependence structure. As was pointed out in the introduction, in contrast to many statistical situations, observations in time series are usually dependent and it is this dependence that enables us to forecast future values. The usual way of examining this dependence is by displaying the autocorrelation or autocovariance function. The autocorrelation function (acf) at lag k measures the correlation between pairs of values k apart in the series, that is (x_1,x_{k+1}), (x_2,x_{k+2}), . . ., (x_{n-k},x_n) where n is the number of observations in the series. A plot of the acf against the time lag is called the correlogram. This is very useful for distinguishing between different types of series and for choosing appropriate models. The command ACF in *Minitab* computes the autocorrelation function. For example, the command ACF 20 C1 would calculate the acf for lags 1,2,. . .,20 for the series in column C1 and give a simple plot in low resolution. The autocovariance function records the covariances rather than the correlations and is obtained simply by multiplying the autocorrelation function by the variance of the series.

To interpret the correlogram we need to know how large values must be to be important. As with ordinary correlation coefficients, values must lie between -1 and $+1$, with values near these extremes indicating a high degree of linear dependency. Values close to zero suggest that values are more or less independent. Approximate 95% confidence limits for the values of the acf for a series of n independent values are $-2/\sqrt{n}$ and $2/\sqrt{n}$. If a series has almost all of the values of its acf within these limits, then the observations can be regarded as independent. If many of the values are much larger than these limits, then the dependence is significant. The macro AUTOCF (*Appendix 7.16*) calculates the acf as indicated earlier, plots a correlogram using high resolution graphics, and draws these confidence limits, so that the correlogram can be easily interpreted. We find generally that periodic behaviour in the series is reflected by similar periodic behaviour in the acf, while trend in the series is reflected in an acf which dies away very slowly indeed. *Figure 5* shows the correlograms of the EEG series of *Figure 1a*, the heart deaths example of *Figure 1b* and an artificial series of white noise, that is a series of independent observations. The EEG series shows values of the acf which are certainly non-zero, but with no striking pattern other than the fact that they gradually die away, sufficiently quickly for us not to worry about non-stationarity. The heart deaths example reflects the fact that periodic behaviour in the series is usually reflected in the acf. The last example shows that for a random series of independent observations, the correlations are very small in general. A glance at the correlogram readily distinguishes between these types of series in many cases. Note that in this figure a common scale from -1 to 1 has not been used; in order to show detail the full scale has been used in each case. Thus the values in *Figure 5c* are much smaller than in the other two cases.

Protocol 1 summarizes the order in which the investigations described in Sections 2 and 3 should be done.

Protocol 1. Initial investigation of a time series

1. Plot the series—use TPLOT[a] or SCTPLOT.
   - TPLOT plots the series using default scales and axes
   - SCTPLOT allows the user to choose which part of a series to plot and what vertical scale to use
2. Are there any obvious features?
3. Is the variability constant? If not consider a logarithmic transformation.
4. Plot the correlogram, using AUTOCF, to help in identifying obvious features causing non-stationarity. These include:
   - trend, identifiable by the acf dying away very slowly
   - periodicity, often recognizable by regular peaks in the acf
5. Choose smoothing or differencing as a technique for producing a stationary series. Smoothing gives a simple graphical picture of the non-stationary nature of the series but it cannot be easily incorporated into a model or extrapolated for forecasting.
6. If smoothing is to be used and if there is no obvious seasonality, use SMOOTH1 to estimate and remove the trend. Otherwise use SMOOTH to remove both trend and seasonality.
7. If differencing is to be used, use DFF to choose the necessary differences. Simple first differences should remove trend, while seasonal ones will be needed for the periodic effect.
8. Plot the resulting series and its correlogram to check that it seems stationary, looking for features as in 4.

[a] *Minitab* macro names are in capital letters

4. Analysis in the frequency domain

4.1 Introduction to the frequency domain

Sometimes a series contains a very obvious seasonal component; we have already seen several examples of such series. In these there is no doubt that seasonality exists and the number of observations in a cycle is obvious either from the context, as in the heart deaths series, or from a quick look at the observations and the correlogram. In other cases the existence of a periodic component is not so obvious. In *Figure 6* two series of hand tremor measurements are shown. In the study in which these were recorded, a subject was monitored for approximately 10 seconds and recordings of the acceleration of the hand were made at the rate of 50 per second. The series are listed in

Appendices 7.5 and 7.6. The examples shown are from different individuals with different physiological conditions. Any periodic components in the series were of particular interest, since it was believed that the nature of these would give useful diagnostic information about the condition of the individual. There is clearly a periodic component in the first series; a study of the data suggests that the number of observations in a cycle is about 10. What about the second series? We may suspect that there is such a component, but it is not clear. To see how this may be investigated we now consider briefly the analysis of time series in the frequency domain. The aim of this analysis is to identify variation in the series at different frequencies to see which contribute most to the overall variation of the series. At first it seems an unnatural approach but it does have a lot of useful properties other than those considered here; for our purposes it is merely a useful diagnostic tool.

Fourier analysis is an important mathematical technique which allows any periodic function to be represented as a sum of sine or cosine waves. It can also be applied to time series recorded at discrete time points and it can be shown that a series of length n (taken to be an even number for convenience) can be represented as a sum of $n/2$ sine waves of different frequencies. A sine wave at frequency ω takes the form

$$c \sin(\omega t + \varphi)$$

where c is the amplitude and φ the phase. As the sine function repeats itself every time its argument increases by 2π, this wave is periodic with period $2\pi/\omega$. The amplitude is the height of the peak of the wave above the average value, while the phase measures the distance between the start of a cycle and the time origin; it indicates how advanced the cycle is at time 0. *Figure 7* shows the graph of a sine wave and the amplitude and phase are indicated on it.

The Fourier decomposition in fact represents the series as a sum of waves of the form

$$c_k \sin(\omega_k t + \varphi_k), \qquad k = 1,2,\ldots,n/2,$$

where $\omega_k = 2\pi k/n$. These are sometimes called the Fourier frequencies. Now the period of the kth such frequency is $2\pi/\omega_k = n/k$. This is the number of observations in a complete cycle of that frequency. The square c_k^2 of the amplitude of this wave is a measure of its importance in the representation of the series. Thus a particularly large value at ω_k might indicate that the series contains a periodic component at, or near, this frequency. The periodogram of the series is essentially a plot of this squared amplitude against frequency. Unfortunately, the statistical properties of the periodogram are very poor; its variance does not decrease as the series length increases and a better method is needed to smooth it and give more reliable estimates of the underlying function, the spectrum.

Note that the frequencies ω_k range from $\omega_1 = 2\pi/n$, with period n, to

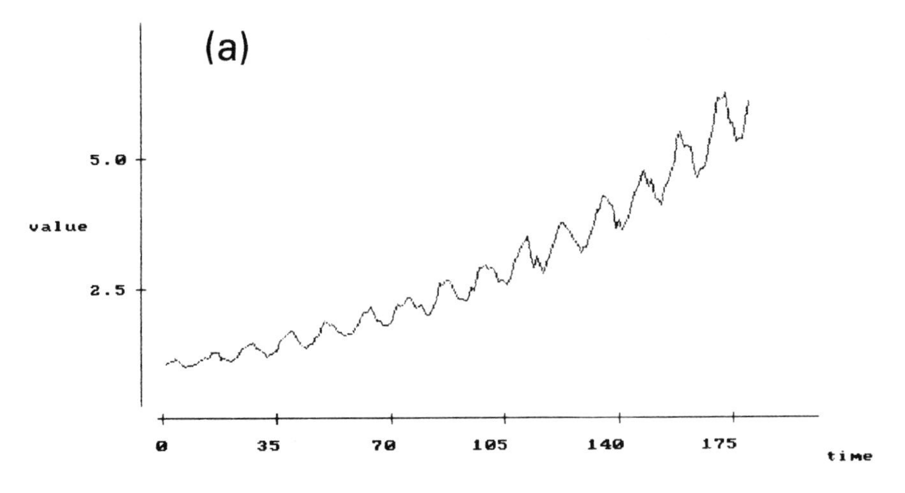

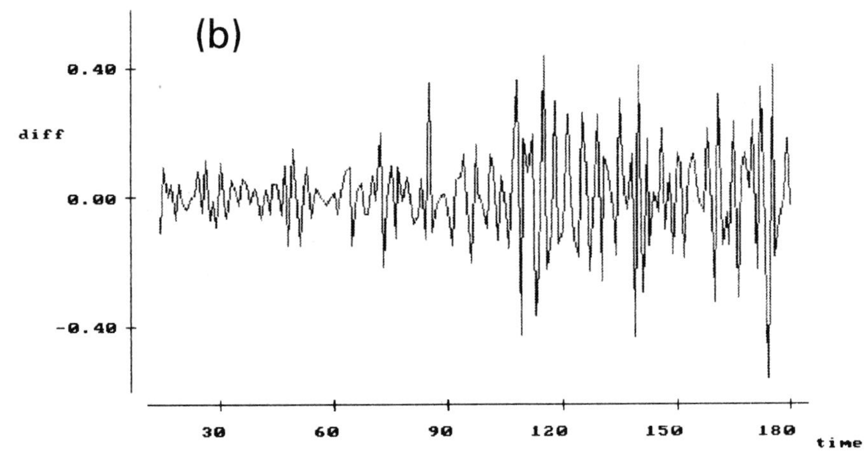

Figure 4. Series (a) showing multiplicative trend and seasonality, (b) after first and seasonal differencing, (c) of logarithms of original values, and (d) loged after first and seasonal differencing of logarithms.

$\omega_{½n} = \pi$, which has period 2. This is the practical range which can be investigated. If there is an annual period say, but we have daily data for three months only, then we cannot sensibly estimate the annual effect. Indeed it may appear as a trend if the observations all come from near one extreme of the cycle. Similarly, if we have weekly data, then we cannot investigate any daily cycles as the data are not sufficiently detailed. The longest cycle that we can consider is one in which the length is the whole series since we must have information from the whole cycle. The shortest cycle that we can consider is one with two observations. If we record temperature daily, then we have no

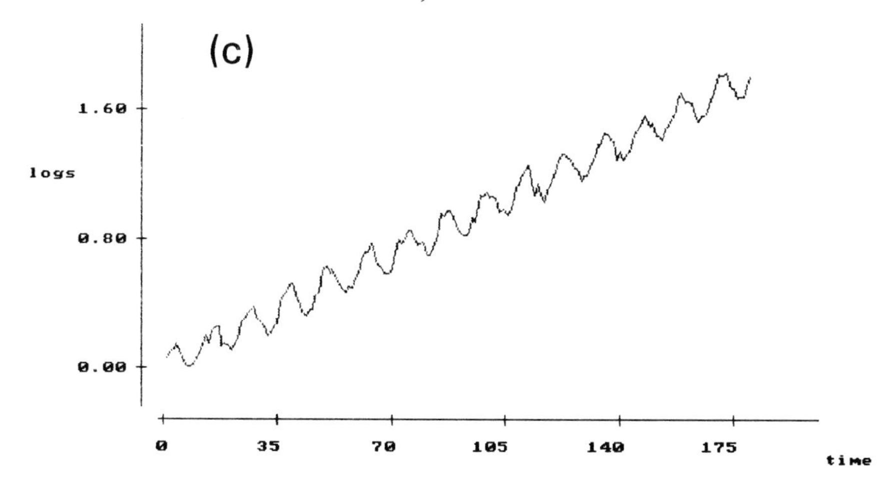

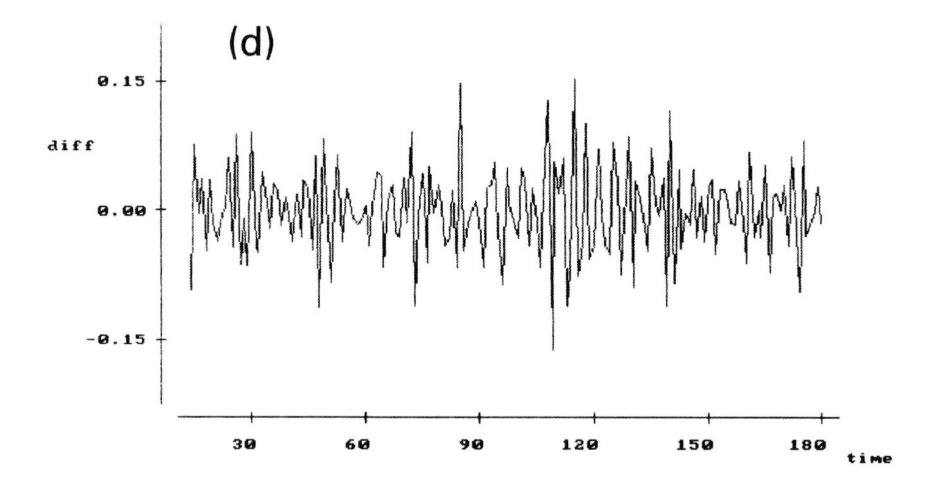

idea about variation within a day. If we record it at noon and at midnight, then at least we know it is hotter during the day than at night.

4.2 Estimating the spectrum

We want, therefore, to be able to estimate the importance of frequencies up to π, not necessarily just at the Fourier frequencies. Much work has been carried out on this problem, recently concentrating on using the Fast Fourier Transform (FFT), a technique for calculating the c_ks very easily and rapidly, and smoothing the resulting values. *Minitab* does not contain a routine for calculating this transform and the facilities available are not suitable for construction of a macro for this purpose. Nor does it provide an alternative

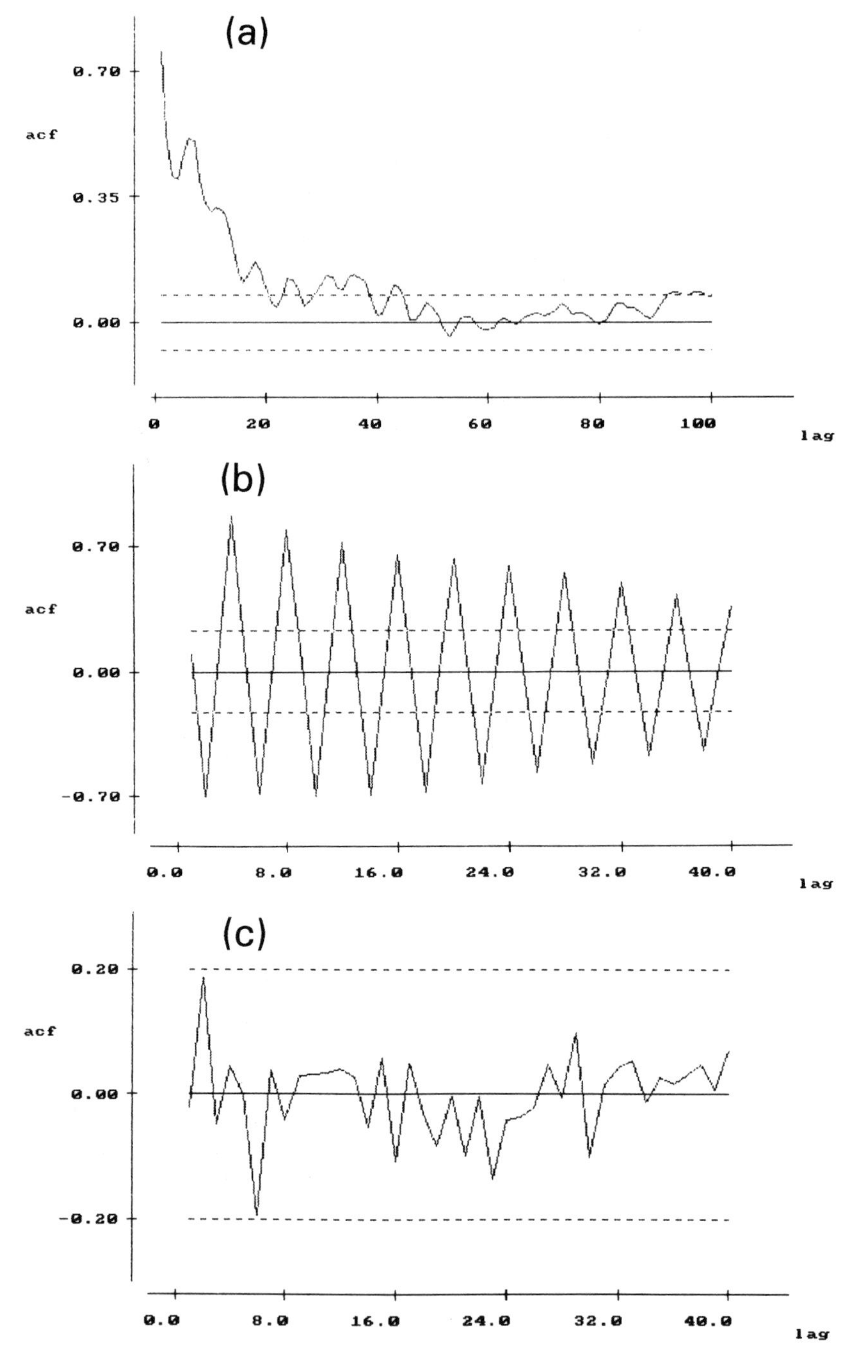

Figure 5. Correlograms of (a) EEG series, (b) heart deaths series, and (c) white noise series.

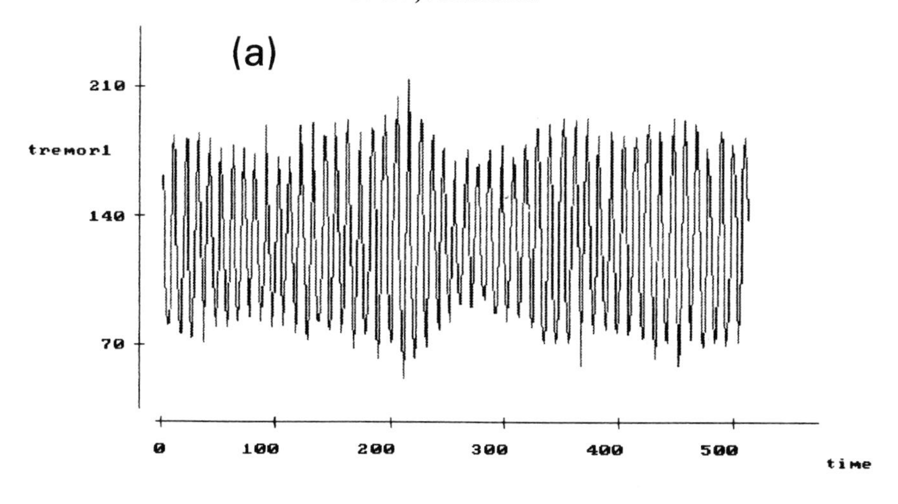

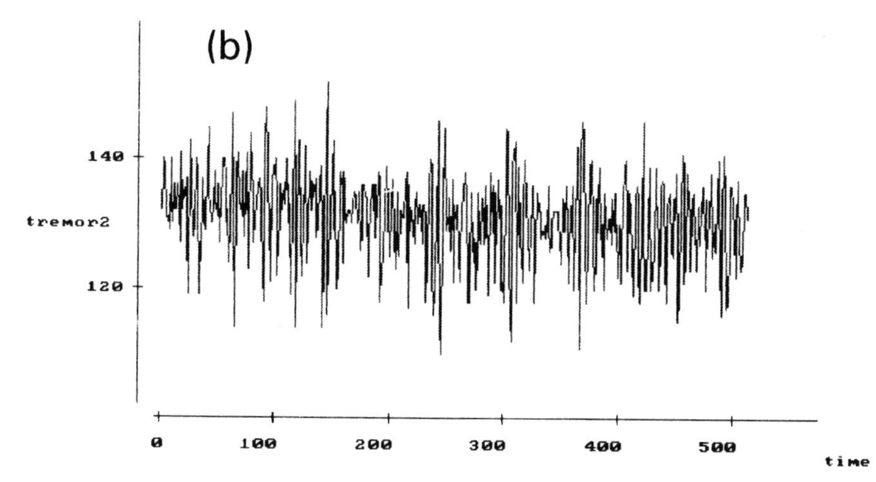

Figure 6. Two series of 512 readings of hand tremor from (a) a patient with essential tremor and (b) a healthy subject.

method for computing the required estimates. We have provided, therefore, a macro to calculate estimates by a different method. This is equivalent to using an FFT and smoothing the results, but is computationally greatly inferior. It involves calculating, for any frequency ω, spectral estimates as a weighted combination of autocorrelations, namely

$$\frac{4\pi}{n} c(0) \left(1 + 2 \sum_{k=1}^{m} r(k)\lambda(k)\cos(k\omega)\right), \tag{1}$$

where $r(k)$ denotes the value of the acf at lag k, $\lambda(k)$ is a weighting function described shortly, and $c(0)$ is the series variance. The number m of terms in

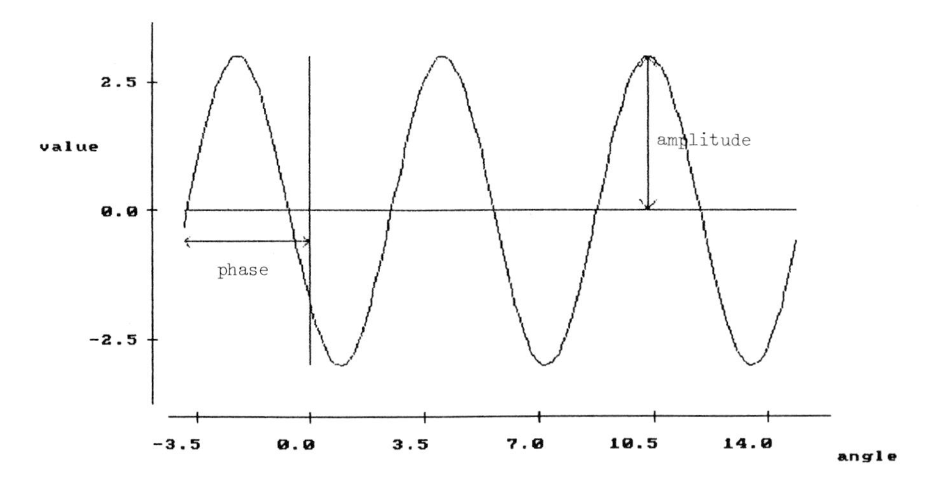

Figure 7. A sinusoidal wave showing the amplitude and phase.

the sum is called the *truncation point*. This is generally chosen to be large, but much smaller than n. The function $\lambda(k)$ is called a lag window. Historically much work has gone into investigating different forms of this. Two of the most commonly used ones are:

$$\text{Bartlett:} \quad \lambda(k) = 1 - k/m \qquad 1 \leqslant k \leqslant m;$$

and

$$\text{Parzen:} \quad \lambda(k) = \begin{cases} 1 - 6u^2 + 6\,u^3 & 1 \leqslant k \leqslant m/2; \\ 2(1 - u)^3 & m/2 \leqslant k \leqslant m; \end{cases}$$

where $u = k/m$. Although this seems to have little connection with the c_k^2 described earlier, the values produced are equivalent, apart from a scaling factor, to those produced by an appropriate smoothing of the periodogram. Applying (1) is very easy from a computational point of view, although it is not a fast procedure. This procedure has been implemented in a *Minitab* macro, SPECT (see *Appendix 7.17*). This uses the Bartlett window above but could be trivially modified to apply a different one, such as Parzen's window. All the user need specify are the column number of the series and the truncation point m. There is no firm rule for this. Essentially the point is that small values of m lead to a very smooth plot with estimates of the true values possibly biased but with small variance, while a large value preserves more detail but has larger variance. A rough guide is that m should be, for series of moderate length, between $n/5$ and $n/10$, say.

We have stated that a large peak indicates some periodic component at about that frequency, but interpretation is not always so simple. If the periodic variation is not sinusoidal in nature—for example it could have a sawtooth pattern—then a peak will still occur at about the correct frequency ω, say, but there are likely to be peaks at harmonics, that is frequencies which are multiples of ω. It does not mean that there are necessarily periodic components at these frequencies, but they are the product of the process of representing the periodic component in terms of sine waves. This is illustrated by the graphs in *Figure 8*. Here the series appears to have a period of about 21, that is it repeats itself after 21 time units have elapsed. This means that its frequency is $\omega = 2\pi/21 \approx 0.3$ and that is indeed where the peak occurs in the spectrum. There are other smaller peaks at frequencies approximately 0.6, 0.9, and 1.2, i.e. at harmonics of 0.3. If the series contains a trend then this tends to show up in the spectrum via a large value at the lowest frequencies; it is being interpreted as the relevant part of a sine wave of very low frequency.

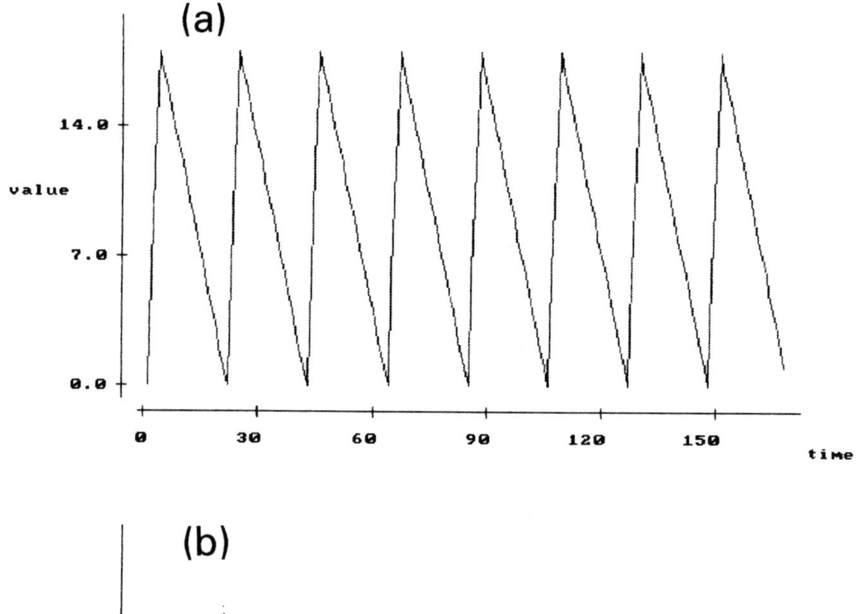

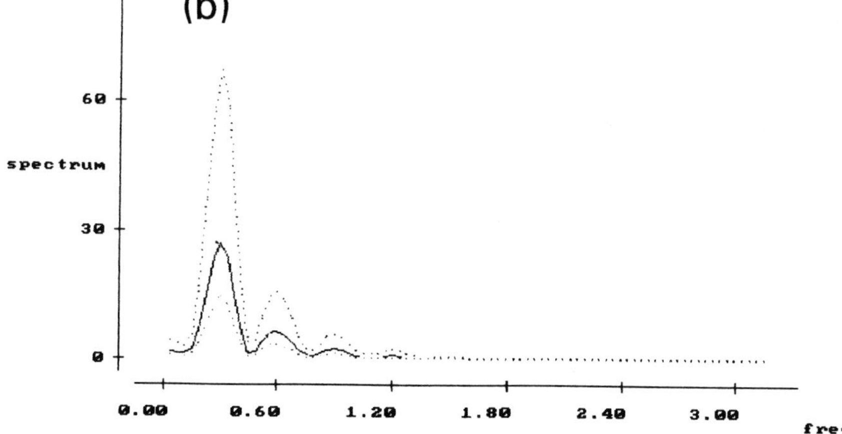

Figure 8. Plots of (a) saw tooth series and (b) its spectral estimate.

To illustrate the use of the frequency domain, *Figure 9* contains the spectral estimates of three series. Firstly shown is that of a series of length 100 of independent observations, white noise. Then we have the spectra of the two hand tremor series referred to earlier. The white noise spectrum (*Figure 9a*) shows no particular features—theoretically it should be constant. Although there are some peaks and troughs, these are not particularly large compared with the general variability of the spectrum. For the series with a clear periodic component the result is a very large peak corresponding to the frequency of the obvious periodicity (*Figure 9b*). For the other tremor series there is a clear peak (*Figure 9c*), showing evidence of a periodic component which was not entirely obvious from the data. For the latter two series, of length 512, the truncation point was taken to be 64, in line with the rule of thumb given earlier. For the white noise series it was 20. It is possible to derive confidence limits for the true values of the spectrum, that is the underlying function which we are estimating here. These are based on the χ^2 distribution, the number of degrees of freedom depending on the window used and on the values of m and n. 95% confidence limits are plotted by the macro SPECT, using dotted lines. It is also possible to test to see if a peak which occurs in the estimated spectrum is actually significant, although such tests are generally not very powerful. An account of them is contained in Diggle (3).

5. Model fitting

5.1 Autoregressive–moving average models

Consider first a series which does not appear to contain a periodic component. Suppose that, by means of differencing, the series has been reduced to apparent stationarity. Let d be the number of differences taken (in practice this will rarely exceed 2). To this stationary series we fit a model from the class of so-called autoregressive–moving average models (abbreviated to ARMA). These models relate the current value of the series to earlier values and also to values of a series of random errors, often referred to as a white noise series. An ARMA(p,q) model expresses the current series value as a linear combination of the preceding p values, together with an error term for the current time and a linear combination of the q most recent errors. Let x_t denote the current series value and y_t be that obtained after differencing (so $y_t = x_t$ if $d = 0$). If ε_t is the error at time t, then the ARMA(p,q) model for y_t takes the form

$$y_t = c + \varepsilon_t + \varphi_1 y_{t-1} + \ldots + \varphi_p y_{t-p} - \theta_1 \varepsilon_{t-1} - \ldots - \theta_q \varepsilon_{t-q}, \quad (2)$$

where $c, \varphi_1, \ldots, \varphi_p, \theta_1, \ldots, \theta_q$ are constants to be estimated by the fitting process. This model has been expressed in terms of the series obtained after differencing. In terms of the original variable x_t, we say it is an autoregressive,

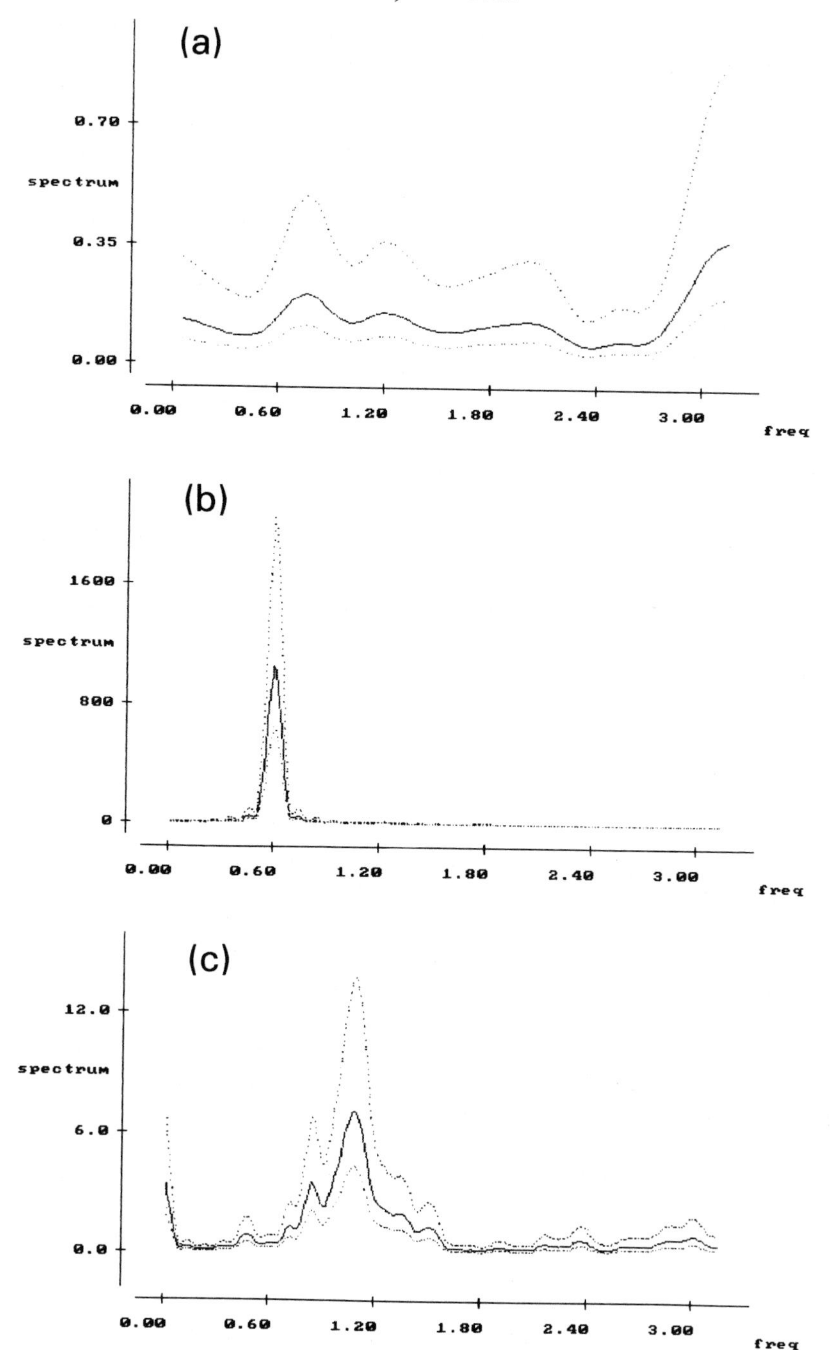

Figure 9. Spectral estimates of (a) white noise series, (b) series of hand tremor from *Figure 6a*, and (c) series of hand tremor from *Figure 6b*.

integrated, moving average process, abbreviated to an ARIMA(p,d,q) process. The constant c is not, in general, equal to the mean, but is related to it and to the other parameters. Although such a model appears rather daunting, in most practical cases the values of p and q are small and fitting such a model is easy in *Minitab*. If $q = 0$ the model is said to be an autoregressive process of order p (abbreviated to AR(p)), while if $p = 0$ it is a moving average model of order q (MA(q)). The autoregressive model is very like a standard multiple regression model, except that the explanatory variables are past values of the actual series. The procedure for fitting an autoregressive model is very like that for a regression model, but when there is a moving average component, there are considerable theoretical and practical difficulties.

Using *Minitab* an ARIMA model can be fitted to a series in column C1 with the single command

```
ARIMA p d q C1
```

By default, a fair amount of output is generated and this requires some explanation. First, however, consider the problem of deciding on appropriate values of p and q. Fortunately there are some simple diagnostic tools which, in some cases at least, give an indication of possible values. Later we shall see an automatic, if rather time-consuming, method for selecting their values.

We shall later consider non-stationary series, but suppose first that no differencing has been necessary so that $d = 0$. There is no obvious trend or other non-stationarity and the acf dies away gradually but reasonably rapidly. First consider the correlogram. In many series the acf gradually dies away, but in some series there is a cut-off, that is a point after which the values of the acf are small in magnitude. If the last value which is substantially different from 0 is at lag q, then this points to an appropriate model being a moving average process of order q. It is not always easy to decide, in a practical case, if a cut-off exists and, if so, at what point. The 95% confidence limits for the acf of white noise given earlier can give a guide to this; if virtually all values after a given lag are within these limits, then there is evidence of a cut-off. The correlogram of such a series is shown in *Figure 10*. For this series there seems to be a cut-off at lag 2, as the acf values are small after that, and an MA(2) model might therefore be appropriate. For that whose acf is shown in *Figure 5a*, while the acf falls to values around the upper confidence limit by about lag 20, it continues to hover around that limit until beyond lag 40. Even after that there is no sudden decrease in magnitude and there is therefore no real evidence of a cut-off; a model other than an MA one is appropriate here.

5.2 The partial autocorrelation function

The correlogram does not give information directly about p but there is another function, the partial autocorrelation function (pacf), which can convey information about its value. The pacf at lag k is a measure of the correlation

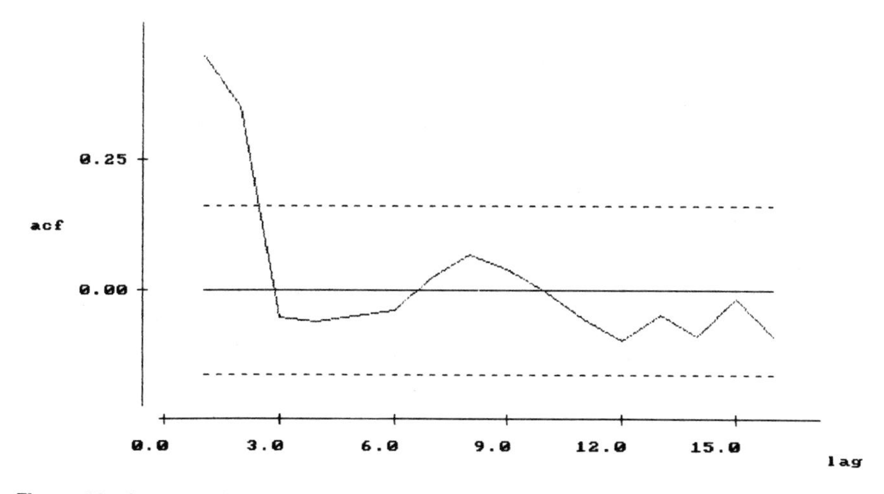

Figure 10. Autocorrelation function showing behaviour typical of an MA(2).

which exists between values k apart in the series which is not due to the intermediate values. If the current value is always correlated with the previous one, then this induces correlation between values two apart; the pacf is a measure of the correlation between these values not induced via the intermediate value. It is easily calculated in *Minitab* using the command PACF. The macro PAUTOCF (see *Appendix 7.17*) plots this in a similar way to that in which AUTOCF plotted the acf. Dotted lines are plotted to indicate the limits beyond which it is reasonable to conclude that values are significantly different from 0; these again lie at $-2/\sqrt{n}$ and $2/\sqrt{n}$. The really useful feature of this plot is that if a series really is an AR(p), then there should be a cut-off in the pacf after lag p; after that all values should be small in the fashion described above for the acf of a MA(q) model. This helps us to identify an autoregressive model. The pacf of a typical such series is shown in *Figure 11*; the graph suggests that an AR(2) model might be appropriate since there seems to be a cut-off in the pacf at lag 2.

These diagnostic tools are useful because it is often difficult to identify the type of model from a plot of the actual series values. To illustrate this, in *Figure 12* three series are plotted. Each has been computer generated using an AR(2) model but with different parameters in the three cases. In the first case the parameters were $\varphi_1 = 1.6$ and $\varphi_2 = -0.8$; here the behaviour for the first part of the series appears to have some periodic characteristics. In the second case $\varphi_1 = 0.6$ and $\varphi_2 = 0.3$. This leads to a strong positive correlation and there are often long runs of observations above or below the mean. In the last case $\varphi_1 = -0.7$ and $\varphi_2 = -0.2$. This time there is negative correlation and consecutive values are often on opposite sides of the mean.

It is quite possible that neither the graph of the acf nor that of the pacf has an obvious cut-off, but both gradually die away. This is indicative of the fact

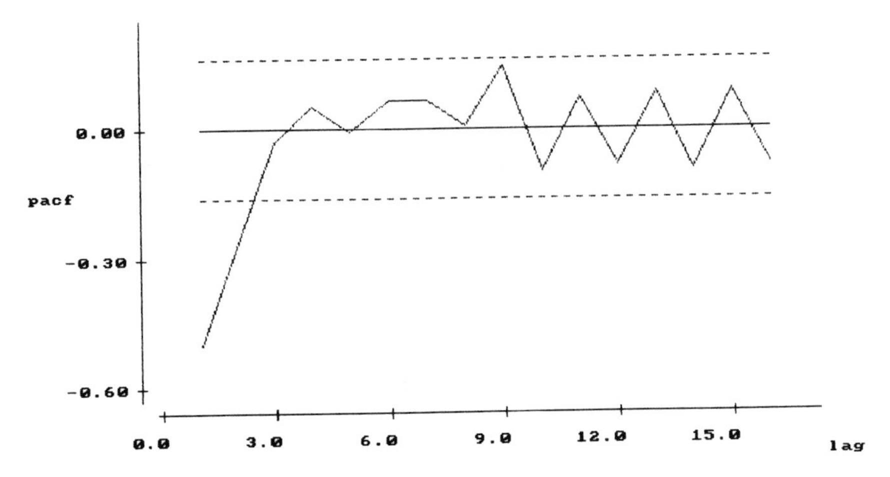

Figure 11. Partial autocorrelation function showing behaviour typical of an AR(2).

that an ARMA model with both p and q at least 1 is appropriate; unfortunately there is no easy way of determining from a simple plot sensible values to take for p and q. We therefore have to find some criterion for deciding appropriate values. Essentially this is done by fitting a number of different models and then examining how well they fit, choosing that which gives the best fit. Before discussing the details of the method, a description of the output from the ARIMA command is needed.

5.3 Fitting the model using *Minitab*

To illustrate the process consider fitting a model (*Protocol 2*) to a series of 99 observations recording weekly the logarithm of the number of heterotrophic bacteria per ml in a pond. The data are listed in *Appendix 7.7*. A graph of the series, together with the correlogram and plot of the pacf, is shown in *Figure 13*. There is no obvious non-stationarity, so we will try $d = 0$. The acf gradually decreases, but the pacf seems to be rather small after the first value. Therefore an AR(1) model may be appropriate. Such a model is fitted with the command

```
ARIMA 1 0 0 C1
```

assuming the data are contained in column C1.

The algorithm for fitting the model is an iterative one and in this case six iterations were needed for the method to converge. The first part of the output, which is shown in *Figure 14*, lists the results of each iterative step and is not needed for the final model. Next are shown the final estimates of, in this case, the AR parameter φ_1 and of the constant (c in the model; equation (2)) together with estimates of their standard deviations. An estimate of the series

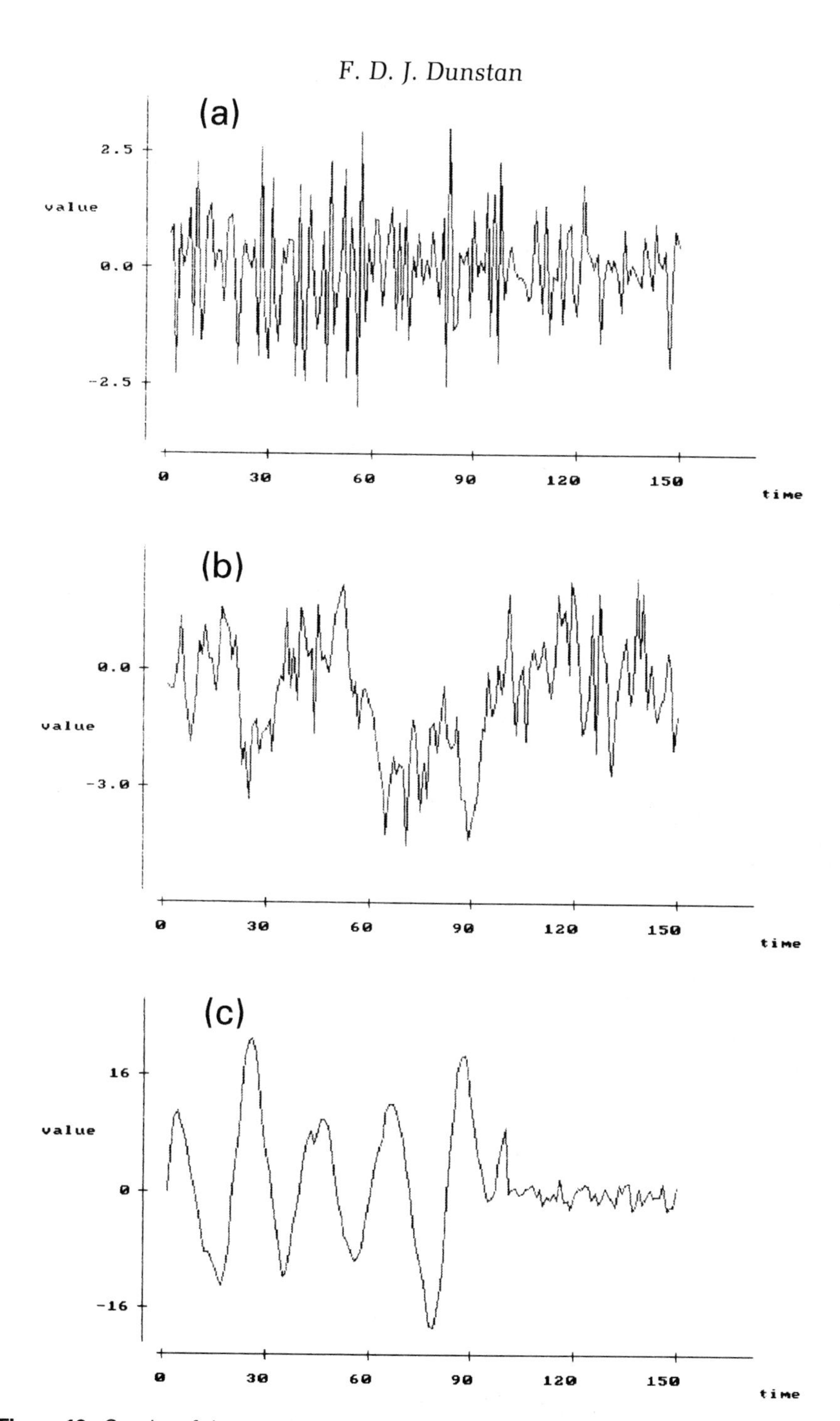

Figure 12. Graphs of three series all generated from AR(2) models; (a) $\varphi_1 = 1.6$, $\varphi_2 = -0.8$; (b) $\varphi_1 = 0.6$, $\varphi_2 = 0.3$; (c) $\varphi_1 = -0.7$, $\varphi_2 = -0.2$.

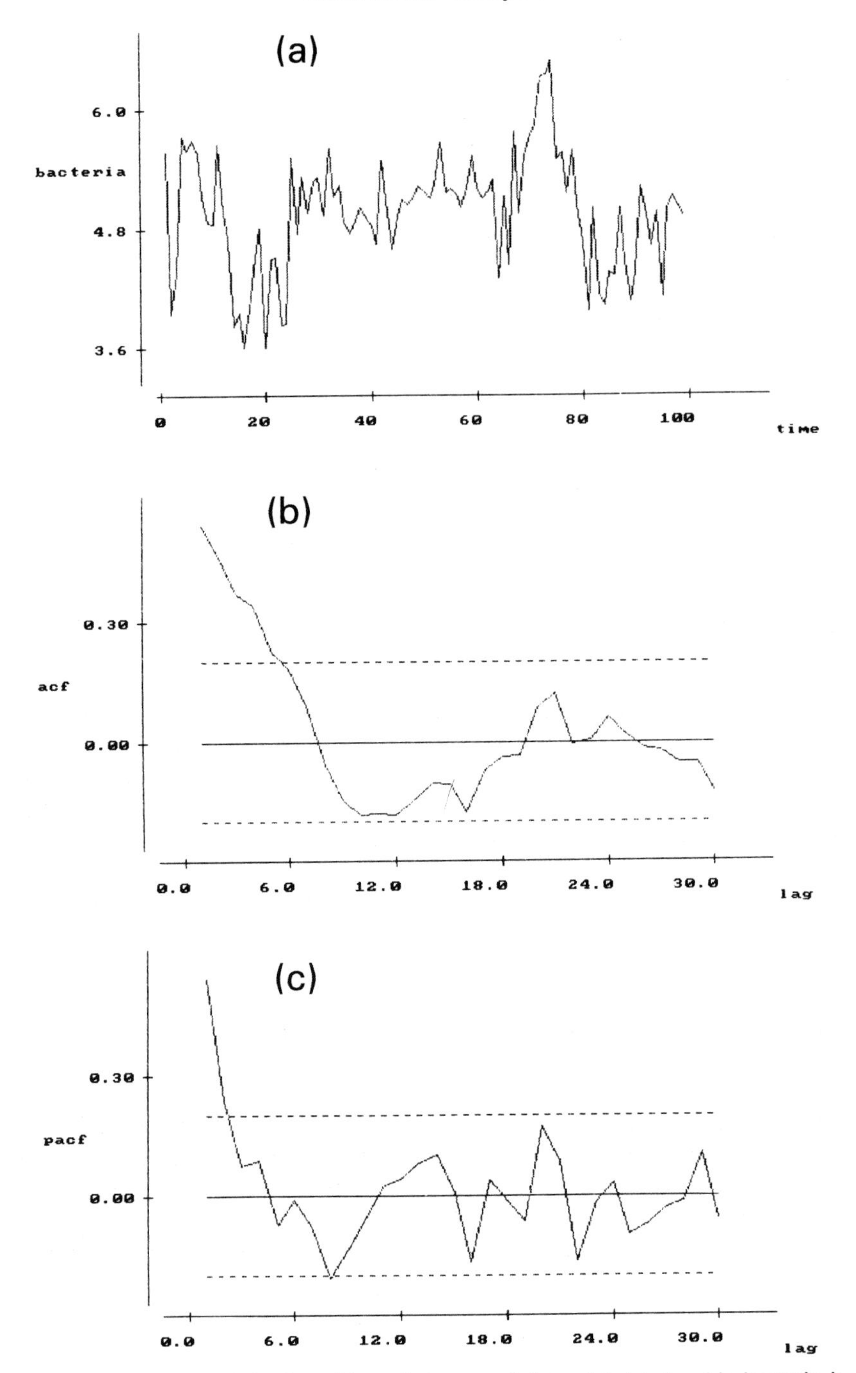

Figure 13. (a) Series of the logarithm of the population of heterotrophic bacteria in a freshwater pond, with its (b) correlogram and (c) partial autocorrelation function.

```
MTB > arima 1 0 0 c1

Estimates at each iteration
Iteration          SSE       Parameters
    0           31.2131      0.100      4.557
    1           27.0463      0.250      3.784
    2           24.5484      0.400      3.012
    3           23.7170      0.538      2.300
    4           23.7106      0.548      2.247
    5           23.7106      0.548      2.244
    6           23.7106      0.548      2.244
Relative change in each estimate less than  0.0010

Final Estimates of Parameters
Type         Estimate       St. Dev.   t-ratio
AR    1        0.5485        0.0848       6.47
Constant     2.24424        0.04961      45.24
Mean           4.9702        0.1099

No. of obs.:    99
Residuals:      SS = 23.6316   (backforecasts excluded)
                MS =  0.2436   DF = 97

Modified Box-Pierce chisquare statistic
Lag                     12              24             36              48
Chisquare     12.0(DF=11)    24.4(DF=23)    30.8(DF=35)    44.8(DF=47)
```

Figure 14. *Minitab* output from fitting an AR(1) model to the series of *Figure 13a*.

mean is also shown. This is related to, but not the same as, the constant c. The 't-ratio', simply the ratio of each estimate to its standard deviation, is also shown. This can be compared with percentiles of the t-distribution with degrees of freedom equal to the series length minus the number of fitted parameters, in this case 97. These percentiles are listed in *Appendix B.6*. The program automatically calculates the residuals. These are analogous to the residuals in a regression model. The model fitted in this case, an AR(1) model, is of the form

$$x_t = c + \varepsilon_t + \varphi_1 x_{t-1}.$$

If the estimates of c and φ_1 are denoted by $\hat{c}$ and $\hat{\varphi}_1$, then the residual at t is

$$e_t = x_t - \hat{c} - \hat{\varphi}_1 x_{t-1}$$

(with a slight modification for $t = 1$). The sum of squares of the residuals is shown as 'SS = 23.6316' and also listed is the mean sum of squares, i.e. this sum divided by the degrees of freedom. This fitting process is straightforward, but how do we know if the model is appropriate? One way is to plot the residuals to see if any obvious pattern exists. The residuals can be stored by adding to the previous command and using

```
ARIMA 1 0 0 C1 C2
```

This command will work as before but will also store the residuals in column C2, so they can be inspected and plotted if required. A test has been formulated to consider whether or not a fitted model was the correct one. It uses the fact that the residuals should (if the model was correct) have little autocorrelation, and the test uses the acf of the series of residuals. The test is sometimes called the Ljung–Box test, but *Minitab* refers to it as a modified Box–Pierce test. It is based on a number, k say, of the squared autocorrelations of the residuals. The statistic produced has, under the hypothesis of the model fitted being correct, an approximate χ^2 distribution, with degrees of freedom equal to $k - p - q$, that is the number of autocorrelations included minus the total number of φs and θs in the model. *Minitab* actually gives the values for k = 12,24,36, and 48. In this case, if we take $k = 24$, the value of the statistic is 24.4 with 23 degrees of freedom. We can find the P-value from *Appendix B.8* or, more accurately, by using the *Minitab* CDF command, i.e.

```
CDF 24.4 K1;
CHISQUARE 23.
LET K2 = 1 - K1
PRINT K2
```

Here the value is $P = 0.382$, which is clearly not significant at conventional levels; to be significant at a level of 5%, for example, P must be less than 0.05. It is perhaps a little dangerous to look at all four values given, for different values of k, as there is a much greater chance of one exceeding a critical value and being significant if all four are considered. It is probably wisest to choose in advance to consider the value of the statistic for a given value of k and to base the test on that result. There is no accepted 'best' value of k to take here; usually it should be chosen to be reasonably large, but small compared with the series length. Here its value has been taken to be 24. Having carried out such a test it is advisable to make a visual inspection of the residuals and their correlogram. These are shown in *Figures 15a* and *15b*. There is no obvious pattern in the residuals and the acf values all lie well within the white noise limits, apparently confirming the appropriateness of the model selected.

Protocol 2. Fitting an ARMA model to a stationary series

1. Examine the acf (using AUTOCF[a]) and pacf (using PAUTOCF) of the series to try to determine the values of p (in pacf, as the AR order) and q (in acf, as the MA order) by identifying cut-offs, if they exist.
2. Use the *Minitab* command

   ```
   ARIMA p 0 q C1
   ```

   with the column containing the data being C1 in this example.
3. Check that the Box–Pierce value is not significant.
4. Plot the residuals (using TPLOT) and their acf (using AUTOCF) to see if there is any obvious pattern

- random residuals and acf inside confidence bands indicates a good model
- pattern in residuals and/or acf outside confidence bands indicates a poor model

[a] Unless stated otherwise *Minitab* macro names are in capital letters.

5.4 Determining the order of the model

In practice the fact that a model passes this test does not necessarily mean that it is the unique correct model, but rather that it provides a satisfactory fit. A

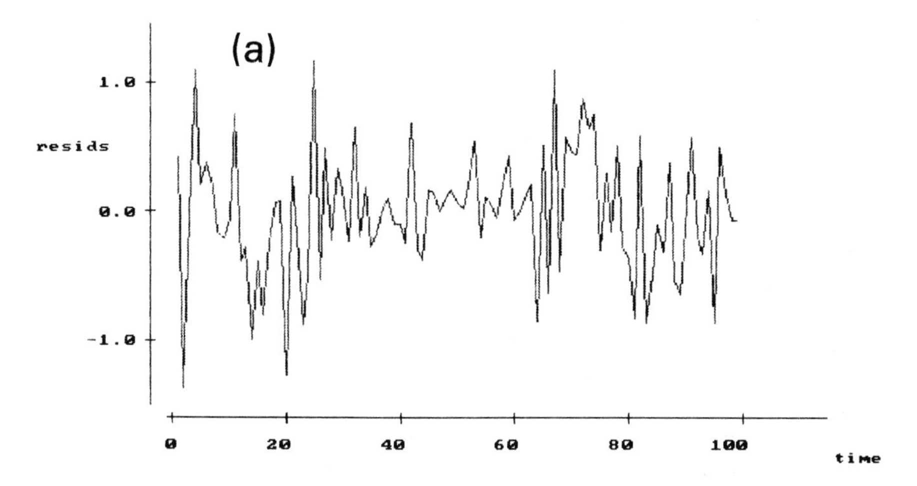

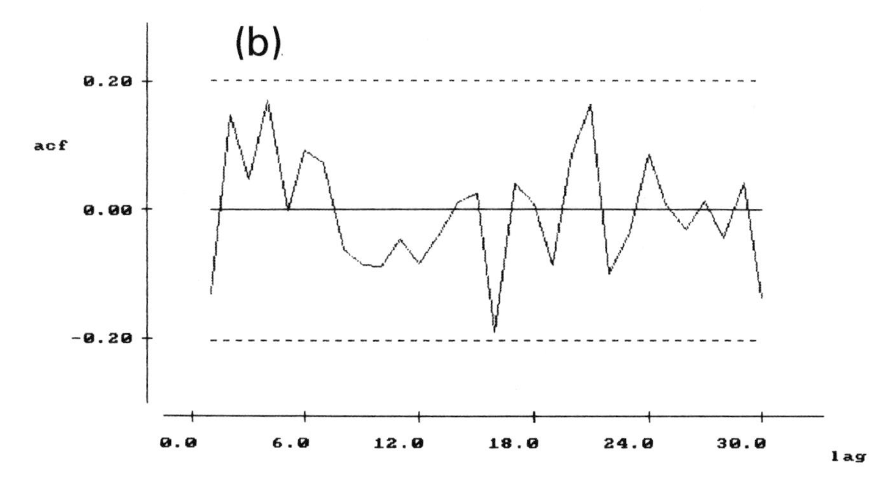

Figure 15. (a) Residuals from fitting an AR(1) model to the series of *Figure 13a* and (b) the correlogram of the residuals.

number of different models might pass the test, and we have to find a way of choosing between them. In a way the situation is rather like that in multiple regression, where adding extra terms to a model leads to a better fit, but sometimes the improvement is very small and does not justify the inclusion of extra parameters (see Chapter 4, Section 6). To help in model selection, methods based on what are called information criteria have become popular. This involves calculating, for each model fitted, a function which takes into account the goodness of fit and the number of parameters fitted. For normal time series this criterion reduces to the form

$$n \times \log_e \text{(residual variance)} + \text{no. of fitted parameters} \times \text{penalty}$$

Here n is the series length and the residual variance is the mean residual sum of squares (MS in the *Minitab* output). The number of fitted parameters is simply $p + q + 1$ (remembering that c has to be estimated). The idea behind the criterion is that a better fit gives a smaller residual variance, reducing the first term, but if this occurs because extra parameters have been included, then a penalty is incurred. The method involves choosing the model which minimizes the value of this criterion. The hope is that it gives a trade-off between the conflicting demands of a good fit and the use of few parameters. Different suggestions have been put forward for the penalty to be attached to each parameter. Akaike (8) suggested a penalty of 2 per parameter and for a time this was very popular; it does tend to give models containing a lot of parameters, however, and has been shown to tend to overfit. Schwarz's criterion (9) uses a penalty of $\log_e n$ for each parameter and that is what is used here, in the macro FIT (see *Appendix 7.19*). This fits a range of models, specified by the user, and chooses that which minimizes the value of the criterion. The user specifies the maximum values of p and q and the program fits all models whose AR order is at most p and whose MA order is at most q, listing at the end, the models fitted, together with the associated values of Schwarz's criterion:

$$\text{SCH} = n \times \log_e \text{(residual variance)} + (p + q + 1) \times \log_e n.$$

For the bacterial series considered above the results are as follows. The maximum value of p was taken to be 4 and that of q was taken as 1. The values of the criterion were:

p	q	SCH
1	0	−137.23
2	0	−138.02
3	0	−133.83
4	0	−130.19
0	1	−123.70
1	1	−138.48
2	1	−134.04
3	1	−129.45
4	1	−126.05

If we select the model which minimizes this criterion, the chosen one is an ARMA(1,1), with the minimum value of −138.48. For that model the revised Box–Pierce statistic was 23.4 based on 22 degrees of freedom, a value which is definitely not significant; its *P*-value was 0.379. It is definitely advisable to examine the value of this statistic even for the selected model as it could be that none of those considered is appropriate. Note that for almost all of the models fitted, the Box–Pierce statistic was not significant. This shows the usefulness of a criterion for model selection. Note that the fact that the values of SCH are negative here need not cause concern; they simply reflect the fact that the residual variance here is less than 1, giving negative logarithms.

5.5 Fitting models to non-stationary series

5.5.1 Series with no periodic component

The method presented above applied to series which appeared to be stationary so that no differencing had taken place. Suppose now that a series appears to have a trend but no seasonal effect, so that some first differences should produce stationarity. Suppose that d such differences have been taken (in practice d will rarely exceed 2). We can fit an ARMA model to the differenced series, but it is easier to simply use the value of d in the ARIMA command. Thus to fit an ARMA(3,2) to a series of first differences we would simply type

```
ARIMA 3 1 2 C1
```

The form of the Schwarz criterion changes slightly. Firstly a differenced series will generally have no constant term included (forming $x_t - x_{t-1}$ removes the term c) and *Minitab* assumes no constant unless requested. Hence there is one parameter fewer to estimate. Also, the series contains one fewer observation than before for each difference taken. To accommodate this the criterion becomes

$$\text{SCH} = (n - d)\log_e(\text{residual variance}) + \frac{n}{n - d} \times (p + q)\log_e n.$$

The macro FIT will calculate this automatically and this enables models involving differences to be compared with those which do not.

5.5.2 Series with a periodic component

Suppose now that a series contains a periodic component. How do we model this? The family of ARIMA models can be extended to cover these. Suppose that the period of the component has length s. As has been indicated, it is useful to take an sth difference to produce a stationary series. It has been found that even after that, there tends to be correlation remaining at lags which are multiples of s. To deal with this, some further seasonal terms are incorporated into the model.

Suppose the series x_t under consideration has a periodic component with period s. We may take d first differences and D seasonal differences (that is perform the operation of the form $x_t - x_{t-s}$ D times). We write the new series as $\nabla^d \nabla_s^D x_t = y_t$ say. To this new series, which we hope is stationary, we fit a seasonal ARIMA model. To explain this it is simplest to introduce some new notation. The backshift operation B is defined by

$$\mathrm{B}x_t = x_{t-1}.$$

So the effect of applying B is to change the time by one unit. In this notation the first difference is

$$\nabla x_t = x_t - x_{t-1} = x_t - \mathrm{B}x_t = (1 - \mathrm{B})x_t.$$

Similarly a seasonal difference is

$$\nabla_s x_t = x_t - x_{t-s} = x_t - \mathrm{B}^s x_t = (1 - \mathrm{B}^s)x_t.$$

The ARMA model introduced earlier can be written as

$$x_t - \varphi_1 x_{t-1} - \ldots - \varphi_p x_{t-p} = \varepsilon_t - \theta_1 \varepsilon_{t-1} - \ldots - \theta_q \varepsilon_{t-q}.$$

Using the backshift notation this is

$$(1 - \varphi_1 \mathrm{B} - \ldots - \varphi_p \mathrm{B}^p)x_t = (1 - \theta_1 \mathrm{B} - \ldots - \theta_q \mathrm{B}^q)\varepsilon_t.$$

So we have two polynomials of orders p and q in B corresponding to the autoregressive and moving average parts of the model. A seasonal ARMA model incorporates also polynomials of orders P and Q with argument B^s, these multiplying the ordinary polynomials above. So the full model would be

$$(1 - \varphi_1 \mathrm{B} - \ldots - \varphi_p \mathrm{B}^p)\,(1 - \alpha_1 \mathrm{B}^s - \ldots - \alpha_P \mathrm{B}^{Ps})\nabla^d \nabla_s{}^D x_t$$
$$= (1 - \theta_1 \mathrm{B} - \ldots - \theta_q \mathrm{B}^q)\,(1 - \beta_1 \mathrm{B}^s - \ldots - \beta_Q \mathrm{B}^{Qs})\varepsilon_t.$$

This is called, both in the literature and by *Minitab*, an ARIMA$(p,d,q) \times (P,D,Q)s$ model. The s refers to the period of seasonality and the upper case letters to the orders of the various seasonal components. Thus D is the number of seasonal differences taken and P and Q are the numbers of terms in the polynomials of the seasonal part of the model. This looks very daunting in its full form, so we consider two simple special cases.

An ARIMA $(0,1,1) \times (0,1,1)4$ model would have the form

$$\nabla \nabla_4 x_t = (1 - \theta\mathrm{B})(1 - \beta\mathrm{B}^4)\varepsilon_t, \qquad (3)$$

i.e.

$$\nabla \nabla_4 x_t = \varepsilon_t - \theta\varepsilon_{t-1} - \beta\varepsilon_{t-4} + \theta\beta\varepsilon_{t-5}.$$

This has been found to be very useful for modelling many seasonal series. An ARIMA $(1,0,0) \times (1,1,1)12$ model would have the form

$$(1 - \varphi\mathrm{B})\,(1 - \alpha\mathrm{B}^{12})y_t = (1 - \beta\mathrm{B}^{12})\varepsilon_t,$$

or, in longhand,

$$y_t = \varepsilon_t - \beta\varepsilon_{t-12} + \varphi y_{t-1} + \alpha y_{t-12} - \varphi\alpha y_{t-13}, \tag{4}$$

where $y_t = \nabla_{12}x_t = x_t - x_{t-12}$. The notation is very complicated, but without it there is no easy way of writing the models and interpretation of *Minitab* output becomes very difficult, as this notation is implicit in the *Minitab* commands and output. In spite of this the fitting of such models is easy. To fit a model of this type the command is simply of the form

ARIMA *p d q P D Q s* C1

where C1 is the column containing the data. For example, the model defined by Equation 4 will be fitted by the command

ARIMA 1 0 0 1 1 1 12 C1

Note that the command has the same form as for non-seasonal models, but with extra parameters. If the seasonal component is not included explicitly, it is omitted.

To illustrate the procedure (for summary see *Protocol 3*), consider the data on deaths due to heart disease (*Figure 1b*). There is a very obvious seasonal effect, the data being quarterly with an annual period. There is some slight evidence of a downwards trend—certainly the values at the end of the series are a little less than at the start. These remarks suggest that we could take $d = D = 1$ with $s = 4$. The correlogram of the resulting differenced series (by lags of 1 and 4 with macro DFF) is shown in *Figure 16a*. The most noticeable features are the large absolute values at lags 1 and 4, together with the fact that there is no evidence of gradually declining terms characteristic of an AR component. Thus we take $p = P = 0$. There still seems to be some evidence of periodicity and so a term should be included to represent this. The large value of the acf at lag 1 suggests an MA term of lag 1 and so we take $q = 1$. To deal with the remaining periodicity we select a seasonal MA term with $Q = 1$. We therefore fit a model using the command

ARIMA 0 1 1 0 1 1 4 C1

if the data are in column 1. The resulting output is shown in *Figure 17*, omitting the iterative steps. The two parameters are referred to as MA 1 and SMA 4; these refer respectively to the parameter of an ordinary MA(1) model (θ in Equation 3 above) and a seasonal moving average term of lag 4 (β in Equation 3). Their standard errors are also shown, together with the *t*-ratio which gives a measure of the importance of their inclusion. The output confirms that an ordinary (termed regular here) and a seasonal difference of order 4 were both applied and gives the residual and mean sums of squares.

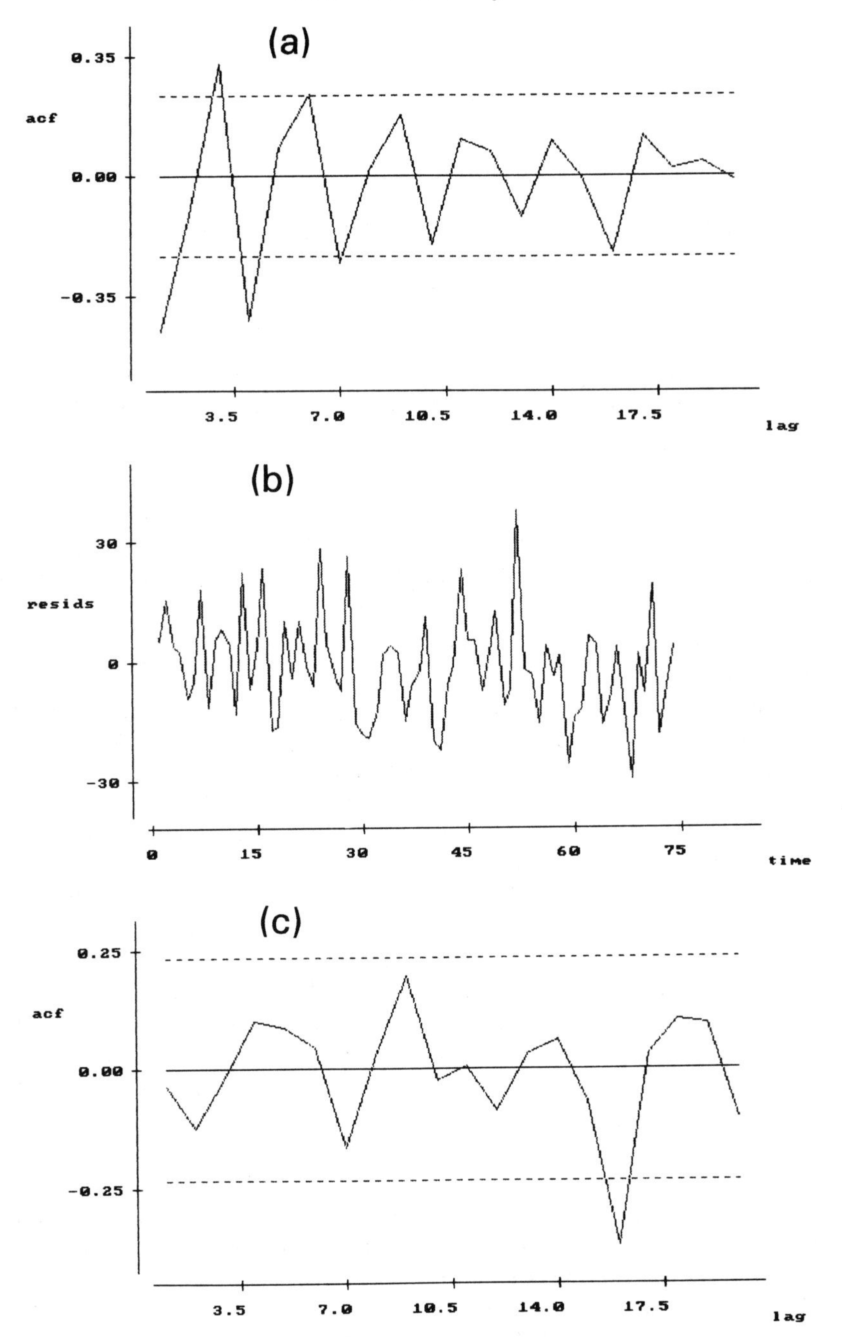

Figure 16. (a) The correlogram of the series of heart deaths after an ordinary and a seasonal difference have been calculated, (b) the residuals after the specified ARIMA model has been fitted, and (c) the correlogram of the residuals.

```
MTB > arima 0 1 1 0 1 1 4 c1

Final Estimates of Parameters
Type        Estimate      St. Dev.    t-ratio
MA   1       0.7157        0.0831       8.61
SMA  4       0.9080        0.0697      13.02

Differencing: 1 regular, 1 seasonal of order 4
No. of obs.:  Original series 79, after differencing 74
Residuals:    SS = 13041.6  (backforecasts excluded)
              MS =   181.1  DF = 72

Modified Box-Pierce chisquare statistic
Lag                 12              24              36              48
Chisquare     9.2(DF=10)     28.0(DF=22)     36.2(DF=34)     57.1(DF=46)
```

Figure 17. *Minitab* output, without iterative steps, from fitting a seasonal ARIMA 0,1,1,0,1,1,4 model to the series of deaths from heart disease shown in *Figure 1b*.

Finally the modified Box–Pierce statistics are shown. In this case the value for 22 degrees of freedom is 28.0; the *P*-value of this is 0.260 and so there is no reason to doubt the validity of the model. Again a visual inspection of the residuals and of their correlogram is valuable. These are shown in *Figures 16b* and *16c* respectively and suggest that the model is satisfactory.

Choosing the orders of the various components of the model is rather harder in the seasonal case; there are more parameters to be specified and fewer readily available diagnostic tools. It is possible to use an automatic criterion, such as that of Schwarz described earlier. This is easy to adapt to the more general case. A macro has not been provided since the range of models that might be specified is potentially so large that the execution time would be prohibitive. One pragmatic approach is to choose and fit a plausible model, as we did above, and then to deliberately overfit by trying a different model containing the same parameters but with extra ones too. So in the above case, for the heart deaths data, we might fit a second model containing autoregressive terms, such as a $(1,1,1) \times (1,1,1)4$ model or even include extra moving average terms. If the values of the extra parameters are small, and if the residual sum of squares has changed little, then the larger model is not justified. In this case if the AR terms are included the resulting estimates (in the above notation) are

$$\varphi = -0.0065 \quad \alpha = 0.1158 \quad \theta = 0.7316 \quad \beta = 0.9122,$$

with residual sum of squares 12 865.1 (compared with 13 041.6 for the simpler model). Thus there is no real evidence that the extra terms are worth including and the simpler model is adopted. It is also worthwhile plotting the residuals, as was done above, to check that no obvious pattern exists which was not detected by the value of the Box–Pierce statistic. For example, the macro SPECT could be applied to the residuals to investigate any remaining periodicities.

Protocol 3. Fitting a general ARIMA model

1. As a result of the initial investigation, decide on the differencing and any transformations which are needed to produce a stationary series (see *Protocol 1*).
2. Examine the acf (using AUTOCF[a]) and pacf (using PAUTOCF) to try to identify p and q (from cut-offs in pacf and acf, respectively) in the ARIMA model.
3. If there is no periodic component use the macro FIT, choosing maximum values for p (as order of AR) and q (as order of MA) in line with the results of step 2.
4. The macro FIT will identify the model with the minimum of Schwarz's criterion:
   - check that the Box–Pierce statistic is not significant by examining its *P*-value
   - plot the residuals, as an extra check, looking for any obvious pattern as remaining non-stationarity.
5. If there is a periodic component of period s fit an ARMA $(p,d,q) \times (P,D,Q)s$ model, trying low values of P and Q:
   - use *Minitab* command

     ```
     ARIMA p d q P D Q s C1
     ```

     where C1 contains the original time series.
   - check the Box–Pierce statistic again
6. Test overfitting with extra parameters, which should be very small if the model is suitable. If model is unsuitable fit a new model (step 5).

[a] Unless stated otherwise *Minitab* macro names are in capital letters.

6. Prediction

In many contexts it is of great interest to try to predict future values of a series. This is most unlikely to be of interest in a case like an EEG or hand tremor series, but could be of great interest in the series of deaths due to heart disease or in series recording the numbers of certain organisms in a particular area. The full details of the methodology involved are beyond the scope of this chapter, but there is no difficulty in obtaining the predictions, or forecasts as they are often referred to, and confidence limits for them. The basic rationale behind the method can be explained by a very simple example. Consider a seasonal ARIMA model (1,1,0) × (0,1,0)4 model; that is

$$(1 - \varphi B)\nabla\nabla_4 x_t = \varepsilon_t.$$

Written in longhand this appears to be much more complicated, and is

$$x_t = (1 + \varphi)x_{t-1} - \varphi x_{t-2} + x_{t-4} - (1 + \varphi)x_{t-5} + \varphi x_{t-6} + \varepsilon_t.$$

Suppose we have observations recorded up to $t = 100$, say. To forecast the 101st, we set $t = 101$ on the right-hand side. As ε_{101} will be independent of previous values, we can best predict it to be 0. The remaining terms are all known and the prediction can be evaluated. Thus the predicted value is

$$\hat{x}_{101} = (1 + \varphi)x_{100} - \varphi x_{99} + x_{97} - (1 + \varphi)x_{96} + \varphi x_{95}.$$

For the 102nd observation we apply the same argument, except that the value x_{101} now appears. As this is not known we replace it by its predicted value, and continue in this way, obtaining

$$\hat{x}_{102} = (1 + \varphi)\hat{x}_{101} - \varphi x_{100} + x_{98} - (1 + \varphi)x_{97} + \varphi x_{96}$$

and so on. The details are much more complicated if moving average terms are involved, but fortunately *Minitab* does all the work and can calculate forecasts and confidence limits. To obtain them a sub-command is needed. In this the number of steps ahead for which forecasts are needed must be specified, and column numbers can be given for storing the forecasts and their confidence limits. Thus the command

```
ARIMA 0 1 1 0 1 1 4 C1 C2;
FORECASTS 16 C3 C4 C5.
```

would fit an ARIMA (0,1,1) × (0,1,1)4 model to data in column 1, store the residuals in column 2, and would store forecasts of the next 16 values in column 3, putting the lower and upper 95% confidence limits in columns 4 and 5. If the columns are not specified in the FORECASTS sub-command, then the values are printed automatically.

To demonstrate the method, we use the example on deaths due to heart disease. Rather than fitting a model to the whole series, we fit a model to the data from the first 17 years, i.e. 68 observations, and use this to forecast values for the next 16 quarters. For the first 11 of these the actual values are known, so that the quality of the forecasts can be judged. The model fitted is of the same form as before, that is an ARIMA (0 1 1) × (0 1 1)4, but with slightly different parameters. The forecasts are listed in *Figure 18*, together with the lower and upper 95% confidence limits and the actual values for the first 11 lead times, the lead time being simply the time between the current time and the observation being predicted, i.e. the number of steps ahead.

As can be seen the forecasts for rows 5 and 9 are too high; in both cases the observed value actually lies below the lower limit of the confidence interval. There is some evidence from the graph of the data (*Figures 1b, 2a*) that there is a decline in the number of deaths towards the end of the series. It is possible that in fitting a model to the reduced data set, this has not been accounted for fully; it could be that a different model is needed for the last part of the series

```
MTB > arima 0 1 1 0 1 1 4 c1 c2;
SUBC> forecasts 16 c3 c4 c5.
```

Lead	quarter	lower	forecast	upper	actual
1	69	384.576	410.429	436.283	392
2	70	327.698	354.320	380.943	340
3	71	282.327	309.697	337.066	305
4	72	338.278	366.375	394.471	347
5	73	381.415	410.611	439.806	367
6	74	324.539	354.502	384.465	335
7	75	279.166	309.878	340.590	282
8	76	335.113	366.556	397.999	362
9	77	378.267	410.792	443.317	369
10	78	321.386	354.683	387.980	323
11	79	276.008	310.059	344.111	287
12	80	331.947	366.737	401.527	
13	81	375.110	410.973	446.837	
14	82	318.221	354.864	391.507	
15	83	272.835	310.241	347.647	
16	84	328.765	366.918	405.072	

Figure 18. Forecasts and their confidence limits for the series of heart deaths for 16 quarters using a model fitted to the first 17 years of the series.

from that for the first part. The other forecasts are quite close to the actual values, while tending on the whole to be a little too high, possibly for the above reasons. It can be seen that the width of the confidence interval increases with the lead time.

Note that *Minitab* will only produce 95% confidence limits. If other limits are required, then a little work must be done. For example suppose a 99% interval is required for the forecast at row 5. Both intervals are centred on 410.611 and to find the 99% limits we simply note that the estimated standard deviation will be multiplied by 2.576 rather than 1.96 (from Student's t at df = ∞ in *Appendix B.6*). So the upper limit will be 410.611 + (439.806 − 410.611) × 2.576/1.96 = 448.982. Similarly the lower limit is 372.240. No macro has been supplied for calculating the forecasts as it merely involves a single sub-command in addition to the necessary ARIMA command.

7. Regression models

The analysis carried out so far for non-stationary series has assumed the use of either smoothing or differencing to produce a stationary series. Both methods have associated difficulties. The process of smoothing with a moving average can be shown to distort the autocorrelation function and, as we have seen, it is not easy to extrapolate with this method. Differencing works well if the seasonal effect is fairly regular but, if it is a little erratic, then the resulting series often contains a residue of periodicity. Further, by removing it, we are often unable to look at the seasonal effect in detail to see if it can be given a physical interpretation. This is often of great interest in a practical application.

Whether the periodic effect is smoothly sinusoidal or looks like a saw-tooth, if it is regular it will disappear on differencing.

Another way of dealing with a systematic component is to model it explicitly by, say, a regression method (*Protocol 4*). To illustrate this, consider the series in *Figure 19a*. This series, listed in *Appendix 7.8*, consists of 288 measurements of the skin temperature on the breast of a female patient, readings being taken every 15 minutes for 3 days. It is to be expected that there is a daily, or circadian, rhythm leading to a periodic component of period 24 hours, i.e. 96 observations. If we remove this by differencing, then

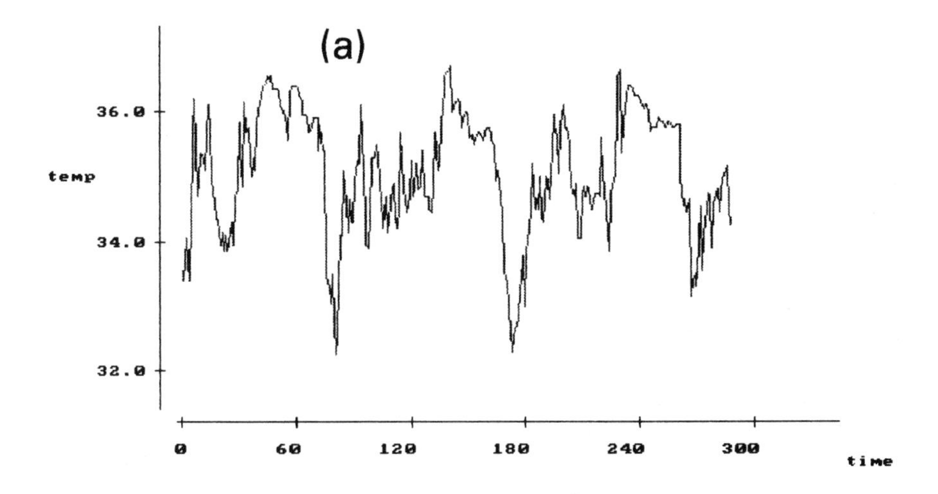

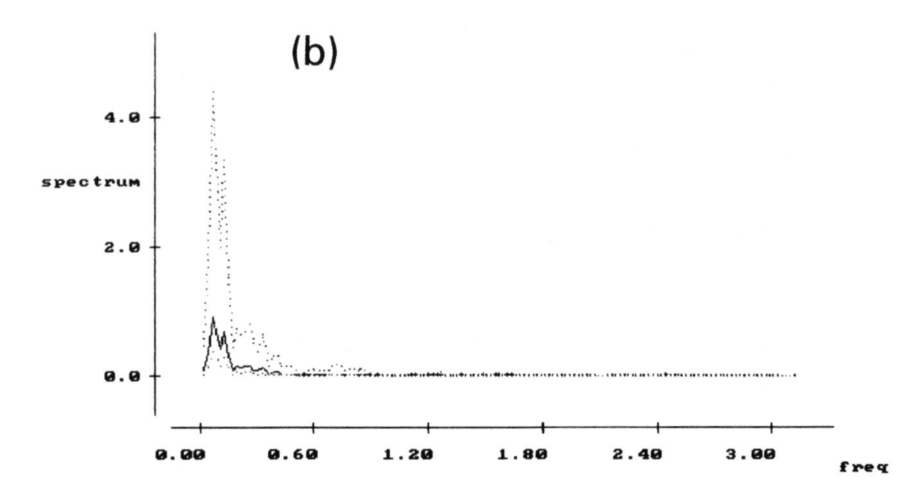

Figure 19. (a) Series of breast skin temperatures recorded every 15 minutes for 72 hours and (b) its spectral estimate.

a third of the data would be lost. Moreover, one of the features of interest in this study, which was related to the possible diagnosis of breast cancer, was the nature of this daily rhythm. By differencing, all information on the nature of this effect would be lost. The estimated spectrum is shown in *Figure 19b*; the main peak corresponds to the daily rhythm and we notice also a second peak, corresponding to a 12 hour period. This does not necessarily reflect a genuine 12 hour period. As was indicated earlier in Section 4, this is probably a harmonic.

In this case, therefore, we might try to model the daily rhythm with two sine waves, one of period 24 hours, i.e. 96 observations, and one of period 12 hours, i.e. 48 observations. Now any sine wave can be expressed as a combination of a sine and cosine wave, each of zero phase, and so we can always write $\sin(\omega t + \varphi)$ as $\alpha \sin \omega t + \beta \cos \omega t$ for suitable α and β.

For the two components in question, $\omega = 2\pi/96$ and $2\pi/48$ respectively and so an appropriate model would be

$$x_t = \beta_0 + \beta_1 \sin(\pi t/48) + \beta_2 \cos(\pi t/48) + \beta_3 \sin(\pi t/24) + \beta_4 \cos(\pi t/24) + z_t,$$

where z_t is an error term and $\beta_0, \ldots, \beta_4$ are parameters to be estimated. This can be fitted by regression methods, and the residuals stored (see Chapter 4). Suppose the data x_t are in column C1 and that the times at which the temperatures were recorded are in column C2. (On this occasion the actual times were used, rather than 1,2,. . .,288, because it is easier to interpret the final results, particularly with regard to the phase.) Then the following sequence of *Minitab* commands is used:

```
LET K1=3.14159/12
LET C3=SIN(K1*C2)
LET C4=COS(K1*C2)
LET C5=SIN(2*K1*C2)
LET C6=COS(2*K1*C2)
REGRESS C1 4 C3 C4 C5 C6 C7 C8;
RESIDUALS C9.
```

This stores the fitted values in C8 and the ordinary residuals in C9. If we plot the fitted values on the same graph as the actual series, we can see that the combination of trigonometric functions gives quite a good fit; this is shown in *Figure 20a*. If we look at the acf of the residuals, shown in *Figure 20b*, we see that it contains high values for small lags, gradually tailing off. Clearly the residuals are not independent. In a less clear-cut case, the Durbin–Watson test (see Chapter 2, Section 2.3.2 and Chapter 4, Section 4.1.1) could be used to check this. This means that although the process of estimating the parameters is valid, the standard errors will not be correct, since their calculation assumes independence. We can continue to fit an ARIMA model to the residuals—an AR(1) is chosen by the macro FIT. If we use the command

```
ARIMA 1 0 0 C9 C10
```

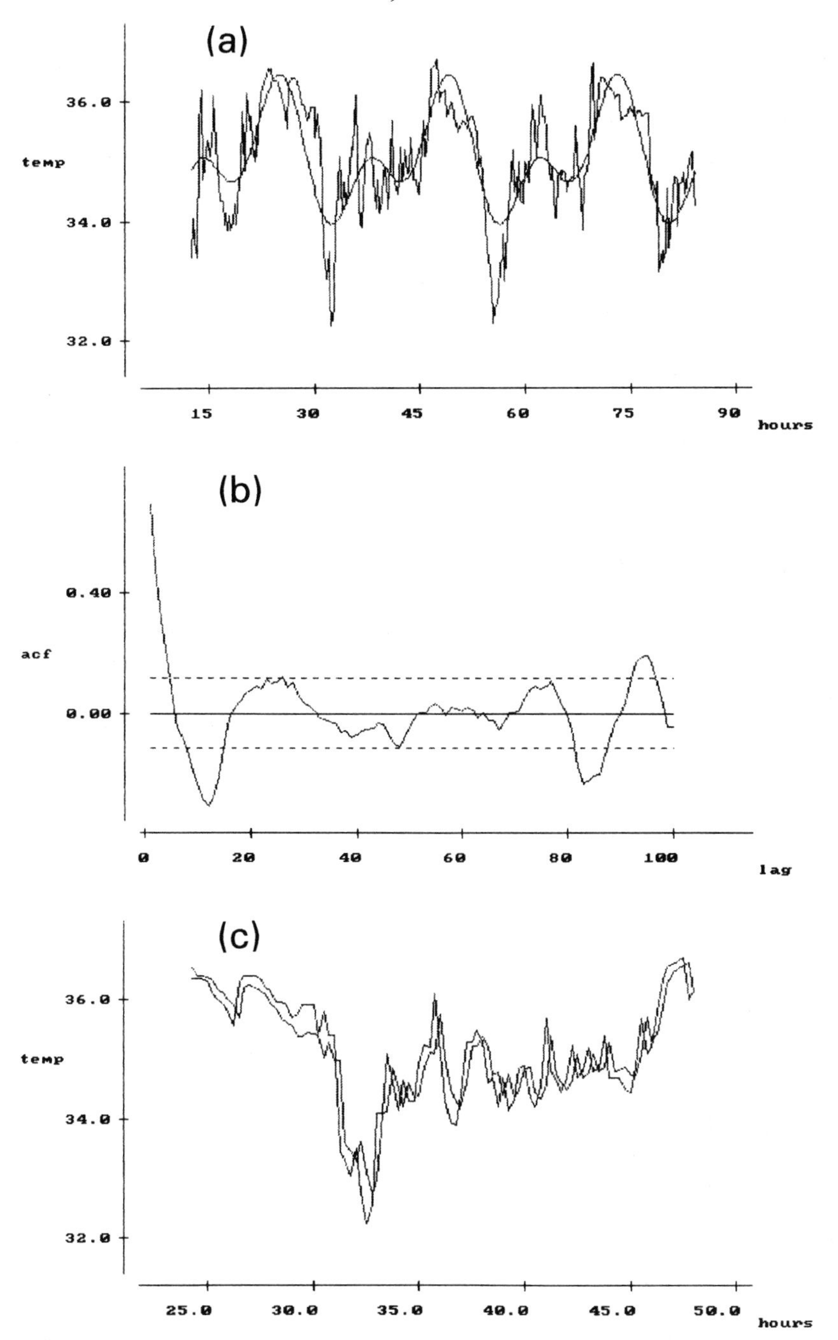

Figure 20. (a) Fitted regression mean for breast skin temperature series of *Figure 19a*, (b) the correlogram of residuals from the regression model of Section 7, and (c) the actual temperatures and fitted values for the first 24 hours in the series in *Figure 19a*.

then the new residuals will be placed in C10. Following this with

```
LET C7=C1-C10
```

will give us new fitted values and they can be plotted by

```
GPLOT;
LINES 0 2 C1 C2;
LINES 0 3 C7 C2.
```

The result is shown in *Figure 20c*, where it can be seen that we seem to have a good model for the data. For reasons of clarity only a relatively short part of the series is shown there. This procedure is not ideal—certainly we cannot use the standard errors produced by the package—but it gives us a model which we can explore. We can calculate the amplitude and phase of each of the waves fitted. For example the amplitude of the 24 hour wave is estimated as $\{\hat{\beta}_1^2 + \hat{\beta}_2^2\}^{1/2}$ and the phase by $\tan^{-1}(\hat{\beta}_2/\hat{\beta}_1)$. In this case their values turn out to be 0.792 and 1.64 radians. This value of the phase in fact means that the peak of the daily rhythm is just before midnight. (The phase $1.64 \approx \pi/2$ indicates how advanced the cycle is at $t = 0, 24, 48. . .$, and since the peak occurs at $\pi/2$, this is at about times 0,24,. . ., that is at midnight.) In the study in which this series was collected, the times of such peaks were felt to be of importance and it was essential to explicitly model the periodic variation. Full details of a method which leads to correct standard errors, including those of the amplitude and phase, are in Dunstan (10).

Protocol 4. Fitting a regression model for the mean of a time series (see Section 7 for details)

1. To model a changing mean explicitly, choose a suitable model:
   - if the trend is linear, then a linear term in time will be included
   - if there is periodic variation, some trigonometric terms could be included
2. Define columns to contain the values of the explanatory variables.
3. Carry out a multiple regression to estimate the coefficients of the explanatory variables.
4. Plot the correlogram of the residuals. If there is much correlation, they are not independent and the estimated standard errors are incorrect.
5. Fit an ARIMA model to the residuals and calculate new residuals and fitted values.
6. Check the new residuals for any obvious pattern.

---

8. Several time series

In many contexts a number of variables are recorded at each time point, leading to several simultaneous series. For example in the study in which the EEG series was recorded, eight electrodes made recordings simultaneously. In a study on breast skin temperatures, devised to investigate possible early detection of breast cancer, readings were taken simultaneously from 14 sensors on the breasts of a patient. In a study on bacterial activity in a pond over 40 variables were measured at weekly intervals. Sometimes it is reasonable to model these individually but in other cases it is interesting to consider joint properties of several series. Sometimes series will be related by what we can think of as an input–output mechanism. For example, the temperature affects the demand for energy; as the temperature falls the demand increases. Here we can think of demand as an output and temperature as an input. In the EEG example this is clearly not the case. Outside influences may affect two series in a similar way, but the two series have a similar status. The first case is an example of a linear system which is beyond the scope of this chapter. It is an example of a problem best handled in the frequency domain. A reasonably elementary introduction to the topic is given in Chatfield (2). *Minitab* does not have facilities for handling such problems.

In the second type of example, suppose that we have two series under consideration. The first step is to plot them. A simple plot for series in columns C1 and C2, assuming they are of the same length, would be produced by

```
SET C3
1:COUNT(C1)
END
GPLOT;
LINES 0 2 C1 C3;
LINES 0 3 C2 C3.
```

From such a plot we can examine the behaviour of the two series. The only command supplied by *Minitab* for examining them jointly calculates the cross-correlation function. If the two series are denoted by $\{x_t\}$ and $\{y_t\}$ then the cross-correlation at lag k measures the correlation $r_{xy}(k)$ between x_t and y_{t+k}. This is not a symmetric function; $r_{xy}(k)$ is not necessarily equal to $r_{xy}(-k)$. Moreover, $r_{xy}(0)$ is not necessarily 1, though it cannot exceed 1. It is therefore harder to interpret than the acf of a single series. It has been found that if this function is calculated for two quite unrelated series, each of which has a high degree of correlation, then high values of the cross-correlation function can be produced spuriously. For this reason it is generally recommended that the series be pre-whitened or filtered before the calculations are performed. This filtering simply means that an appropriate ARIMA model should be fitted, and the residuals formed, for each series. The cross-correlation function is then calculated for the two series of residuals with a command

```
CCF 20 C1 C2
```

This will compute the cross-correlation function for lags -20, -19, . . ., $-1,0,1,. . .,20$ between the series of residuals in columns C1 and C2. Unfortunately release 7 of *Minitab* does not store the results, so that it is difficult to follow this up in any serious way. We can note that if the two series are uncorrelated and have been filtered, then theoretically the cross-correlations should have mean 0 and standard deviation $1/\sqrt{n}$, where n is the series length. Thus 95% of values should lie between $-2\sqrt{n}$ and $2/\sqrt{n}$ and any values far outside these limits indicate significant values. If there is a large value at 0, then it means that the series are tending to vary in the same way at the same time. If there is a large value at lag d, say, then the values of the second series seem to depend on those of the first series d time points earlier.

An example of a pair of series is shown in *Figure 21*. These are from a study of a freshwater pond in which bacterial activity was observed over a period of some 90 weeks. A large number of variables were observed and in *Figure 21* are plotted the values of two, namely the logarithms of the numbers of xylanase-producing bacteria and paraquat-resistant bacteria per ml, measured weekly. These are listed in *Appendices 7.9* and *7.10*. The cross-correlation function for these series is shown in *Figure 22a*. There is little structure but it is noticeable that all values are positive. Models were selected, using the macro FIT. Those selected were an ARIMA(1,1) for the xylanase-producing bacteria and an AR(1) for the paraquat-resistant bacteria. Using these the series were filtered and the cross-correlation function of the resulting series is shown in *Figure 22b*. It can be seen that almost all of the values lie within the limits at $\pm 2/\sqrt{n}$, but that there is a large positive value at about lag 0 (actually 0.53). This emphasizes that there is a strong correlation between the numbers of the two types of bacteria in the same week, but that there is no evidence that the number of one type in a given week directly affects the number of the other type in a different week. The class of ARIMA models has been extended to vector processes, that is ones consisting of several simultaneous series, but details are not included here.

9. Missing values

The problem of missing values is a serious one in time series analysis. All the above methods require a full set of values and it is only recently that methods have been devised for handling series in which there are gaps. These are not easy, however, and are not described here. We have provided a macro MAUTOCF (see *Appendix 7.20*) for estimating the acf of such a series in a

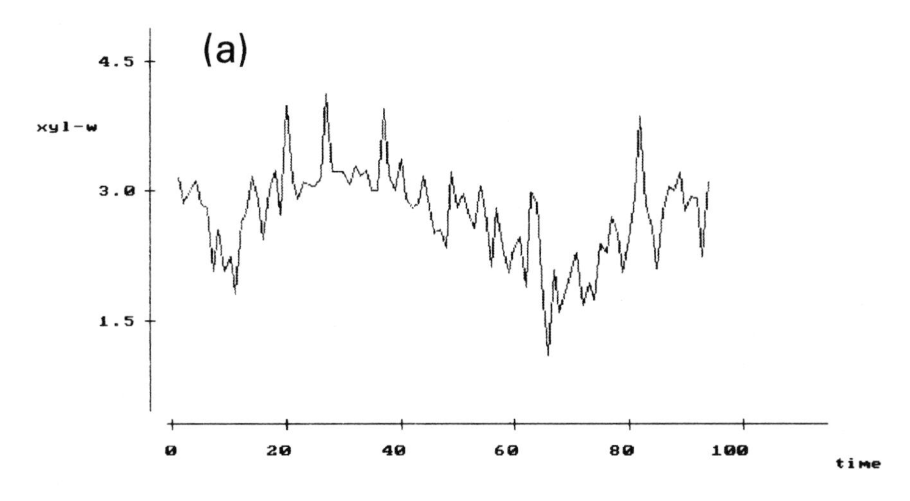

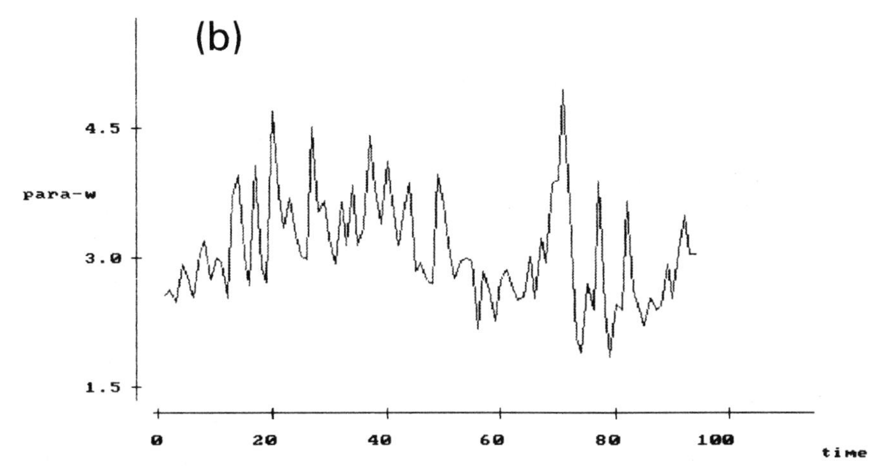

Figure 21. Logarithms of populations of (a) xylanase producing bacteria and (b) paraquat-resistant bacteria in a freshwater pond, recorded weekly.

sensible way, and the macro TPLOT used earlier will plot a series with gaps. If there is only a very occasional missing value than a simple interpolation will probably suffice and a model could be fitted as usual. If they are reasonably common, or if there are blocks of missing values, then a more sophisticated approach is needed. Methods that have been devised include the EM algorithm, an iterative approach, and the method of the Kalman filter. Details are contained in Barham and Dunstan (11). To apply these methods a more specialized computer package is needed.

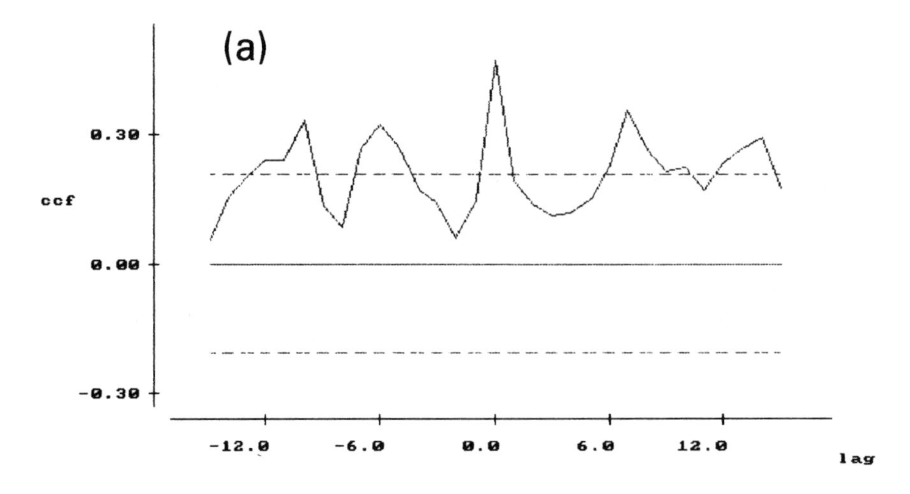

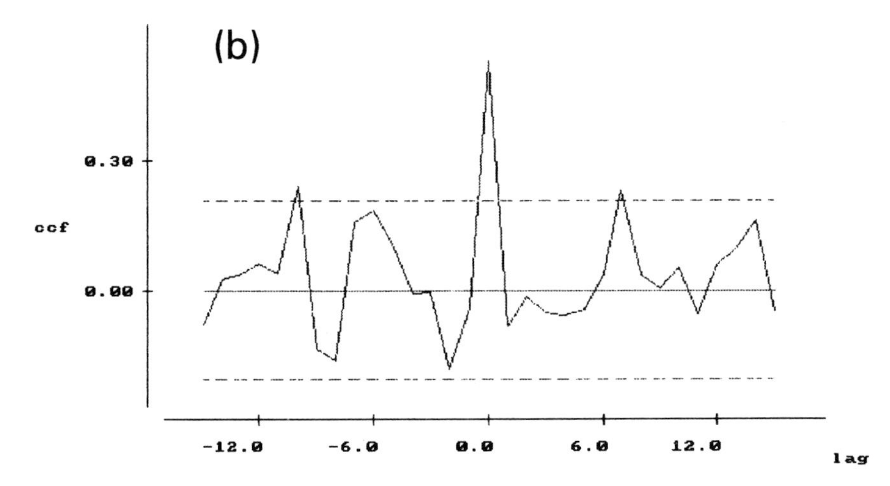

Figure 22. The cross-correlation functions of the two series in *Figure 21*, showing results for (a) the original and (b) the pre-whitened series.

References

1. Priestley, M. (1981). *Spectral analysis and time series*. Academic Press, London.
2. Chatfield, C. (1989). *The analysis of time series*. Chapman & Hall, London.
3. Diggle, P. J. (1990). *Time series: A biostatistical introduction*. Oxford University Press, Oxford.
4. Cryer, J. D. (1986). *Time series analysis*. PWS-Kent, Boston.
5. Box, G. E. P. and Jenkins, G. W. (1976). *Time series analysis, forecasting and control*. Holden Day, San Francisco.

6. Kenny, P. B. and Durbin, J. (1982). *Journal of the Royal Statistical Society A* **145,** 1.
7. Kendall, M. G. and Stuart, A. (1966). *The theory of advanced statistics,* Vol. 3. Griffin, London.
8. Akaike, H. (1974). A new look at the statistical model identification. *IEEE Transactions on Automatic Control* **AC-19,** 716.
9. Schwarz, G. (1978). Estimating the dimension of a model. *Annals of Statistics* **6,** 461.
10. Dunstan, F. D. J. (1982). In *Time series analysis: Theory and practice*, Vol. I (ed. O. D. Anderson), pp. 111–22. North-Holland, Amsterdam.
11. Barham, S. Y. and Dunstan, F. D. J. (1983). In *Time series analysis: Theory and practice*, Vol. II (ed. O. D. Anderson), pp. 25–41. North-Holland, Amsterdam.

Appendix 7.1. EEG data: file EEG.DAT

This data set consists of 640 EEG readings from a sensor attached to the scalp of a patient. The data were recorded at the rate of 640 per second for 10 seconds. The initial recordings were measured in microvolts but a calibration formula has been applied to the original values

1988	2096	2105	2235	2144	2227	2083	2094
2295	2282	2244	2269	2276	2359	2206	2279
2413	2454	2532	2318	2167	2034	2053	2128
2211	2299	2412	2307	2140	2052	1872	1898
1923	1993	1951	1964	2054	2076	2017	2060
2053	2088	2013	1997	2008	2090	2157	2052
2027	2138	2144	2123	2092	2010	2075	2037
1952	1956	2050	2066	2069	2107	2081	2002
1966	1940	1860	1856	1857	1830	1904	1988
1988	1987	1931	1843	1958	1984	1952	1849
2041	1993	2055	2062	2089	2104	1968	1992
2002	2076	2141	2061	2021	1946	1923	2076
2117	2088	2084	2020	1990	2050	2067	2031
2033	1940	1968	1988	2055	2074	2207	2140
2165	2030	1970	1987	2012	2106	2060	2094
2051	2073	2079	2044	2091	2068	1995	2005
1971	1945	2009	1975	2033	2076	1987	2069
2079	2063	2046	1992	2025	2023	2060	2090
2130	1996	2028	2081	2040	2179	2155	2047
1844	1990	2090	2204	2297	2255	2189	2091
2092	2031	2202	2289	2221	2098	2068	2192
2140	2102	2078	2089	2169	2312	2267	2138
2124	2095	2075	2112	2158	2131	2166	2108
1931	2088	2180	2127	2108	2051	2076	2178
2201	2220	2096	2030	2008	2107	2214	2221
2195	2061	1996	1944	2088	2202	2292	2266
2164	2057	2077	2090	2148	2151	2097	2154
2083	2117	2151	2092	2067	1988	1959	2063
2107	2100	2093	2079	2037	2115	2223	2169
1987	2022	1880	1938	2110	2015	1992	1891
1856	1992	2172	2184	2113	1966	1814	2052
2139	2119	2026	1984	1904	1934	1923	2029
2026	2028	1901	1897	1833	1912	2123	2082
2106	2059	1887	1935	1987	1936	1891	1994
1911	1955	1920	1980	2048	2057	2038	2026
2055	2062	2108	2044	2055	2045	2060	2083
2018	1935	2017	1988	2056	2060	2112	2053
1982	2000	2014	2095	2039	2058	2012	1938
2045	1984	1930	1904	1856	2006	2047	1931
1861	1797	1843	1818	1964	1936	1800	1851
1928	1900	1896	1942	1801	1842	1963	1941
1838	1975	1924	1960	1845	2065	1935	1828
1767	1770	1916	1943	1860	1892	1832	1711
1790	1917	1867	1997	1899	1911	1861	1766
1944	1908	1964	1980	1865	1832	1887	2054

Appendix 7.1. (*contd.*)

1974	2005	1960	1900	2019	2028	1894	1824
1873	1939	1930	2038	1868	1983	1876	1900
1936	2042	1941	1849	1936	1918	2091	2115
1912	1877	2018	2077	2105	2133	2416	2306
2323	2568	2360	2128	2121	2254	2243	2188
2158	2238	2116	2148	2178	1926	2003	2026
1962	1920	1927	1870	1822	1796	1838	1738
1761	1813	1923	1927	1846	1935	1961	1869
1863	2025	1954	1824	1801	1833	1860	1994
2158	2115	1986	1910	2013	2203	2074	1928
1914	1951	1997	2039	2027	1952	1865	1920
2015	2021	2104	2045	2017	1925	1959	2012
2081	2008	1972	2016	2001	2052	2038	2000
1942	1952	2052	2081	2148	2153	1967	1956
2016	2081	2125	2074	2009	2001	2080	2173
2122	2022	1944	2019	2153	2223	2208	2133
1984	1912	2083	2220	2132	2005	1982	1959
2086	2222	2154	2138	2088	2042	1954	2094
2250	2224	2080	1988	1984	1988	2049	1973
1880	1945	2000	2010	1980	2082	2060	2018
1929	1867	1904	1958	2076	2152	2117	2156
2060	2021	2051	2134	2149	2177	2154	2146
2070	2107	2011	1995	2037	2016	2111	2166
2022	1960	1904	1997	2183	2118	2080	2140
2166	2190	2073	2093	2119	2090	2030	2074
2100	2026	2069	1940	1866	1804	1879	2058
1999	1964	1970	1895	1935	1979	2118	1934
1993	1951	1991	2061	2037	2175	2244	2213
2058	2116	2118	2157	2072	2091	2061	2121
2154	2131	2230	2119	2075	2077	2203	2067
2016	2097	2132	2117	2148	2198	2099	2110
2062	2202	2093	2215	2183	2061	2108	2124
2124	2111	2131	2066	2013	2151	2147	2210
2027	2156	2238	2180	2022	2089	2134	2088
2172	2032	2069	1996	2185	2133	1958	2103

Appendix 7.2. Heart deaths data: file DEATHS.DAT

These are quarterly figures for the numbers of deaths per hundred thousand population from ischaemic heart disease in British males, 1971–1990

389	345	303	362	412	356	325	375
410	350	310	388	399	362	325	382
399	382	318	385	437	357	310	391
413	377	325	381	446	382	331	387
454	370	318	372	412	370	327	386
408	361	318	390	399	340	305	369
427	364	321	371	415	373	309	370
450	369	321	368	424	363	321	353
400	343	312	368	392	340	305	347
367	335	282	362	369	323	287	

Appendix 7.3. Protozoal growth data: file PROTOZOA.DAT

These figures give the number of the protozoan *Paramecium aurelium* in a closed colony; the numbers were recorded daily

17	29	39	63	185	258	267	392
510	570	650	560	575	650	550	480
520	500						

Appendix 7.4. Airline data: UKAIR.DAT

These data are monthly figures for the numbers of passengers carried on scheduled services by UK airlines, 1977–1990. The values are shown in thousands

1174	1101	1411	1109	1519	1719	1854	1688
1582	1372	1277	1280	1249	1150	1547	1585
1762	1904	2155	2108	2064	1817	1515	1417
1263	1237	1591	1875	1986	2111	2357	2441
2281	2058	1599	1513	1471	1404	1714	1791
1894	2076	2272	2368	2161	1942	1541	1537
1490	1371	1613	1802	1762	1856	2136	2262
2157	1928	1571	1414	1497	1321	1594	1742
1736	1875	2136	2059	1995	1785	1440	1430
1396	1256	1614	1636	1738	1876	2046	2007
2042	1818	1482	1477	1443	1359	1623	1816
1952	2106	2243	2257	2288	2080	1739	1651
1616	1477	1927	2019	2189	2383	2509	2521
2429	2179	1824	1755	1724	1556	1921	1971
2043	2201	2409	2540	2498	2313	1926	1896
1775	1702	2107	2333	2462	2565	2860	2912
2808	2655	2191	2127	2063	2015	2458	2494
2651	2792	3025	3018	3033	2893	2426	2356
2335	2216	2715	2777	2974	3117	3357	3395
3405	3302	2817	2644	2641	2557	3076	3278
3382	3510	3774	3730	3679	3498	2759	

Appendix 7.5. First tremor data set: file TREMOR1.DAT

This is a set of measurements of hand tremor from a patient suffering from essential tremor, recorded at the rate of 50 per second for 10.24 seconds. The values measured were accelerations which were then scaled to the present values

162	145	112	89	81	82	96	124
158	176	184	168	137	109	89	76
76	88	124	157	182	181	164	129
90	74	75	77	114	151	177	185
164	130	102	84	71	77	104	146
167	182	178	144	112	89	80	88
92	127	162	177	174	151	126	95
81	80	87	120	156	176	178	156
126	97	83	87	91	118	152	177
168	151	126	97	85	91	94	118
156	173	170	150	125	102	83	93
91	113	139	169	189	159	133	105
92	80	90	107	145	169	172	159
129	103	89	81	95	116	146	170
172	156	129	99	86	77	86	108
138	165	189	169	145	112	94	79
73	94	133	163	191	180	149	106
87	84	83	92	120	149	184	183
157	123	104	81	79	89	125	159
191	176	153	109	98	77	85	94
121	150	179	192	167	125	100	88
68	83	109	146	167	185	171	142
108	93	76	78	95	125	158	187
185	164	123	100	82	63	79	117
147	172	194	177	146	110	84	72
74	83	119	157	180	204	173	134
97	81	52	72	110	152	177	214
178	140	106	83	63	73	91	135
169	192	188	158	123	97	79	69
80	111	152	178	184	168	139	104
86	78	78	105	147	175	177	168
136	102	92	82	94	119	151	170
160	148	124	104	93	93	96	120
147	168	176	161	133	103	91	91
96	111	146	166	168	159	131	106
97	96	95	111	143	164	176	170
141	112	88	89	88	95	131	158
176	178	156	128	100	83	87	95
116	153	167	172	164	136	107	87
88	85	102	134	162	175	179	162
131	103	90	80	85	105	142	169
188	188	152	115	87	74	72	85
125	160	185	190	177	139	107	82
71	76	92	134	163	182	193	173
138	104	82	71	75	92	130	162

Appendix 7.5. *(contd.)*

185	192	173	142	105	73	59	69
97	143	176	193	185	155	115	85
77	84	91	124	165	184	175	158
130	108	81	83	79	98	134	166
186	177	156	122	98	81	77	87
113	150	171	184	172	139	111	86
76	81	93	123	157	174	183	171
138	111	87	74	75	90	126	159
181	190	175	138	109	83	63	76
98	135	170	186	175	152	121	93
73	72	79	114	150	176	193	189
162	123	90	73	59	71	109	165
192	191	171	132	92	73	76	74
110	151	179	190	183	148	116	83
73	69	86	130	161	177	167	158
122	95	86	72	76	106	154	175
186	178	150	122	89	70	76	89
124	166	179	170	156	124	95	72
77	86	122	157	176	183	162	138

Appendix 7.6. Second tremor data set: file TREMOR2.DAT

This is a set of measurements of hand tremor from a normal person, recorded at the rate of 50 observations per second for 10.24 seconds. The values measured were accelerations which were then scaled to the present values

132	138	140	139	131	130	132	129
140	133	130	136	132	132	136	132
127	141	132	135	134	137	134	129
119	143	137	136	128	130	140	138
135	119	129	131	136	137	130	129
139	145	134	133	130	133	138	133
133	131	136	127	132	131	140	140
137	130	132	124	130	139	147	133
131	114	139	138	141	133	133	131
138	128	135	141	123	132	126	144
138	135	127	131	133	136	137	137
134	120	128	118	143	148	140	126
132	121	137	138	140	133	122	128
130	136	133	132	135	133	140	130
136	130	119	135	142	149	132	114
128	141	143	128	122	132	137	142
124	130	138	135	133	132	136	135
137	128	130	136	139	128	114	125
144	152	140	116	125	130	139	143
129	135	120	123	135	138	136	138
124	137	133	130	132	132	131	130

Appendix 7.6. (*contd.*)

133	135	134	130	132	132	135	126
129	136	136	134	134	122	128	132
136	136	128	128	136	131	138	137
118	123	125	133	138	139	132	125
133	135	133	137	128	123	135	127
125	132	131	131	131	136	138	131
117	136	129	132	129	127	133	135
130	133	129	132	127	133	133	131
118	124	136	140	139	123	116	120
135	137	146	134	114	110	131	133
145	129	131	129	134	126	137	121
133	132	131	133	125	121	126	132
135	138	134	136	118	118	125	133
135	126	128	120	135	123	132	127
134	131	127	136	128	133	123	119
138	132	136	121	135	127	137	131
133	127	120	121	118	139	145	144
125	115	112	139	141	143	121	118
118	139	128	125	121	133	140	133
129	123	126	127	136	133	129	118
127	135	132	132	128	129	129	128
132	129	136	130	126	127	130	132
132	132	132	130	128	124	134	133
133	129	136	129	121	128	130	136
120	134	126	142	126	114	111	141
146	144	126	120	118	128	139	140
129	127	120	125	134	129	134	139
128	130	120	135	131	128	131	129
131	127	134	130	135	129	130	122
130	121	125	134	139	140	131	125
123	135	132	125	125	119	134	136
134	123	118	132	143	146	130	120
120	130	139	136	120	123	126	139
133	133	126	120	128	136	137	136
124	118	133	134	135	126	125	134
133	131	138	126	115	119	133	141
139	121	125	138	133	132	126	123
134	135	128	131	123	133	127	133
132	136	128	134	120	124	129	130
138	128	125	129	126	135	140	135
124	116	131	141	141	135	117	118
127	136	136	133	129	122	130	137
135	128	123	125	124	135	135	131

Appendix 7.7. Data set of heterotrophic bacteria: file HETBACT.DAT

These numbers are the logarithms (to base 10) of the number of heterotrophic bacteria per ml in a pond, recorded weekly for 99 weeks

5.583	3.937	4.367	5.740	5.591	5.695	5.562	5.134
4.859	4.845	5.661	4.968	4.697	3.831	3.959	3.613
3.996	4.512	4.806	3.616	4.496	4.519	3.839	3.854
5.522	4.751	5.342	4.956	5.292	5.322	4.940	5.613
5.134	5.253	4.859	4.752	4.884	5.021	4.906	4.835
4.650	5.484	4.960	4.591	4.932	5.097	5.049	5.134
5.230	5.182	5.111	5.253	5.672	5.167	5.196	5.146
5.017	5.215	5.538	5.212	5.111	5.185	5.301	4.303
5.121	4.431	5.777	4.952	5.531	5.736	5.839	6.318
6.352	6.474	5.504	5.562	5.146	5.585	5.033	4.659
3.974	5.013	4.137	4.029	4.352	4.326	5.000	4.462
4.061	4.352	5.217	4.921	4.621	4.957	4.100	4.992
5.124	4.997	4.919					

Appendix 7.8. Skin temperature data set: file SKINTEMP.DAT

These data are skin temperatures recorded using a special sensor placed on the breast of a patient suffering from breast cancer. The values were recorded every 15 minutes for 72 hours, starting at 10.30 a.m.

33.4	34.0	33.7	33.4	35.4	35.7	36.2	34.7
35.0	35.3	35.3	35.1	35.7	36.1	35.7	35.0
34.6	34.3	34.3	34.0	34.2	33.8	34.1	33.8
34.0	34.3	34.0	34.7	34.8	35.8	35.4	34.8
36.2	35.7	35.8	35.3	35.0	35.4	35.1	35.8
36.2	36.3	36.4	36.5	36.5	36.5	36.5	36.3
36.3	36.3	36.3	36.1	36.0	35.9	35.8	35.5
36.3	36.4	36.4	36.4	36.3	36.2	36.2	36.0
36.0	35.9	35.7	35.8	35.9	35.9	35.9	35.4
35.8	35.4	35.4	33.5	33.3	33.0	33.5	32.8
32.3	32.5	34.1	34.1	35.1	34.6	34.2	34.7
34.3	34.3	35.0	35.3	35.2	36.1	35.1	34.3
34.0	33.9	34.4	35.3	35.3	35.5	35.3	34.6
34.7	34.2	34.7	34.2	34.3	34.8	34.9	34.3
34.2	34.5	35.7	34.8	34.7	34.5	34.7	35.3
34.7	34.8	35.2	34.8	34.8	35.4	34.7	34.7
34.7	34.5	34.5	34.9	35.7	35.1	35.2	35.8
36.3	36.5	36.6	36.7	36.7	36.0	36.2	36.2
36.2	36.1	35.8	35.9	36.0	36.0	35.6	35.7
35.5	35.6	35.7	35.7	35.7	35.5	35.7	35.8
35.8	35.7	35.5	35.5	35.0	35.1	34.7	34.4
33.5	33.3	33.4	33.0	32.3	32.5	32.7	32.8
33.3	33.4	33.8	33.0	33.8	34.2	34.5	35.2
34.5	34.7	34.5	35.0	34.3	34.3	35.0	35.0
34.7	35.4	36.0	35.8	35.6	35.0	35.8	36.1

Appendix 7.8. (*contd.*)

35.8	35.8	35.5	35.3	34.8	34.7	34.9	34.0
34.0	34.8	34.8	34.7	34.8	34.8	34.5	34.7
34.8	34.8	34.7	35.6	35.0	34.8	34.5	33.8
34.8	34.8	35.0	36.0	36.5	36.7	35.3	35.8
36.3	36.4	36.4	36.3	36.3	36.3	36.3	36.2
36.2	36.0	36.1	36.1	36.0	35.7	35.8	35.8
35.8	35.9	35.8	35.8	35.8	35.8	35.8	35.8
35.8	35.8	35.8	35.8	35.8	35.0	34.5	34.7
34.5	34.7	33.2	33.4	33.5	33.3	33.5	34.5
33.5	34.1	34.5	34.8	34.7	33.9	34.6	34.7
34.8	34.5	34.8	35.0	35.1	35.2	34.5	34.3

Appendix 7.9. Data set of xylanase-producing bacteria: file XYLBACT.DAT

This is a series of the logarithms of the number of xylanase-producing bacteria per ml in a pond, recorded weekly for 94 weeks

3.146	2.860	3.000	3.124	2.845	2.813	2.079	2.544
2.072	2.243	1.813	2.653	2.740	3.176	2.885	2.439
2.995	3.243	2.720	3.978	3.124	2.916	3.114	3.079
3.061	3.146	4.130	3.225	3.225	3.212	3.072	3.286
3.176	3.238	3.000	3.000	3.954	3.190	3.000	3.380
2.916	2.813	2.860	3.170	2.824	2.512	2.544	2.344
3.212	2.813	2.978	2.760	2.574	3.061	2.778	2.124
2.813	2.367	2.061	2.352	2.477	1.903	2.989	2.879
1.740	1.097	2.097	1.603	1.845	2.114	2.301	1.688
1.936	1.751	2.398	2.301	2.699	2.512	2.068	2.439
2.936	3.860	2.838	2.574	2.111	2.778	3.045	3.004
3.225	2.772	2.936	2.929	2.243	3.114		

Appendix 7.10. Data set of paraquat-resistant bacteria: file PARABACT.DAT

This is a series of the logarithms (to base 10) of the number of paraquat-resistant bacteria per ml in a pond, recorded weekly for 94 weeks

2.566	2.626	2.470	2.929	2.769	2.522	3.045	3.204
2.743	2.990	2.944	2.542	3.697	3.963	3.021	2.670
4.057	2.875	2.714	4.699	3.723	3.332	3.686	3.348
3.029	2.979	4.516	3.525	3.667	3.225	2.919	3.633
3.134	3.842	3.143	3.350	4.415	3.789	3.386	4.124
3.667	3.134	3.597	3.878	2.847	2.932	2.747	2.702
3.971	3.626	3.021	2.766	2.959	2.985	2.958	2.161
2.851	2.636	2.262	2.739	2.865	2.648	2.512	2.554
3.009	2.531	3.223	2.942	3.854	3.894	4.951	3.575
2.064	1.903	2.699	2.403	3.889	2.394	1.845	2.462
2.394	3.667	2.638	2.400	2.212	2.535	2.398	2.455
2.921	2.531	3.076	3.489	3.053	3.049		

Note for *Appendices 7.11–7.20*

The appendices which follow contain listings of the *Minitab* macros referred to in the chapter. Some of the main macros call others and it is assumed that all have been loaded on the current drive; if not then a failure will occur in some cases. They require the series to have been read into a column and sometimes require other constants to be input. They use constants and columns as working space. These are usually deleted at the end, except where the end-product is useful for further work. Generally columns c90–c99 and constants k90–k99 are used as workspace, but in a few cases extra ones, with high numbers, are used; those required are indicated in each macro. These columns should be avoided when entering data as this would be overwritten.

Appendix 7.11. Macro TPLOT in file TPLOT.MTB

This macro plots a time series, joining up successive values. It will work even if there are missing data points

```
noecho
note
# macro tplot
note
note Enter the number of the column containing the series
note This will still work even if there are missing values
note Workspace used: columns c91–c93 and constants k92,k93
note
note Enter the number of the column containing the series
set 'terminal' c93;
nobs=1.
copy c93 k93
let k92=count(ck93)
set c91
1:k92
end
copy ck93 c92;
omit ck93='*'.
copy c91 c91;
omit ck93='*'.
name c91 'time'
gplot;
lines 0 2 c92 c91.
erase c91 c92 c93 k92 k93
echo
```

Appendix 7.12. Macro SCTPLOT in file SCTPLOT.MTB

This macro plots a portion of a time series, to be selected by the user, who can also select the vertical scale. It is not designed to deal with a series with missing values

```
noecho
note
# macro sctplot
note
note This macro enables you to plot part of a series
note or to plot on a scale other than the default
note First enter the number of the column holding the series
note Workspace: columns c90–c93 and k90–k94
set 'terminal' c90;
nobs=1.
let k90=c90(1)
count ck90 k95
describe ck90
note Enter the first and last time points that you require
set 'terminal' c91;
nobs=2.
let k91=c91(1)
let k92=c91(2)
note Now enter the smallest and largest values that you
note require on the y-axis
set 'terminal' c92;
nobs=2.
let k93=c92(1)
let k94=c92(2)
set c93
k91:k92
end
copy ck90 c90;
use k91:k92.
name c93 'time'
gplot;
ystart k93 k94;
lines 0 4 c90 c93.
erase c90–c93 k90–k95
echo
```

Appendix 7.13. Macro SMOOTH in file SMOOTH.MTB

This macro uses moving average methods to remove trend and seasonal effects from a time series. It stores the final residuals for further analysis. It calls other macros listed below

```
noecho
# macro smooth
oh=0
note
note This computes a simple moving average designed to estimate
note a seasonal effect and removes this seasonal effect
note Workspace: Columns c90–c99 and constants k81–k99
note The final residuals are stored in column c92
note The first graph shows the original values and the trend
note The second graph shows the detrended values
note The final graph shows the residuals after removing the seasonality
note
note Enter the number of the column containing the series
set 'terminal' c99;
nobs=1.
let k81=c99(1)
note Now enter the number of observations per cycle
set 'terminal' c99;
nobs=1.
let k82=c99(1)
let k83=round((k82–2)/2)
let k90=count(ck81)
set c90
1:k90
end
copy c90 c91
name c90 'time'
copy ck81 c94
copy ck81 c95
copy ck81 c96
exec 'add' k83
let k84=(2*k83<k82–1)
exec 'addl' k84
let c96=c96/k82
erase c94 c95
let k85=round((k82–1)/2)
copy ck81 c97
let k98=count(c91)
let k97=k98–k85+1
delete 1:k85 k97:k98 c91 c96 c97
gplot;
lines 0 2 ck81 c90;
lines 0 3 c96 c91.
let c98=c97–c96
name c91 'times'
name c98 'values'
```

Appendix 7.13. (*contd.*)

```
gplot;
lines 0 2 c98 c91.
let k91=round(k90/k82)-1
let k92=k91*k82
let k93=k90-k92
set c94
1:k93
end
set c92
k91(1:k82)
end
stack c92 c94 c92
exec 'chop' k85
let k93=0
exec 'macl' k82
let c94=c93
let k91=k91+1
exec 'stck' k91
let k97=count(c91)+k85+1
let k98=count(c94)
delete 1:k85 k97:k98 c94
let c92=c98-c94
name c92 'resid'
gplot;
lines 0 2 c92 c91.
erase c90 c91 c93-c99 k81-k99
oh=24
echo
```

```
# macro add
lag 1 c94 c94
let k99=count(c95)
let c94(1)=0
delete 1 c95
let c95(k99)=0
let c96=c96+c94+c95
```

```
# macro addl
let k99=count(c95)
lag 1 c94 c94
let c94(1)=0
delete 1 c95
let c95(k99)=0
let c96=c96+(c94+c95)/2
```

```
# macro chop
let k99=count(c92)
delete k99 c92
delete 1 c92
```

Appendix 7.13. (*contd.*)

```
# macro mac1
let k93=k93+1
copy c98 c95;
use c92=k93.
let c93(k93)=mean(c95)
erase c95
```

```
# macro stck
stack c94 c93 c94
```

Appendix 7.14. Macro SMOOTH1 in file SMOOTH1.MTB

This macro calculates a 9-point moving average used to estimate the trend of a non-seasonal time series. The residuals are stored for further analysis

```
noecho
# macro smooth1
oh=0
note
note This macro carries out a simple smoothing based on a nine-point
note moving average due to Henderson. It is not suitable for series
note with a periodic component. The resulting smoothed series is stored
note in column c90. Values are not returned for the first four and
note last four time points.
note Workspace: Columns c88–c99 and constants k90–k92.
note
note Enter the column number of the series
set 'terminal' c90;
nobs=1.
let k90=c90(1)
copy ck90 c91
let k91=count(c91)
set c89
1:k91
end
lag 1 c91 c92
let c92(1)=0
lag 1 c92 c93
let c93(1)=0
lag 1 c93 c94
let c94(1)=0
lag 1 c94 c95
let c95(1)=0
copy c91 c96;
omit 1.
let c96(k91)=0
copy c96 c97;
```

Appendix 7.14. (*contd.*)

```
omit 1.
let c97(k91)=0
copy c97 c98;
omit 1.
let c98(k91)=0
copy c98 c99;
omit 1.
let c99(k91)=0
let c90=0.33*c91+0.267*(c92+c96) +0.119*(c93+c97)-0.01*(c94+c98)
let c90=c90-0.041*(c95+c99)
let k92=k91-3
copy c89 c88
delete 1:4 k92:k91 c89 c90
name c90 'smoothed' c88 'time'
gplot;
lines 0 2 ck90 c88;
lines 3 3 c90 c89.
erase c88 c89 c91-c99 k90-k92
oh=24
echo
```

Appendix 7.15. Macro DFF in file DFF.MTB

This enables the user to take a number of ordinary and seasonal differences to try to reduce a series to stationarity. The final residuals are stored for subsequent analysis

```
noecho
# macro dff
oh=0
note
note This macro enables the user to take a number of
note differences to try to reduce a series to stationarity
note Each newly differenced series is plotted
note It allows you to take up to 4 differences. The final differenced
note series is stored in column c93.
note Workspace: columns c90-c99 and constants k90-k99
note
erase c90-c99
note Enter the number of the column containing the data
set 'terminal' c90;
nobs=1.
let k91=c90(1)
let k92=count(ck91)
set c91
1:k92
end
name c91 'time'
```

Appendix 7.15. *(contd.)*

```
gplot;
lines 0 2 ck91 c91.
copy ck91 c93
exec 'header'
exec 'draw' k94
exec 'header' k94
exec 'draw' k94
exec 'header' k94
exec 'draw' k94
exec 'draw' k94
erase c90–c92 c94–c99 k90–k99
echo
```

```
# macro header
note  Enter the lag of any difference you require
note  Enter 0 if no difference is needed
note  Enter 1 if a first difference is required
note  Enter 12, for example, if a difference of lag 12 is needed
set 'terminal' c92;
nobs=1.
let k93=c92(1)
let k94=(k93>0)
```

```
# macro draw
diff k93 c93 c93
exec 'del' k93
name c93 'diff'
gplot;
lines 0 2 c93 c91.
```

```
# macro del
delete 1 c91
delete 1 c93
```

Appendix 7.16. Macro AUTOCF in file AUTOCF.MTB

This calculates the autocorrelation function of a time series and plots values. The values are stored for further use

```
noecho
note
# macro autocf
note
note  This macro produces a graph of the autocorrelation function (acf)
note  of a time series, first printing the values. 95% limits for the acf
note  of white noise are shown. The acf is stored in column c96.
note  Workspace: Columns c90–c95 and constants k90–k93
note
oh=0
```

Appendix 7.16. *(contd.)*

```
erase c90–c99
note  Enter number of column containing series
set 'terminal' c93;
nobs=1.
copy c93 k92
note  Enter number of lags required
set 'terminal' c93;
nobs=1.
copy c93 k93
acf k93 ck92 c96
set c95
1:k93
end
let k90=count(ck92)
let k91=2/sqrt(k90)
set c90
k91 k91
end
set c91
1 k93
end
let c92=–c90
set c94
0 0
end
name c96 'acf'
name c95 'lag'
gplot;
lines 0 3 c96 c95;
lines c94 c91;
lines 3 2 c90 c91;
lines 3 2 c92 c91;
erase c90–c95 k90–k93
oh=24
echo
```

Appendix 7.17. Macro SPECT in file SPECT.MTB

This macro estimates the spectrum of a time series using the lag window method with Bartlett's window. It plots the resulting estimate and 95% confidence limits, storing the estimates for future use

```
noecho
# macro spect
note
note  This macro calculates an estimate of the spectrum
note  It uses the Bartlett window to smooth the estimate
note  The user must specify a truncation point; this should be much smaller
note  than the series length but still be moderately large
note  The final estimates of the spectrum are stored in column c99 with the
note  corresponding frequencies in c96.
```

Appendix 7.17. (*contd.*)

```
note  The spectral estimates are plotted and the 95% confidence limits for
note  the true values are shown by dotted lines.
note  Workspace columns c90–c99 and constants k90–k99
note
note  Enter the number of the column containing the series
oh=0
set 'terminal' c90;
nobs=1.
copy c90 k91
let k90=count(ck91)
note  Enter the truncation point
set 'terminal' c90;
nobs=1.
copy c90 k92
acf k92 ck91 c93
let k94=stdev(ck91)
let c93=c93*k94*k94
note  The calculations will take some time!
set c94
1:k92
end
let c95=1–c94/k92
let c95=c95*c93
let k96=round((k90–1)/2)
set c96
1:k96
end
set c97
k96(0)
end
let c98=c97
let c96=6.28318*c96/k90
let c90=cos(c96)
let k97=k92
let k98=k92–1
name c96 'freq'
name c99 'spectrum'
execute 'loop' k98
let c99=k94*k94+2*(c98*c90–c97)
let c99=c99*12.566/k90
let k95=round(3*k90/k92)
invcdf 0.025 k91;
chisquare k95.
invcdf 0.975 k92;
chisquare k95.
let c91=k95*c99/k91
let c92=k95*c99/k92
gplot;
title 'Plot of estimated spectrum';
lines 0 2 c99 c96;
```

Appendix 7.17. (*contd.*)

```
lines 4 3 c91 c96;
lines 4 5 c92 c96.
erase k90–k99
erase c90–c95 c97 c98
echo
```

```
# macro loop
let k97=k97–1
let k99=c95(k97)
let c99=2*c90*c98–c97+k99
let c97=c98
let c98=c99
```

Appendix 7.18. Macro PAUTOCF in file PAUTOCF.MTB

This macro calculates and plots the partial autocorrelation function of a time series. The values are stored for future use

```
noecho
# macro pautocf
note
note This macro plots the partial autocorrelation function (pacf) of a
note times series, having first printed out the values. It also plots 95%
note limits beyond which it is reasonable to conclude that values are
note different from 0. The pacf is stored in column c93
note Workspace: c90–c92 c94 c95 k90–k95
note
oh=0
erase c90–c99
note Enter number of column containing series
set 'terminal' c91;
nobs=1.
copy c91 k93
note Enter number of lags required
set 'terminal' c91;
nobs=1.
copy c91 k94
pacf k94 ck93 c93
set c95
1:k94
end
let k90=count(ck93)
let k91=2/sqrt(k90)
set c90
k91 k91
end
set c91
```

Appendix 7.18. *(contd.)*

```
1 k94
end
let c92=-c90
set c94
0 0
end
name c93 'pacf'
name c95 'lag'
gplot;
lines 0 3 c93 c95;
lines 3 2 c94 c91;
lines 3 2 c90 c91;
lines 3 2 c92 c91.
erase c90-c92 c94-c95 k90-k95
echo
```

Appendix 7.19. Macro FIT in file FIT.MTB

This macro uses Schwarz's criterion to select the optimal ARMA model for a given time series within a range of models specified by the user

```
noecho
# macro fit
oh=0
brief 1
note
note This chooses the optimal model using the Schwarz criterion
note It applies to non-seasonal series only
note If non-seasonal differences are required, the number
note should be specified now
note
note Enter the number of first differences that are to be taken
set 'terminal' c90;
nobs=1.
let k90=c90(1)
note Enter the column of the data containing the series
set 'terminal' c91;
nobs=1.
let k91=c91(1)
let k92=count(ck91)
let k93=k92-k90
note Enter the maximum AR order and the maximum MA order required
set 'terminal' c90;
nobs=2
let k94=c90(1)
let k97=c90(2)
let k95=-1
let k99=-1
let k98=loge(k92)
let k96=k97+1
execute 'loop1' k96
name c93 'AR'
name c94 'MA'
```

Appendix 7.19. (*contd.*)

```
name c95 'SCHWARZ'
print c93 c94 c95
note  The model for which the minimum value of the criterion
note  occurs indicates a likely good model.
note  Checks should be made with the modified Box–Pierce
note  Minimum value of criterion
minimum c95
erase c90–c95 k83–k99
echo
noecho
```

```
# macro loop1
let k99=k99+1
let k95=–1
let k89=k94+1
execute 'loop2' k89
noecho
```

```
# macro loop2
let k95=k95+1
let k88=(k95+k99>0)
execute 'model' k88
noecho
```

```
# macro model
arima k95 k90 k99 ck91 c92
let k87=ssq(c92)
let k86=loge(k87/k92)
let k85=(k90>0)
let k86=k93*k86+k98*(k95+k99+k85)*k92/k93
let k84=k99*k89+k95
let c93(k84)=k95
let c94(k84)=k99
let c95(k84)=k86
```

Appendix 7.20. Macro MACF in file MACF.MTB

This macro calculates estimates for the autocorrelation function for a time series with missing values. The estimates are stored for future use. If many values are missing, the estimates may be poor

```
noecho
# macro for the acf with missing values
note
oh=0
note  This computes an estimate of the acf when there are missing values
note  in the series and plots the usual 95% confidence limits for the
note  acf of a white noise series. The estimated acf is stored in column c95.
note  Workspace: columns c90–c99 and constants k90–k99
note
note  Enter the number of the column containing the series
```

Appendix 7.20. (*contd.*)

```
set 'terminal' c90;
nobs=1.
let k91=c90(1)
note  Enter the maximum lag required
erase c90–c99
set 'terminal' c90;
nobs=1.
let k99=count(ck91)
let k92=c90(1)
let c90=ck91–mean(ck91)
let k96=ssq(c90)
copy c90 c93
copy c90 c90;
omit c90='*'.
let k90=count(c90)
erase c90
let c90=c93
let k96=k96/k90
let k93=0
exec 'lac' k92
let c95=c95/k96
erase c90
set c90
1:k92
end
name c90 'lag'
name c95 'acf'
print c90 c95
set c96
0 0
end
let c97=c96+1/sqrt(k99)
let c98=–c97
set c99
0 k92
end
gplot;
lines 0 2 c95 c90;
lines c96 c99;
lines 3 5 c97 c99;
lines 3 5 c98 c99.
erase c90–c94 c96–c99 k90–k99
echo
```

```
# macro lac
let k93=k93+1
lag c93 c93
let c94=c90*c93
let k94=sum(c94)
copy c94 c94;
omit c94='*'.
let k95=count(c94)
let k97=k94/k95
let c95(k93)=k94/k95
erase c94
```

PART
2

Modelling

8

Dynamic models of homogeneous systems

DAVID W. BOWKER

1. Introduction

This chapter provides instructions for the development of simple mathematical models which simulate the dynamics of single species populations of organisms in cultures and natural environments. These models are particularly suitable for biologists with limited previous experience in modelling because they are conceptually straightforward, mathematically tractable, and easy to implement on a computer. They consist of equations which recur frequently in modelling to describe fundamental processes such as exponential growth and decay, and they serve as a starting point from which the beginner can acquire sufficient expertise to progress to more complex modelling problems such as those described in Chapter 9.

1.1 Definitions

The models considered here are classified as dynamic models of homogeneous systems. Dynamic models are defined as abstractions of reality expressed as ordinary differential equations in which time is the independent variable. Homogeneous systems are conceived as physically uniform environments which operate as single entities and which contain discrete populations of functionally identical organisms evenly distributed in space.

1.2 The purpose of modelling

Some biologists distrust mathematical models because of the need for simplifying assumptions which ignore much of the inherent variablity and complexity observed in reality. Such criticism shows a lack of understanding of the main purpose of modelling in biology, which is to gain insight into the operation of natural systems by describing their structural and functional properties in the simple language and concepts of mathematics. Verbal descriptions of natural systems may be over-elaborate, ambiguous, confusing, and difficult to verify. Mathematical models, on the other hand, are concise, unequivocal, and explicit statements which can be verified against reality by means of computer simulation.

The power of modelling in biology does not come necessarily from its mathematical elegance, analytical precision, or predictive abilities, but from its facility to create a theoretical framework which improves our conceptual awareness and understanding of reality.

2. The modelling procedure

The rigorous following of a set of rules is not necessarily the best procedure for developing a mathematical model. Nevertheless, modelling must be learnt by active participation, and a set of guidelines within which to operate is presented in *Protocol 1*. Similar guidelines are presented in most texts on mathematical modelling, of which Burghes and Borrie (1), Edwards and Hamson (2), Jeffers (3), Jorgensen (4), Patten (5), and Spain (6) are recommended.

The development of a mathematical model is not always a linear series of steps as outlined in *Protocol 1*. Many steps may have to be re-traced along the way and enthusiasm has to be sustained throughout these excursions. This circular approach has been aptly called the 'modelling cycle' (2).

Protocol 1. General guidelines for the development of a dynamic model of a homogeneous system

1. State the aim of the project.
2. Obtain background information.
3. Conceptualize the model system.
4. Specify the components of the model system.
5. Construct a conceptual flow-chart.
6. Construct equations in words and symbols.
7. Calibrate the equations with numerical data.
8. Implement the model on a computer using an appropriate high-level language or simulation package.
9. Generate simulation data and plot graphs.
10. Verify and/or validate the simulation data. If the model is untenable then return to step 2.
11. Perform a sensitivity analysis.
12. Return to step 2 to develop the model further.

2.1 Aim

The aim of this chapter is to improve conceptual awareness and understanding of the factors and processes which control the dynamics of single species populations of organisms in nature. This aim will be achieved by means of the development of mathematical models which simulate temporal variations in the population densities of algae, bacteria, and fish in homogeneous systems.

2.2 Background information

Mathematical models are based upon fact rather than fantasy and the modelling procedure must begin with observations from reality. Examples of background information from the literature on the population dynamics of algae, bacteria, and fish are therefore supplied here.

Data from Macan (7) on the population densities of the planktonic diatom *Asterionella formosa* and the concentration of dissolved silicate in the surface waters of Lake Windermere for 100 days between March and June are shown in *Figure 1*. At first the cells multiplied rapidly by asexual division whilst they removed silicate from the surrounding water. Then the population suffered a 'crash', coincident with the depletion of silicate to a critically low concentration. Thereafter, only a small residual population of diatoms was sustained. A similar event, commonly known as the 'spring bloom', occurs annually in most lakes and oceans at temperate latitudes.

A population of micro-organisms developing under controlled laboratory conditions in a chemostat exhibits similar dynamic behaviour. A chemostat is

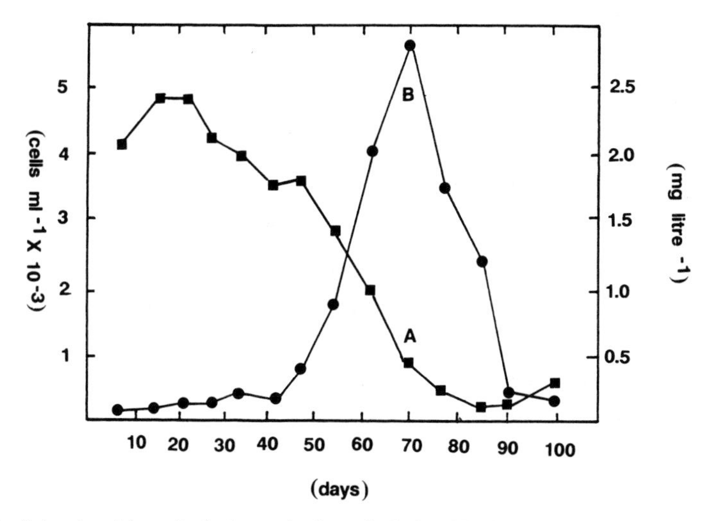

Figure 1. A 'spring bloom' of phytoplankton in Lake Windermere. A = concentration of dissolved silicate (mg/1); B = population density of the diatom *Asterionella formosa* (cells/ml).

a culture vessel through which a continuous and uniform flow of a well-mixed liquid growth medium is pumped from an external reservoir. All the nutrients in the medium are in excess, except for one, termed the growth limiting nutrient. Data from Herbert *et al.* (8) on the dynamics of a chemostat containing an axenic culture of the bacterium *Aerobacter cloacae* growing for 10 hours in a basal salt medium with glycerol as the limiting carbon source are illustrated in *Figure 2*. At first the bacterial cells multiplied and the nutrient concentration declined, a stage known as equilibration. Then the biomass of bacteria and the limiting nutrient concentration reached constant values. At this stage the chemostat was in a stable equilibrium or a steady state.

The biomass of a cohort of fish rises and falls during its lifespan like a 'bloom' of algae. *Figure 3* illustrates data from Jones (9) on the change in the biomass of a cohort of the haddock, *Melanogrammus aeglefinus*, over a period of nine years in the North Sea. In the first few years, the increase in biomass was rapid. Thereafter, there was a decline which converged upon zero at the end of the lifespan.

The physical, chemical, and biological processes causing the 'spring bloom' of phytoplankton in a lake, the equilibration of a bacterial population in a chemostat, and the dynamics of a cohort of fish in the sea are clearly not the same. Statistical analysis of the data in *Figures 1–3* would not help to elucidate these processes. They can, however, be identified, described, and analysed by means of the dynamic modelling approach.

2.3 Conceptualization of the system

Conceptualization means the creation of a series of theoretical assumptions about how a system of interest functions in time and space. The assumptions

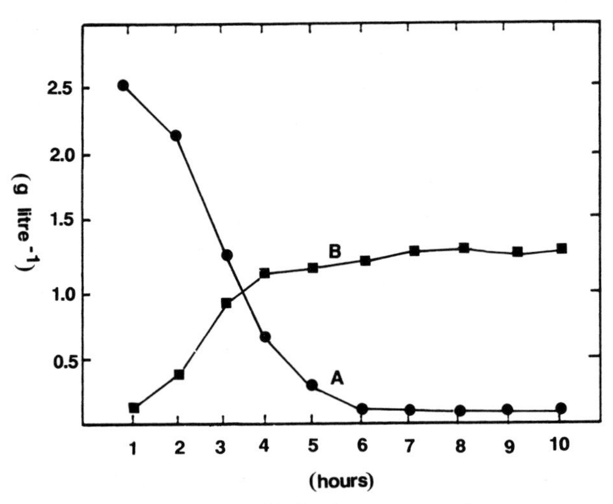

Figure 2. The equilibration of a carbon limited chemostat. A = concentration of glycerol (g/l); B = biomass of the bacterium *Aerobacter cloacae* (g/l).

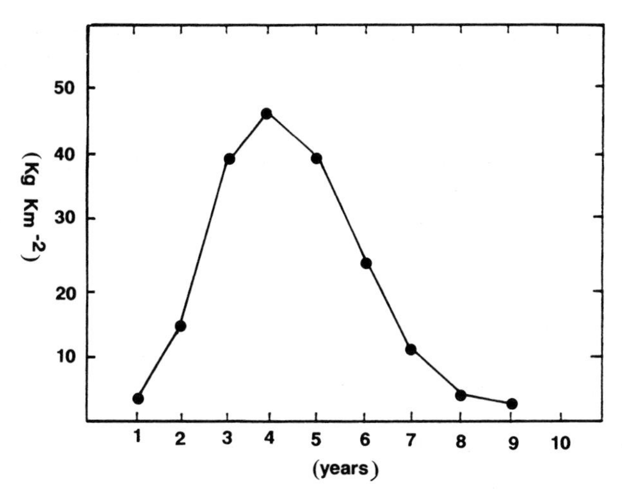

Figure 3. The biomass (kg km^{-2}) of a cohort of Haddock, *Melanogrammus aeglefinus*, in the North Sea.

underlying the construction of dynamic models of homogeneous systems include:

- the principle of mass balance
- the kinetic principle
- the deterministic assumption

2.3.1 The principle of mass balance

The principle of mass balance, which is based upon the law of conservation of energy, assumes that in a homogeneous system, all changes in mass with respect to time must be accounted for by a mass balance equation. This is a differential equation which states that the rate of change of mass equals the rate of gain of mass minus the rate of loss of mass.

2.3.2 The kinetic principle

The kinetic principle assumes that the rate at which a reaction proceeds is proportional to the concentration of its reactants. Therefore, in a mass balance equation, each rate of gain or rate of loss is calculated as the product of a mass and one or more coefficients.

The principle of mass balance and the kinetic principle were originally devised by chemists for modelling reactions between substances in continuously stirred tank reactors. The same principles are adopted by biologists to model the dynamics of homogeneous systems containing biological populations which are typically quantified in units of biomass (e.g. dry or fresh weight) and/or of population density (e.g. numbers of cells or whole organisms) per unit volume or area of environment.

2.3.3 The deterministic assumption

Homogeneous systems are assumed to be deterministic. This means that unexpected perturbations, mutations, or random variations are excluded, and that the state of a system at any given time is predetermined entirely by the state of the system at a previous time. The larger and the more homogeneous the system, the more it will conform to this deterministic ideal.

2.3.4 Violations of the assumptions

Axenic populations of unicellular micro-organisms suspended in liquid media in batch or continuous cultures are probably the best examples of homogeneous systems which exist in nature. Single-species populations of aquatic organisms, such as phytoplankton or fish, evenly dispersed in a lake or ocean are also assumed to constitute natural homogeneous systems. However, these systems are not completely homogeneous in reality. The inherent differences between the individual members of a living population, such as variations in genotype, sex, morphometry, chemical composition, or physiological condition are neglected and random effects, such as uneven spatial distribution and genetic mutation, are ignored. Consequently, for modelling purposes, the variability found in reality is eliminated and attention is focused upon generality at the expense of precision and realism.

2.4 Specification of system components

The components of a homogeneous system include:

- state variables
- driving or forcing variables
- sources and sinks
- processes
- flows

2.4.1 State variables

State variables predict the state of a system at any point in time. They are the dependent variables in the differential equations, otherwise known as state equations, in which time is always the independent variable. The state variables in dynamic models of homogeneous systems typically include the biomass or population densities of the constituent organisms.

2.4.2 Driving variables

Driving variables, otherwise known as forcing variables, are the external environmental factors such as light, temperature, and/or nutrient supply which act upon the system to promote a change in state.

2.4.3 Sources and sinks

Sources and sinks are passive repositories for energy or materials flowing respectively into or out of a system. They do not promote any changes in state.

2.4.4 Flows

There is a continuous flow of energy, materials, and/or information between the state variables, driving variables, sources, and sinks.

2.4.5 Processes

Processes are physical, chemical, or biological mechanisms which act as valves or gates, controlling the magnitude of the flows. Two types of process are distinguished. Gain processes, such as growth, cause the state variables to increase in magnitude whilst loss processes, such as decay, cause the state variables to decrease.

2.5 Construction of a conceptual flow-chart

A conceptual flow-chart illustrates the interrelationships between the different components of a system and acts as a convenient bridge between the conceptualization of a model and the construction of equations. Various symbolic conventions have been proposed for flow-charts. Chapter 9 presents alternative symbols to the convention used in this chapter which is based upon Forrester's symbolism as outlined by Jeffers (3):

- state variables are rectangles or boxes
- driving variables are circles
- flows are lines with arrows
- sources and sinks are polygons or clouds
- processes are valves or gates

Conceptual flow-charts are presented in *Figure 4* to illustrate the four models considered in this chapter. *Figure 4a* conceptualizes a general model of phytoplankton dynamics in a lake or ocean which is developed further in *Figure 4d*. *Figure 4b* describes a general model of a chemostat system and *Figure 4c* conceptualizes a general model of the dynamics of a cohort of fish. The models described in *Figure 4a–d* are referred to according to the names of their originators as O'BRIEN (10), HERBERT (8), BEVERTON (11), and DROOP (12) respectively.

2.6 Construction of equations

Equations are constructed with direct reference to a flow-chart according to the following guidelines:

- there is normally one state equation for each state variable

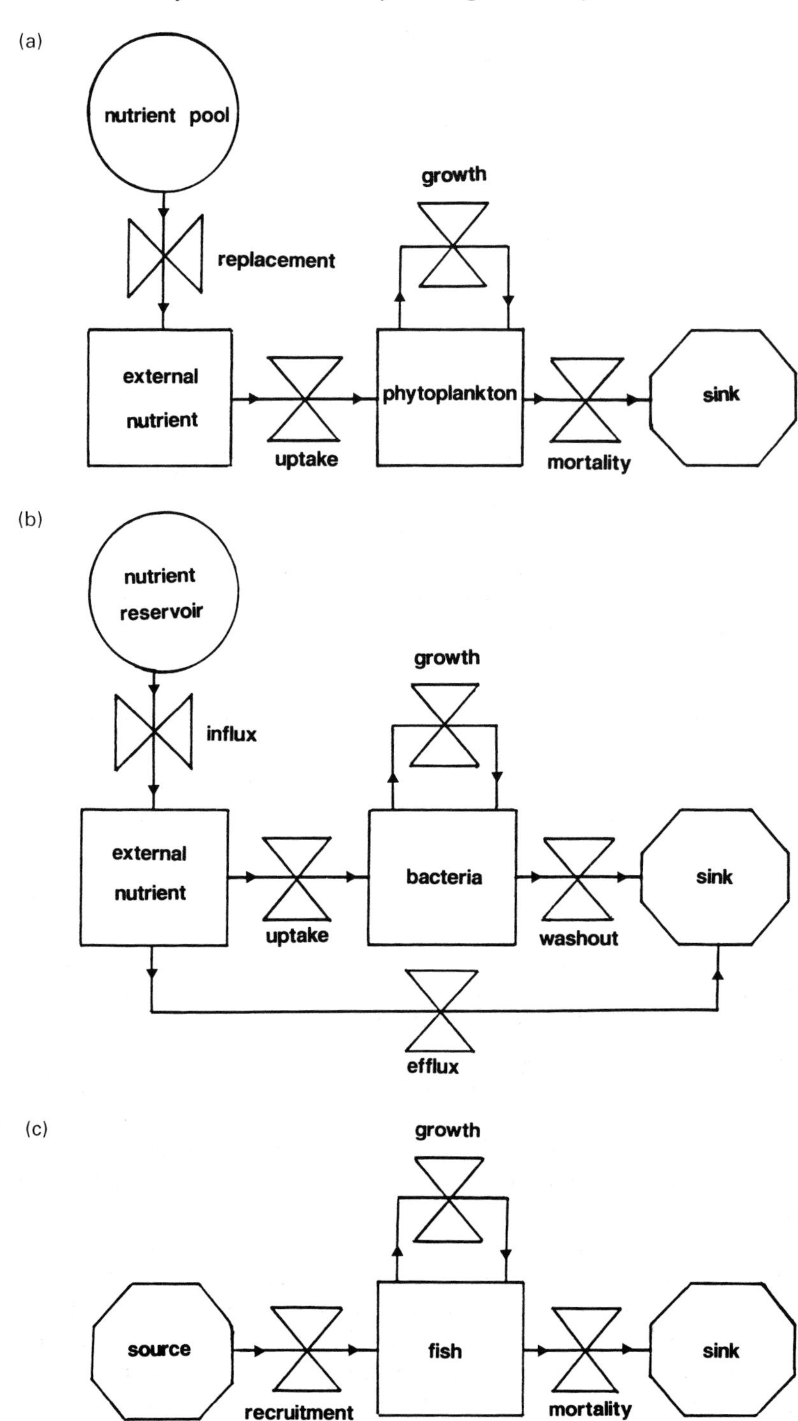
(a)
nutrient pool
replacement
growth
external nutrient
uptake
phytoplankton
mortality
sink
(b)
nutrient reservoir
influx
growth
external nutrient
uptake
bacteria
washout
sink
efflux
(c)
growth
source
recruitment
fish
mortality
sink

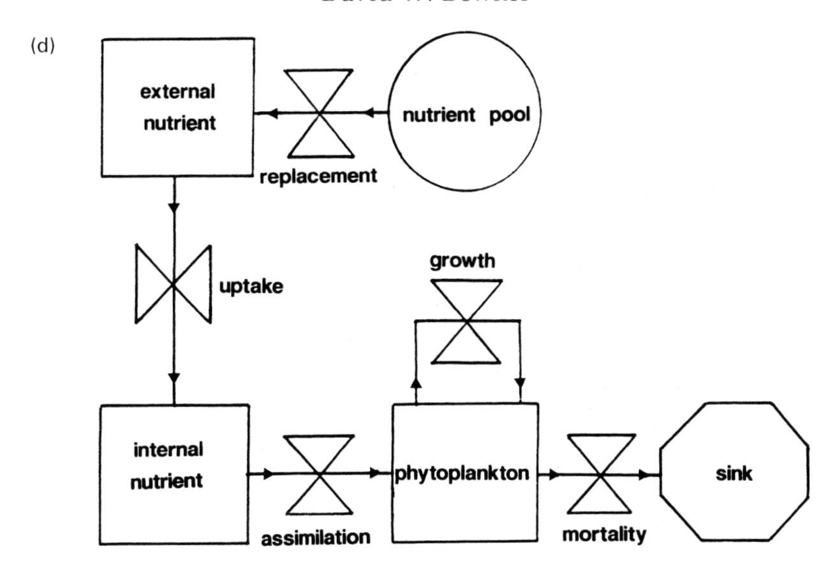

Figure 4. Flow charts of the dynamics of a (a) phytoplankton population in a lake or ocean, (b) population of bacteria in a chemostat, (c) cohort of fish, and (d) population of phytoplankton in a lake or ocean developed from (a).

- the rate of change of a state variable (a box) equals one or more gain processes (a valve controlling a flow which enters a box) minus one or more loss processes (a valve controlling a flow which exits from a box)
- each gain or loss process is generally expressed as the product of a state variable and one or more coefficients

The rate of change of a state variable can be expressed symbolically as $\Delta X/\Delta t$ where X = value of state variable; t = time; and Δ = amount of change. If t is assumed to be infinitely small, then it is possible to describe an instantaneous rate of change in a moment of time, so that $\Delta X = \mathrm{d}X$ and $\Delta t = \mathrm{d}t$. The rate of change term $\mathrm{d}X/\mathrm{d}t$ is called the derivative and may be expressed in shorthand form as X' where $' = \mathrm{d}/\mathrm{d}t$.

The equations described below conform, as far as possible, to those proposed by the originators of each model. The original symbolism has been conserved so that the information given here can be supplemented directly from the literature without confusion. This means, unfortunately, that an identical symbol is sometimes used for different variables, e.g. the symbol N is used in O'BRIEN for the population density of phytoplankton and in BEVERTON for the population density of fish. It also means that different symbols are sometimes used incongruously to define the same variable. For example, g_{m}, μ_{m}, and $\mu_{\max}$ all refer to the nutrient saturated growth coefficient. Chapter 9 presents yet another range of symbols and the modelling literature abounds with examples of confounded mathematical symbolism.

Biologists who are not used to handling equations and symbols should not be deterred by this confusing state of the art.

2.6.1 Equations for O'BRIEN

The flow-chart in *Figure 4a* shows that the state variable (phytoplankton population density) is acted upon by one gain process (growth or asexual multiplication) and one loss process (mortality). It follows that the mass balance equation which defines the rate of change of population density has two terms. The first is a positive term, representing gains caused by growth. The second term is negative, representing losses due to mortality.

Growth is represented in *Figure 4a* by a feedback loop. In modelling terminology, feedback is defined as the return of the effect of a process to its source. The effect of growth is more cells, which in turn produce more cells. Therefore the rate of growth of the population increases in constant proportion to the size of the population. This fundamental biological process is termed exponential growth. In a homogeneous system, each member of a population is assumed to have an equal probability of death and a constant proportion of the total population dies every day. These assumptions result in exponential decay. The mass balance or state equation used to model the rate of change in the population density of phytoplankton in O'BRIEN, is therefore:

$$\text{rate of change} = \text{growth} - \text{mortality},$$
$$N' = (Ng) - (Nd), \tag{1}$$

where N' = rate of change of population density with respect to time, N = population density of phytoplankton, g = growth coefficient, and d = mortality coefficient. Equation 1 may be abbreviated to

$$N' = rN, \tag{2}$$

where r, the instantaneous rate of population growth, is given by

$$r = g - d. \tag{3}$$

Equation 2 is a classical model, first conceptualized by Malthus in 1798 to describe the exponential growth of the human population. It is discussed comprehensively in textbooks on population dynamics, such as Williamson (13), Boughey (14), and Christiansen and Fenchel (15).

The rate of growth of phytoplankton, defined as the product of N and g in Equation 1, is assumed to be limited by the concentration of a single dissolved nutrient in the surrounding water. The growth coefficient, g, is modelled using a classical equation first proposed by Michaelis and Menten in 1913 working on enzyme kinetics and subsequently modified by Monod in 1942 to describe the hyperbolic relationship between microbial growth rate and the external nutrient concentration in the surrounding environment:

$$g = g_m C/(C + K_s), \tag{4}$$

where g = growth coefficient, g_m = nutrient saturated growth coefficient, C = concentration of external limiting nutrient, and K_s = half saturation coefficient (concentration of external nutrient at $g_m/2$). Equation 4 is commonly called the Monod equation.

Figure 4a shows that phytoplankton growth is driven by the uptake of nutrient from the surrounding water and that the state equation which describes the change in nutrient concentration requires two terms. The replacement of nutrient from the external nutrient pool into the water surrounding the algae is a gain process represented by a positive term, whilst nutrient uptake is a loss process represented by a negative term, hence

$$\text{rate of change} = \text{replacement} - \text{uptake},$$
$$C' = R - (qNg), \tag{5}$$

where C' = rate of change of nutrient concentration with respect to time, C = nutrient concentration in water, R = rate of replacement of nutrients, and q = uptake coefficient or depletion factor, which is equivalent to the mass of nutrient per cell. Note that O'Brien (10) proposed the symbol D for the depletion factor. I have substituted q for D to avoid confusion with d in Equation 1 and D in Equations 6, 8, and 9.

2.6.2 Equations for HERBERT

The conceptual flow-chart for HERBERT (*Figure 4b*) displays microbial growth and nutrient uptake processes which are functionally identical to those in O'BRIEN (*Figure 4a*). However, HERBERT includes the additional processes of nutrient influx, nutrient efflux, and washout, which are caused by the continuous flow of growth medium into and out of the chemostat vessel. These processes are defined in exponential terms.

Sterile growth medium is fed into the chemostat at a constant flow rate designated by the symbol f and emerges from it at the same rate. The volume of medium in the culture vessel remains constant, designated by the symbol v. The residence time of medium in the culture vessel is determined by their ratio which is called the dilution rate defined by

$$D = f/v, \tag{6}$$

where D = dilution rate or the number of complete volume changes per unit of time. With complete mixing, every molecule of nutrient and every bacterial cell has an equal probability of leaving the culture vessel within a given time. The rate of efflux of nutrient and the washout rate of bacteria are therefore exponential loss processes defined by the following terms: efflux = $-DS$ where S = limiting nutrient concentration and washout = $-Dx$ where x = biomass of bacteria. Similarly, the replacement rate or rate of influx of limiting nutrient from the external reservoir into the culture vessel is an exponential dilution process modelled by DS_R, where S_R = concentration of nutrient in the reservoir.

The growth rate of bacteria in a chemostat, like the growth rate of phytoplankton in a lake, is assumed to be controlled by the concentration of limiting nutrient in the external medium and the Monod equation is therefore applied for both purposes. This equation, using the symbols proposed by Herbert *et al.* (8), is

$$\mu = \mu_m S/(K_s + S), \tag{7}$$

where μ = growth coefficient, μ_m = nutrient saturated growth coefficient, S = limiting nutrient concentration, and K_s = half saturation coefficient (nutrient concentration at $\mu_m/2$). Note that, apart from the symbolism, Equation 7 is the same as Equation 4 and that the Monod equation appears in different guises with different symbols elsewhere in the literature. Equation 7 may also be described elsewhere (e.g. in Chapter 9) as a Michaelis–Menten function.

In HERBERT, the rate of uptake of limiting nutrient by bacteria in a chemostat is expressed as $-(\mu x)/Y$, where Y = yield coefficient or the amount of bacteria produced divided by the amount of nutrient taken up. Note that q in equation 5 of O'BRIEN is numerically equivalent to $1/Y$.

It follows from the flow chart and the information given above that the two state equations for HERBERT are

rate of change of bacteria = growth − washout

$$x' = (\mu x) - (Dx) \tag{8}$$

and

rate of change in nutrient = influx − efflux − uptake

$$S' = (DS_R) - (DS) - (\mu x)/Y. \tag{9}$$

2.6.3 Equations for BEVERTON

As illustrated in the flow-chart (*Figure 4c*) the rate of change in the biomass of a cohort of fish (the state variable) is modelled in terms of the gain processes of recruitment and growth and the loss process of mortality.

A cohort of fish is initiated when the larve hatch from the eggs produced by their parents. These larvae develop into juvenile fish and the influx of juveniles into the population is known as recruitment. In BEVERTON, a defined number of fish are assumed to be recruited from an undefined source at age zero. The population density then declines continuously with time due to mortality. However, each individual fish grows throughout its lifespan by an increase in biomass, a process which is illustrated in *Figure 4c* by means of a feedback loop. The product of the two processes, growth and mortality, promotes a change in the biomass of the cohort. In BEVERTON this change is expressed as the product of two differential equations.

The mass balance equation first proposed by Von Bertalanffy in 1934 is used to describe fish growth in terms of the increase in biomass caused by the assimilation of food minus the loss in biomass due to respiration and other catabolic processes:

$$\text{rate of growth} = \text{assimilation} - \text{catabolism}$$
$$W' = (HW^{0.6}) - (kW), \qquad (10)$$

where W' = rate of change of biomass with respect to time, W = biomass of individual animal, and H and k are coefficients. The exponent in the assimilation term is based on the assumption that the surface area of intestine is proportional to $W^{0.6}$. Equation 10 implies that food is the driving variable. A relationship between the growth rate of fish and the amount of food available is not included in BEVERTON because food is assumed to be in constant and unlimited supply.

A cohort of fish suffers continuous mortality during its lifespan and the population density declines exponentially with time. In BEVERTON, fish mortality is modelled using the same assumptions required for the death of phytoplankton in Equation 1, washout of bacteria in Equation 8, and efflux of nutrient in Equation 9 to give

$$N' = -ZN, \qquad (11)$$

where N' = rate of change in number of fish with respect to time, N = number of fish, and Z = mortality coefficient. Fish mortality may be natural or caused by the fishing activities of man; therefore it has two components:

$$Z = F + M, \qquad (12)$$

where F = fishing mortality coefficient and M = natural mortality coefficient. Fish are not available for exploitation by man throughout their whole lifespan. For the first period of their life they are only subject to natural mortality because they are too small to be caught. However, from a critical age, known as the age of first capture, they suffer from both fishing and natural mortality. This discontinuity is modelled by means of a step function, i.e. an instantaneous change of a variable to a different value for a definite time. It is described by the logical expression

$$\text{if } t < t_c \text{ then } Z = M \text{ else } Z = M + F, \qquad (13)$$

where t = age of fish and t_c = age of fish at first capture.

The total biomass of a cohort of fish at a given age is the product of the number of individuals and the biomass of each individual:

$$B_t = N_t W_t, \qquad (14)$$

where B_t = biomass of cohort at age t, N_t = number of fish at age t, and W_t = biomass of individual fish at age t. In a real fish population, W_t is a normally distributed variable. Variance around W_t develops because the individual members of a cohort hatch at different times and grow at different rates. In BEVERTON, however, the population is assumed to be homogeneous and W_t is constant.

2.7 Calibration

A model is calibrated by substitution of numerical data for the symbols used in the equations. The following calibration data are usually required:

- the initial values of each state variable
- the starting and ending times
- the time steps
- constants (quantities which are not variable)
- parameters (variables and coefficients)

Models are usually calibrated with reference to empirical research on the system of interest and/or from the literature. The models described so far in this chapter are calibrated with the literature values in *Tables 1–3*.

Parameters are often difficult to quantify and the selection of a single value for a parameter may be virtually impossible. Consequently, different values may have to be tried, adopting a trial and error approach. The units of each parameter must also be carefully considered.

Table 1. Calibration data for O'BRIEN

C	initial nutrient conc.	2000	μg/l
CINT	communication interval	1	day
d	mortality coefficient	0.25	day^{-1}
g_m	maximum growth coefficient	0.35	day^{-1}
K_s	half saturation coefficient	10	μg/l
N	initial population density	10×10^3	cells/l
R	nutrient replacement rate	5	μg/l/day
q	uptake coefficient	8×10^{-5}	μg/cell
TFIN	final value of T	100	days

Table 2. Calibration data for HERBERT

CINT	communication interval	1	h
D	dilution rate	0.5	h^{-1}
K_s	half saturation coefficient	0.0123	g/l
S	initial nutrient conc.	2.5	g/l
S_R	reservoir nutrient conc.	2.5	g/l
TFIN	final value of T	12	h
μ_m	maximum growth coefficient	0.85	h^{-1}
x	initial biomass of bacteria	0.1	g/l
Y	yield coefficient	0.53	—

Table 3. Calibration data for BEVERTON

CINT	communication interval	1	year
F	fishing mortality coefficient	0.6	year^{-1}
H	Von–Bertalanffy coefficient	9.0	year^{-1}
k	Von–Bertalanffy coefficient	0.78	year^{-1}
M	natural mortality coefficient	0.28	year^{-1}
N	initial number of recruits	400	fish km^{-2}
t_c	age at first capture	3	years
TFIN	final value of T	10	years
W	initial biomass of fish	0.1	g

2.8 Implementation and simulation

A dynamic model is of little practical value to a biologist unless it can be implemented on a computer. The solutions to the equations can then be calculated using the procedure known as computer simulation. The numerical data generated by the computer are termed simulation data and these include the values of the state and driving variables at successive intervals of time over a predetermined time period.

A model can be implemented using a high level computer language such as Fortran (5), BASIC (6), or Pascal (16). In Chapter 9 such languages are recommended for serious research purposes. However, the absolute beginner to modelling is advised to start with a specialized simulation package such as *ISIM* (*Appendix A*). *ISIM* incorporates comprehensive and easy to use facilities for handling differential equations and for the graphic display of simulation data. Using *ISIM*, the biologist with limited computing experience can start to solve modelling problems within a few hours. In comparison, considerably more time and effort must be invested to learn and use a high-level programming language for modelling purposes.

Protocols 2–4 provide information for the implementation of O'BRIEN, HERBERT, and BEVERTON with *ISIM*. The protocols give instructions for the reader to translate the numbered equations in the text directly into usable *ISIM* programs as listed in *Appendices 8.1–8.3*. The user manual (17) should be referred to for more details about writing, editing, saving, and loading programs in *ISIM*.

Protocol 2. Implementation and verification of O'BRIEN using *ISIM*. (See *Appendix 8.1* for the program)

1. Input the calibration data (*Table 1*).
2. Input the SIM and DYNAMIC statements.
3. Input the Monod Equation 4 followed by the two state Equations 1 and 5.

Protocol 2. *Continued*

4. Convert the phytoplankton population density from cells/l to cells/ml.

5. Input the OUTPUT and PREPARE statements.

6. Execute the program with the START command.

7. Use the GRAPH command to plot the simulation data (P and C on T) as shown in *Figure 5* and verify the simulation against real data (*Figure 1*).

Protocol 3. Implementation and verification of HERBERT using ISIM. (See *Appendix 8.2* for the program)

1. Input the calibration data (*Table 2*).

2. Input the SIM and DYNAMIC statements.

3. Input the Monod Equation 7 followed by the two state Equations 8 and 9.

4. Input the OUTPUT and PREPARE statements.

5. Execute the program with the START command.

6. Use the GRAPH command to plot the simulation data (x and S on T) as shown in *Figure 6* and verify the simulation data against real data (*Figure 2*).

Protocol 4. Implementation and verification of BEVERTON using ISIM. (See *Appendix 8.3* for the program)

1. Input the calibration data (*Table 3*).

2. Input the SIM and DYNAMIC statements.

3. Input the step function 13 and Equation 12.

4. Input the two state Equations 10 and 11.

5. Input the product of the state Equations 14 and convert the biomass from g km^{-2} to kg km^{-2}.

6. Input the OUTPUT and PREPARE statements.

7. Execute the program with the START command.

8. Use the GRAPH command to plot the simulation data (B on T) as shown in *Figure 7* and verify the simulation data against real data (*Figure 3*).

2.8 Integration

The generation of simulation data from differential equations involves the procedure known as integration. A brief introduction to integration is given here but more comprehensive reviews are provided by Jorgensen (4) and

Patten (5). Two approaches are possible, termed analytical and numerical integration.

2.8.1 Analytical integration

The first and most accurate approach is to find an analytical solution to a differential equation in the form of an algebraic equation. This is only possible if the differential equation is linear, i.e. if the state variable changes linearly with time and/or if the equation can be transformed into a linear relationship. For example, the analytical solution to Malthus's Equation 2 is

$$N_t = N_0\, e^{(rt)}, \tag{15}$$

where N_t = population density at time t, N_0 = initial population density, e = base of natural logarithms, and r = instantaneous rate of growth. Exponential population growth is simulated when constant values of N_0 and r are substituted into Equation 15 at successive values of t.

Similarly, Beverton and Holt's differential Equation 11 for describing the exponential decline in the numbers of a cohort of fish with time integrates to

$$N_t = N_0\, e^{(-Zt)}, \tag{16}$$

where N_t = number of fish surviving at age t, N_0 = initial number of fish, and Z = instantaneous rate of fish mortality.

O'BRIEN and HERBERT contain coupled differential equations with several shared parameters. Such equations cannot be integrated analytically unless the systems are in a steady state. If Equations 1 and 5 from O'BRIEN are set to zero and solved for N and C, then

$$N = R/(qd); \tag{17}$$

$$C = dK_s/(g_m - d). \tag{18}$$

Since at steady state $g = d$, then Equation 17 may be reconstructed to redefine the rate of growth of algae in terms of the rate of nutrient supply:

$$Ng = R/q. \tag{19}$$

However, the natural system is not in a steady state. Both the population density of the phytoplankton and the nutrient concentration are time-varying (see *Figure 1*). Similarly, the equilibration phase of the chemostat (*Figure 2*) is a dynamic process which cannot be simulated by analytical integration of Equations 8 and 9. The steady state condition of the chemostat can, however, be described by means of the following analytical solutions:

$$x = Y(S_R - S); \tag{20}$$

$$S = K_s D/(\mu_m - D). \tag{21}$$

In reality many biologists will need to seek the help of a mathematician to provide analytical solutions to all but the simplest models.

2.8.2 Numerical integration

The dynamics of most biological systems are characterized by non-linear behaviour which cannot be simulated by means of analytical integration. Simulation data must therefore be generated by means of approximation or numerical methods. Computer programs can be written in a high-level language to perform numerical integration, but the biologist who is new to modelling is unlikely to have such expertise. This problem is alleviated by the availability of packages such as *ISIM* which incorporate a range of algorithms for numerical integration. However, there is a danger in using simulation packages without a working knowledge of the mathematics upon which they are based, and the beginner must know something about numerical integration to avoid the simulation of misleading data.

Numerical integration itself is easy to understand intuitively. If a state variable changes during a step in time then its new value at the end of the step equals its old value at the beginning of the step plus any change in value which has taken place during the step. If the change is not linear with respect to time, then error is generated in calculating the new value. This error is proportional to the length of the time step and is cumulative since each new value is dependent on its respective old value.

Euler's rectangular method is the simplest numerical integration procedure. If a state variable X varies with time t as expressed by the derivative X' or $\mathrm{d}X/\mathrm{d}t$, then successive values of X can be predicted from the equation

$$X_{t+\Delta t} = X_t + \Delta X, \tag{22}$$

where $X_{t+\Delta t}$ = new value of the state variable X after time $t + \Delta t$, X_t = old value of X at time t and ΔX = change in X during the time step Δt. Although Equation 22 generates error, it is very useful for computer simulation purposes when a quick and approximate solution is acceptable. For example, Chapter 9 includes a program written in BASIC using Euler's integration method.

More accurate integration procedures are based upon improved estimates of the rate of change of the state variable during each time step, but accuracy is only achieved at the expense of greater computation time.

ISIM incorporates a variable time step Runge–Kutta algorithm which optimizes the time step so that the calculation error is minimized. This default option should always be chosen first. However, circumstances can arise when the variable time step will reduce until it becomes so small that integration ceases to progress and an error message is given. Occasionally the integration algorithm becomes unstable and generates simulation data which are several orders of magnitude higher or lower than the expected data. Under these circumstances it is necessary to consult the *ISIM* user manual (17) and change to another integration option with a fixed step length.

2.9 Verification

Verification means to test whether a model is tenable. A model is verified when the computer program executes without error and when the orders of magnitude and the behaviour of the simulation data approximate those found in reality. If verification is not successful then the modelling cycle must be repeated (see *Protocol 1*).

Verification in *Protocols 2–4* involves the visual comparison of the simulation data against the real data which were used for background information when constructing the models. Note that the simulation data do not reproduce the 'noise' or scatter which invariably surrounds real data. Deterministic models simulate generalized patterns of behaviour created by equations which exclude random variability. They cannot resolve fluctuations caused by violations of the assumptions of homogeneity.

The simulation data generated by O'BRIEN (*Figure 5*) reflect the development and 'crash' of a real spring bloom of phytoplankton with the simultaneous depletion of the growth limiting nutrient (*Figure 1*). HERBERT generates simulation data (*Figure 6*) which reproduce the equilibration stage followed by the steady state which can be observed in a real chemostat (*Figure 2*). BEVERTON generates simulation data describing the rise and fall in biomass of a cohort of fish (*Figure 7*) which can also be verified against real data (*Figure 3*).

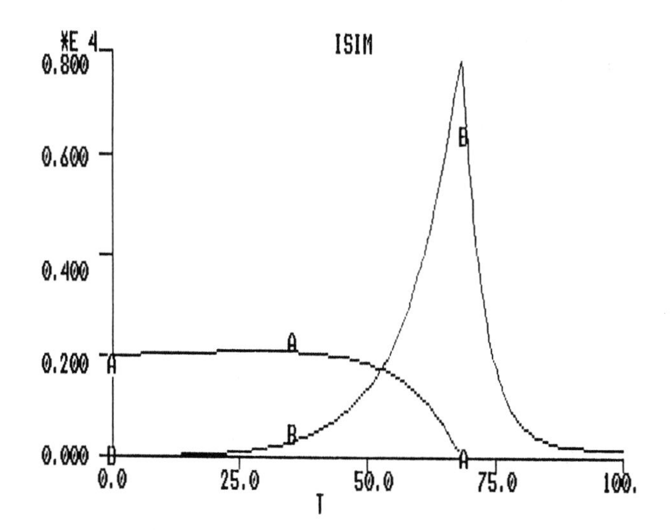

Figure 5. Graphic output from O'BRIEN using the *ISIM* program generated by *Protocol 2* (*Appendix 8.1*). *A* = concentration of limiting nutrient (μg/l); *B* = population density of phytoplankton (cells/ml); *T* = time (days).

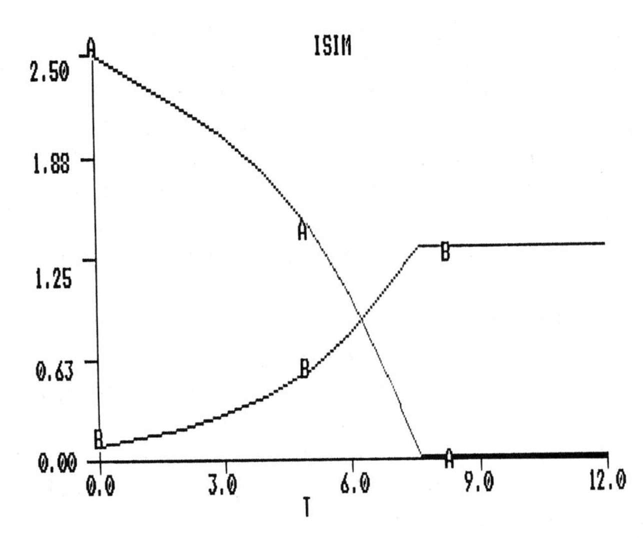

Figure 6. Graphic output from HERBERT using the *ISIM* program generated by *Protocol 3* (*Appendix 8.2*). A = concentration of limiting nutrient (g/l); B = biomass of bacteria (g/l); T = time (hours).

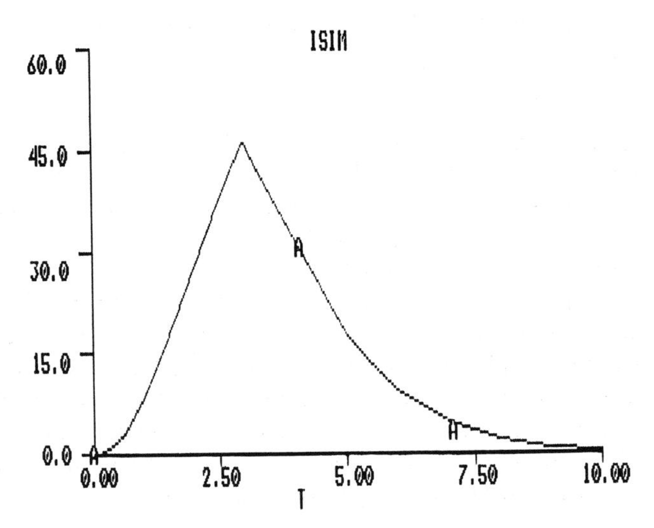

Figure 7. Graphic output from BEVERTON using the *ISIM* program generated by *Protocol 4* (*Appendix 8.3*). A = biomass of fish (kg km^{-2}); T = time (years).

2.10 Validation

Validation means to test the predictive abilities of a model. It usually involves the evaluation of the goodness of fit of the simulation data to a set of independent real data (i.e. data not used for background information during model construction). The classical models described in this chapter have considerable generality and provide insight into fundamental biological processes. However, the application of such simple equations as accurate predictors of reality is questionable and their validation is unwarranted. The models could potentially be further developed, calibrated, and validated to predict population dynamics in specific natural systems such as diatoms in Lake Windermere, bacteria in a laboratory chemostat, or Haddock in the North Sea. However, their powers of generality and tractability would then have to be sacrificed for the sake of precision, realism, and predictive ability.

2.11 Sensitivity analysis

Sensitivity analysis means to determine the effects of parameter manipulation on the behaviour of the simulation data. It does not have to be performed at the end of the modelling pathway as indicated in *Protocol 1*. Sensitivity analysis is useful during model construction to improve the accuracy of the parameters and/or to assist with verification. When a model has been verified, then sensitivity analysis may be applied to:

- test hypotheses
- analyse the stability, resilience and/or resistance of a model (see Chapter 9)
- perform an experiment which would be impossible or very difficult to carry out in reality
- predict events in the future

The simplest sensitivity analysis starts off with a simple question, such as 'What would happen to the simulation data if the value of a particular parameter is changed?'. An elaborate sensitivity analysis, like an elegant laboratory experiment, requires a well planned design in which the user interacts systematically with a model.

The *ISIM* package, as indicated by its name (an acronym of interactive simulator) incorporates facilities for sensitivity analysis. The magnitude of any variable can be monitored and/or altered before, during, or after program execution. The simulation of data can be manually interrupted, the magnitude of one or more program variables altered, and the simulation then continued. Simulation data generated from successive runs of a program can be superimposed on a single graph for comparative purposes.

2.11.1 Sensitivity analysis of O'BRIEN

The *ISIM* programs listed in *Appendices 8.1–8.3* require modification to facilitate sensitivity analysis. An example of an *ISIM* program modified specifically for this purpose is given in *Appendix 8.4*. Instructions for the use of the modified program are given in *Protocol 5*.

Sensitivity analysis demonstrates that O'BRIEN is a very robust model, meaning that its characteristic dynamic behaviour is conserved despite parameter manipulation. A 'bloom' is always simulated, provided that the

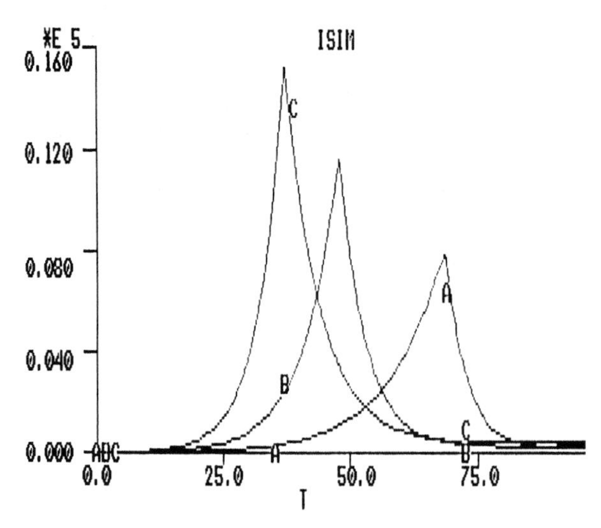

Figure 8. Graphic output from O'BRIEN using the *ISIM* program as described in *Protocol 5* (*Appendix 8.4*). *A, B,* and *C* = population densities of phytoplankton (cells/ml) at $d = 0.25$, $d = 0.2$, and $d = 0.15$ respectively; T = time (days).

growth rate initially exceeds the mortality rate and the population always 'crashes' as a consequence of nutrient depletion (*Figure 8*). This confirms observations from reality about the stability of the 'spring bloom' of phytoplankton.

Sensitivity analysis of O'BRIEN helps to test hypotheses about the ways in which a microbial species may be physiologically adapted to make optimum use of the available nutrient supply. Christiansen and Fenchel (15) for example, suggest that K_s and g_m values may be correlated with the external nutrient concentration. Thus a species with a low K_s and a low g_m is shown to generate greater population densities at low nutrient concentrations than a species with a high K_s and a high g_m (*Figure 9*). However, a species with a high K_s and a high g_m produces higher population densities at higher nutrient concentrations.

Protocol 5. Sensitivity analysis of O'BRIEN

1. Input the program listed in *Appendix 8.4*.
2. Execute the program with the START command.
3. Change the value of the mortality coefficient (d = 0.05–0.75) with the VAL statement (e.g. VAL d = 0.2)
4. Re-execute the program with the GO command.
5. Repeat stages 3–4 with a third value of d.

6. Use the GRAPH command to plot the three sets of simulation data (P on T) on the same axes, as shown in *Figure 8*.
7. Perform an analysis to compare the dynamics of different phytoplankton species which have different maximum growth coefficients (g_m = 0.2 −2.0) and half saturation coefficients (K_s = 1–1000) under different conditions of nutrient supply (R = 1–250; C = 2–2000). See *Figure 9* for an example.

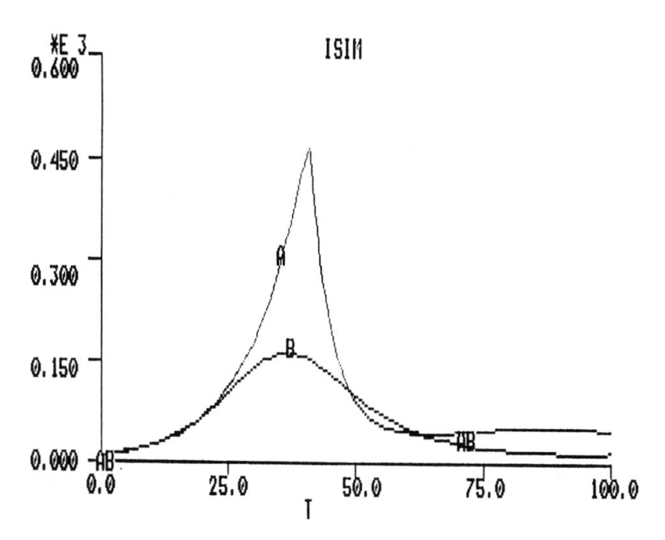

Figure 9. Graphic output from O'BRIEN using the *ISIM* program as described in *Protocol 5* (*Appendix 8.4*). *A* and *B* = population densities of phytoplankton (cells/ml) at K_8 = 1, g_m = 0.35, R = 1, C = 100 and K_8 = 500, g_m = 2.0, R = 1, C = 100 respectively; T = time (days).

2.11.2 Sensitivity analysis of HERBERT

Herbert *et al.* (10) presented experimental data on the relationship between the biomass of *Aerobacter cloacae* produced in a carbon limited chemostat at steady state and the dilution rate of the chemostat. These data (*Table 4*) can be used to verify the model. The values of bacterial biomass produced in reality can be predicted with reasonable accuracy by means of a sensitivity analysis of HERBERT in which the dilution rate is manipulated.

2.11.3 Sensitivity analysis of BEVERTON

Protocol 6 presents instructions for a sensitivity analysis of BEVERTON. This is an example of the use of a model to perform an experiment which could not be performed in reality. In natural systems, the recruitment and mortality of fish are not under the direct control of man, but these processes can be manipulated easily on the computer. The simulated fish population is

Table 4. The biomass of *Aerobacter cloacae* produced in a carbon limited chemostat at steady state

Dilution rate (h^{-1})	**Biomass (g/l)**
0.25	1.30
0.5	1.29
0.72	1.07
0.91	0.72

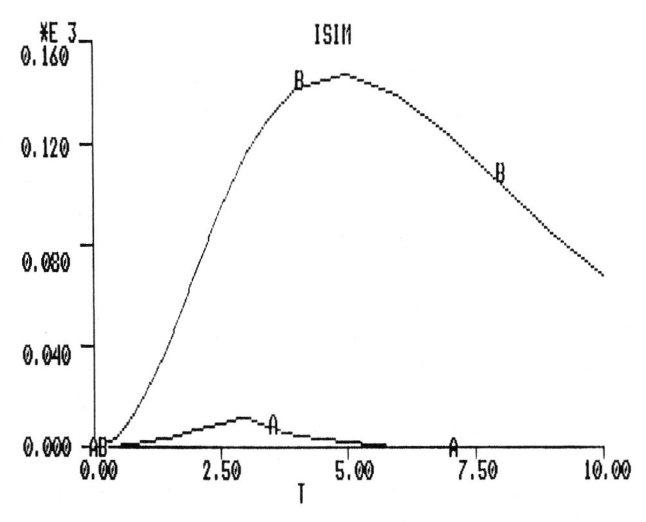

Figure 10. Graphic output from BEVERTON using the *ISIM* program as described in *Protocol 6*. *A* and *B* = biomass of fish (kg km^{-2}) at N_0 = 100, Z = 1.3 and N_0 = 1000, Z = 0.3 respectively; T = time (years).

very sensitive to high mortality and low recruitment. This combination of parameters results in a greatly reduced maximum biomass and a dramatic 'crash' of the cohort well before the end of its natural lifespan (*Figure 10*).

Protocol 6. Sensitivity analysis of BEVERTON

1. Re-write the *ISIM* program (see *Appendix 8.3*) to facilitate sensitivity analysis.
2. Refer to *Protocol 5* for operating instructions.
3. Determine the response of the cohort of fish to:
   (a) low recruitment (e.g. N_0 = 100) and high mortality (e.g. Z = 1.3)

(b) high recruitment (e.g. $N_0 = 1000$) and low mortality (e.g. $Z = 0.3$)

4. Use the GRAPH command to plot the two sets of simulation data (B on T) on the same axes as shown in *Figure 10*.

2.12 Revision

A mathematical model, by definition, is only an abstraction and not an emulator of reality. It is therefore naïve and unrealistic to believe that the multitude of dynamic models found in the literature, including O'BRIEN, HERBERT, and BEVERTON are wholly correct. An incorrect model is beneficial if it leads to new lines of enquiry and the development of a better model which enhances conceptual understanding. The biologist who is new to modelling should therefore not be afraid of making mistakes. The first time a model is constructed, it is likely to be incorrect. Only by further development of the original model can verification be achieved. For example, Droop (12) disproved Monod's assumption, which is implicit in Equation 7, that the growth rate of micro-organisms is controlled directly by the external nutrient concentration. He found experimentally that in some species of algae the growth rate of the cells is controlled by the internal concentration of nutrients stored in the cytoplasm whilst the rate of uptake of nutrients is a function of the external nutrient concentration. DROOP is a revised model of the growth and nutrient uptake kinetics of phytoplankton and is presented here to illustrate how a model such as O'BRIEN can be further developed to include new information. A conceptual flow chart for DROOP is given in *Figure 4d*. The three rectangles in the chart indicate that three state equations are required: one for the external nutrient concentration in the water, one for the internal nutrient concentration within the phytoplankton cells, and one for the population density of the phytoplankton.

DROOP describes the relationship between the rate of uptake of growth limiting nutrient by algal cells and the external concentration of a nutrient in the surrounding water by means of classical Michaelis–Menten kinetics:

$$V = V_{max}\, S/(K_s + S), \tag{23}$$

where V = rate of uptake of external nutrient per cell, V_{max} = maximum rate of uptake, S = external nutrient concentration, and K_s = half saturation coefficient (external nutrient concentration at $V_{max}/2$). The rate of change in the external nutrient concentration is therefore, by development of Equation 5,

$$S' = R - (VN) \tag{24}$$

Note that Droop (12) employed the symbol U for the uptake rate and not V. I have used V to avoid confusion with μ.

The following equation is proposed to simulate the relationship between the growth rate of algae and the intra-cellular concentration of nutrient stored in the cytoplasm:

$$\mu = \mu_{max}\,(1 - kQ/Q), \tag{25}$$

where μ = growth coefficient, μ_{max} = maximum value of growth coefficient, kQ = threshold intra-cellular nutrient concentration required to sustain growth (minimal cell quota), and Q = intra-cellular nutrient concentration (cell quota). It follows that the state equation to describe the rate of change in the population density of phytoplankton, by substitution of μ for g in Equation 1 is:

$$N' = (N\mu) - (Nd) \tag{26}$$

The concentration of nutrients stored in the cytoplasm increases due to uptake from the external medium, but decreases as a result of assimilation processes when the cells are multiplying. The rate of change of intra-cellular nutrient concentration is therefore described by the mass balance equation:

$$\text{rate of change} = \text{uptake} - \text{assimilation};$$
$$Q' = V - (\mu Q), \tag{27}$$

where Q' = rate of change of intra-cellular nutrient concentration with respect to time, Q = intra-cellular nutrient concentration, V = rate of uptake, and μ = growth coefficient.

Protocol 7. Implementation and verification of DROOP *using ISIM*. (See *Appendix 8.5* for the program.)

1. Input the calibration data (*Table 5*).
2. Input the SIM and DYNAMIC statements.
3. Input the algebraic Equations 23 and 25.
4. Input the state equations 24, 26, and 27.
5. Convert the phytoplankton density from cells/l to cells/ml.
6. Input the OUTPUT and PREPARE statements.
7. Execute the program with the START command.
8. Use the GRAPH command to plot the simulation data (S and P on T) as shown in *Figure 11*.
9. Verify the simulation data against reality (*Figure 1*) and compare with O'BRIEN (*Figure 5*).

Protocol 7 gives instructions for the development of O'BRIEN by incorporation of Equations 23–27 to create DROOP. The *ISIM* program, incorporating calibration data from *Table 5*, is listed in *Appendix 8.5* and the simulation data are presented in *Figure 11*. However, the 'spring bloom' simulated by

Table 5. Calibration data for DROOP

CINT	communication interval	1	day
d	mortality coefficient	0.25	day^{-1}
kQ	minimum cell quota	4×10^{-5}	μg/cell
K_s	half saturation coefficient	10	μg/l
N	initial population density	10×10^{3}	cells/l
Q	initial cell quota	8×10^{-5}	μg/cell
R	replacement rate of nutrient	5	μg/l/day
S	initial nutrient concentration	2000	μg/l
TFIN	final value of T	100	days
μ_{max}	maximum growth coefficient	0.5	day^{-1}
V_{max}	maximum rate of uptake	8×10^{-5}	μg/cell/day

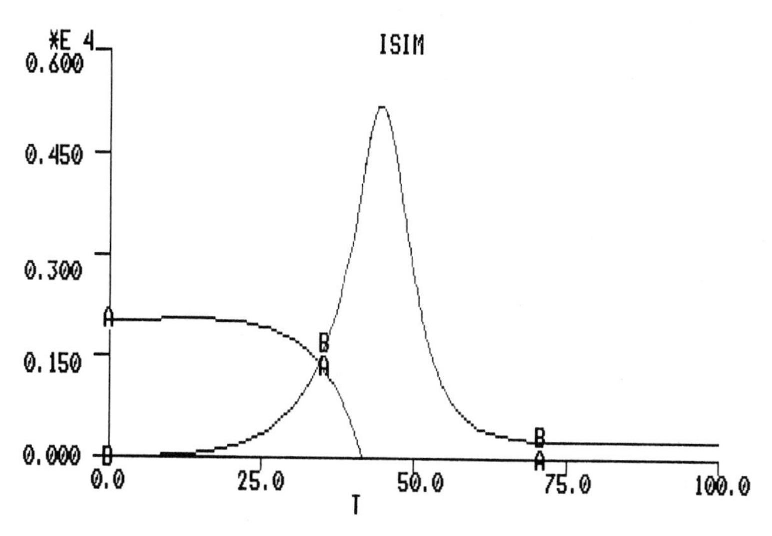

Figure 11. Graphic output from DROOP using the *ISIM* program generated by *Protocol 7* (*Appendix 8.5*). A = concentration of limiting nutrient (μg/l); B = population density of phytoplankton (cells/ml); T = time (days).

O'BRIEN is not very different in behaviour or magnitude to that simulated by DROOP. The question of whether Monod's or Droop's equations should be incorporated for generally modelling phytoplankton dynamics in aquatic systems has not been resolved.

2.13 Further development

The four simple models described in this chapter offer much scope for further development and they provide starting points for the construction of more complex compartment models as shown in Chapter 9. The reader who requires more detailed practical information on the development of dynamic models of homogeneous aquatic systems is recommended to consult Jorgensen (4), Patten (5), Spain (6), Bowker and Randerson (18), and Kremer and Nixon (19).

References

1. Burghes, D. N. and Borrie, M. S. (1981). *Modelling with differential equations*. Ellis Horwood, Chichester.
2. Edwards, D. and Hamson, M. (1989). *Guide to mathematical modelling*. Macmillan, Basingstoke.
3. Jeffers, N. R. (1982). *Modelling*. Chapman & Hall, London.
4. Jorgensen, S. E. (ed.) (1983). *Application of ecological modelling in environmental management, Part A*. Elsevier, Amsterdam.
5. Patten, B. C. (ed.) (1971). *Systems analysis and simulation in ecology*, Vol. I. Academic Press, New York.
6. Spain, J. D. (1982). *BASIC microcomputer models in biology*. Addison-Wesley, Reading, Massachusetts.
7. Macan, T. T. (1970). *Biological studies of the English lakes*. Longman, London.
8. Herbert, D., Elsworth, R., and Telling, R. C. (1956). *Journal of General Microbiology* **14,** 601.
9. Jones, R. (1983). *J. Cons. int. Explor. Mer.* **41,** 50.
10. O'Brien, W. J. (1974). *Ecology* **55,** 135.
11. Beverton, R. J. H. and Holt, S. (1957). *Fishery Investigations, London, Ser. 2* **19,** 7.
12. Droop, M. R. (1974). *Journal of the Marine Biology Association of the UK* **54,** 825.
13. Williamson, M. (1972). *The analysis of biological populations*. Edward Arnold, London.
14. Boughey, A. S. (1973). *Ecology of populations*. Macmillan, New York.
15. Christiansen, F. B. and Fenchel, T. M. (1977). *Theories of populations in biological communities*. Springer, Berlin.
16. Cooke, D., Craven, A. H., and Clarke, G. M. (1985). *Statistical computing in Pascal*. Edward Arnold, London.
17. *ISIM* Simulation (1986). *User's manual*. Simulation Sciences, Manchester.
18. Bowker, D. W. and Randerson, P. F. (1989). *Journal of Biological Education* **23,** 32.
19. Kremer, J. N. and Nixon, S. W. (1978). *A coastal marine ecosystem. Simulation and analysis*. Springer, Berlin.

Appendix 8.1. Listing of the *ISIM* program (OBRIEN1.SIM) for the implementation and verification of O'BRIEN as described in *Protocol 2*

All programs in *Appendices 8.1–8.5* can be transferred from disk to *ISIM* with the READ command and executed with the START command

```
1   C = 2E+03
2   CINT = 1
3   d = 0.25
4   gm = 0.35
5   Ks = 10
6   N = 10E+03
7   R = 5
8   q = 8E-05
9   TFIN = 100
10  SIM
11  DYNAMIC
12  g = ( gm * C ) / ( C + Ks )
13  N' = ( N * g ) - ( N * d )
14  C' = R - ( q * N * g )
15  P = IFIX (N/1000)
16  OUTPUT T,C,P
17  PREPARE T,C,P
```

Appendix 8.2. Listing of the *ISIM* program (HERBERT.SIM) for the implementation and verification of HERBERT as described in *Protocol 3*

```
1   CINT = 1
2   D = 0.5
3   Ks = .0123
4   S = 2.5
5   SR = 2.5
6   TFIN = 12
7   um = 0.85
8   x = 0.1
9   Y = 0.53
10  SIM
11  DYNAMIC
12  u = um * S / ( Ks + S )
13  x' = ( u * x ) - ( D * x )
14  S' = ( D * SR ) - ( D * S ) - (u * x ) / Y
15  OUTPUT T,S,x
16  PREPARE T,S,x
```

Appendix 8.3. Listing of the *ISIM* program (BEVERTON.SIM) for the implementation and verification of BEVERTON as described in *Protocol 4*

```
1  CINT = 1
2  F = 0.6
3  H = 9.0
4  k = 0.78
5  M = 0.28
6  N = 400
7  tc = 3
8  TFIN = 10
9  W = 0.1
10 SIM
11 DYNAMIC
12 IF ( T. LT. tc ) Z = M
13 IF ( T. GE. tc ) Z = M + F
14 W' = ( H * W ** 0.6 ) − ( k * W )
15 N' = − Z * N
16 B = ( N * W ) / 1000
17 OUTPUT T,B
18 PREPARE T,B
```

Appendix 8.4. Listing of the *ISIM* program (OBRIEN2.SIM) for the implementation and verification of O'BRIEN as described in *Protocol 5*

```
1 1 SIM; RESET; INTERACT; GOTO 1
2 DYNAMIC
3 g = gm * c / ( C + Ks )
4 N' = ( N * g ) − ( N * d )
5 C' = R − ( q * N * g )
6 P = IFIX ( N / 1000 )
7 OUTPUT T,C,P
8 PREPARE T,C,P
$VAL C = 2000.0
$VAL CINT = 1.0000
$VAL D = 0.25
$VAL gm = 0.35000
$VAL Ks = 10.000
$VAL N = 10000
$VAL R = 5.0000
$VAL TFIN = 100.00
$VAL q = 0.80000E–04
```

Appendix 8.5. Listing of the *ISIM* program (DROOP.SIM) for the implementation and verification of DROOP as described in *Protocol 7*

```
1   CINT = 1
2   d = 0.25
3   kQ = 4E-05
4   Ks = 10
5   N = 10E+03
6   Q = 8E-05
7   R = 5
8   S = 2E+03
9   TFIN = 100
10  umax = 0.5
11  Vmax = 8E-05
12  SIM
13  DYNAMIC
14  V = Vmax * S / ( Ks + S )
15  u = umax * ( 1 - kQ / Q )
16  N' = ( N * u ) - ( N * d )
17  S' = R - ( V * N )
18  Q' = V - u * Q
19  P = IFIX (N/1000)
20  OUTPUT T,S,P,Q
21  PREPARE T,S,P,Q
```

9

Compartment models

RICHARD G. WIEGERT

1. Introduction

1.1 Definitions

Models are abstractions of reality. They must possess at least some of the attributes of the system of interest, but none possess all or even a large fraction of such attributes. Models are of many kinds: a painting of a landscape, for example, is a model of reality in the sense that it suggests something of the ecosystem it represents. Such models are static—they cannot be used to simulate the changes in a system with time. Dynamic models can simulate changes with time; they were introduced in Chapter 8 by way of simple, single-compartment models.

The basis of compartmental models is the explicit assumption that all within a compartment is the same (homogeneous), but different from the surrounding compartments. Each compartment has dynamic attributes. Thus the dynamic homogeneous models discussed in Chapter 8 are in fact special single-compartmental cases of the models presented here.

A system can, in general, be defined as a collection of parts, interacting with each other to produce some unit behaviour of the whole (1). When it is appropriate to the goals of a model to regard the system as one compartment, the model conveniently reduces to the homogeneous forms presented in Chapter 8. Simple models of population growth and physiological models of whole organisms are among the examples of such models that have produced a wealth of insight into biological processes.

However, in many cases such simplifications will not suffice. The problem is one found throughout the sciences and is hierarchical in nature. In science we seek explanation of observed facts. These explanations or hypotheses then suggest other experiments/observations that may be used to test them. The problem is that the explanation always involves hierarchical level(s) above and/or below that from which the original facts originated. For example, a set of measurements of the metabolic rate of a single resting organism might show a diel pattern of highs and lows. One explanation of such a pattern might involve the stress of seeing other organisms of like or different kinds in the surroundings, a level of organization above that of the organism. Another explanation might be the presence of an endogenous rhythm controlled by the interaction of organ systems, a level below that of the organism.

1.2 Classification

The foregoing discussion assumed a certain type of mathematical model, one that contains rules of operation and in which all the parameters can be defined in biological terms or which have biological meaning. In general, mathematical models can be placed into one of two categories:

- mechanistic, explanatory (causal) models
- empirical, correlative (non-causal) models

The first category, mechanistic models, comprises the kind of model discussed in Part 2 of this volume. Such models are built of equations that contain definable, observable parameters and whose rules involve or invoke levels of organization other than the compartments being modelled, i.e. they are explanations.

The second category, empirical models, contains models with mathematical relationships that serve only to illuminate the relationship between the behaviour of the system and measurements of one or many attributes of the system. Many of the statistical techniques necessary to derive empirical models were discussed in Part 1 of this volume. Empirical models only identify patterns; they do not explain them.

1.3 Historical development

Solution (simulation in time) of differential equations requires that equations have an analytical solution, or else numerical integration methods (cf. Chapter 8, Section 2.8) must be used to solve them. Thus early biological models (prior to the late 1960s) tended to be simple and the number of compartments was small. But most biological processes are in fact non-linear, and for many of these, linear approximations are very poor. Furthermore, biology is rich in threshold behaviour, where the equational rules themselves change. So at best the early models tended to be unrealistic. The situation changed radically following the development of computers.

Analogue computers had a small role in early compartmental model development, but were difficult to program and debug, and their accuracy was usually limited to four decimal places. However, the inexpensive fast digital computer has revolutionized biological modelling. Since the computer excels at just those computations that are required for numerical integration, the biological modeller can explore the consequences of hypotheses that would have been impossible (or too expensive) only a few years ago. One need only peruse the literature to note the change. For example, in 1975, all of the ecological simulation models I could find in the literature could be discussed in one review (2). Today, I couldn't even estimate how many hundreds (likely thousands) of ecological simulation models have been published.

1.4 Model usages

Models differ, depending on the objectives of the modeller. They may be used as:

- predictive tools
- research tools
- theoretical tools

Prediction means the forecasting into the future of some perturbation applied to the biological system of interest. Mechanistic compartmental models are seldom developed for use solely as predictive tools. One reason is the relative expense (in time and needed information) of developing such models compared to an empirical model. If prediction is the only modelling objective, and if data exist on the response of a number of similar systems to a range of values in a particular parameter (or set of parameters) then an empirical model is the best choice. For example, suppose prediction of oxygen consumption of an organism, given body weight, is desired. The procedure would be to measure the oxygen consumption of a number of the organisms, fit an appropriate regression model and use this model for prediction (see Chapter 3). As long as the unknown is within the range of measured weights used in the regression, the possibility of error in the prediction can be assessed. Mechanistic compartment models, when used for prediction, do not provide a comparable level of error assessment.

There is one circumstance, however, where mechanistic models are used for prediction in the manner of an empirical model, and that is where no prior data on the results of system perturbations exist and where it would be too expensive (or socially/environmentally costly) to obtain such data. An example is the case of predicting the impact of increasing the number of mussel rafts on the mussel harvest from a Spanish estuary (3). In this case there existed no other data on the impact of differing concentrations of mussel rafts. The potential social and economic changes as a result of an increase in the number of rafts (and family groups working them) were too important to permit the increase for some test period. Thus the available biological data (supplemented with a five year study) were used to construct a mechanistic compartmental model which enabled a prediction to be made. Other examples of this use of mechanistic compartmental models for prediction can be found in other management situations, such as pollution control, hydrologic manipulations, etc. In all such cases, as in the above example, the data for empirical models do not exist and would be too costly (in either monetary or social terms) to acquire. These situations were relatively few, but they are becoming more common as we face more large-scale and unprecedented changes in the global environment.

One of the most important current uses of a mechanistic compartment model is as a tool to guide biological research. Precisely because such models incorporate the known causal mechanisms governing the dynamics of the system, they can be invaluable in determining the most efficient way to conduct the research. Sensitivity analyses (Section 3.4.2) of the model can suggest which parameter values need more refinement and which may be estimated more crudely (at least initially). Testing the model output against data can reveal weaknesses in the structural and functional attributes that require new or modified hypotheses. As new data are acquired in the course of an investigation, the model is modified to incorporate it and the cycle is repeated.

These compartmental models can also be used to develop and test theory. The model is used to simulate system behaviour under any 'what if?' situation. Theoretical constructs are developed to explain the behaviour and then tested by experiment/observation. For example, mechanistic models exhibiting 'chaotic' behaviour (see Section 3.2) are being used to develop theories about biological processes in fields as disparate as cardiac physiology and ecosystem ecology (4).

2. Model structure and function

Compartment models are described in terms of their structure, interacting with functional components, to produce system behaviour (5). The words *structure* and *function* in this context have a very precise and specialized meaning, different to some degree from the common usage in biology, particularly in ecology. But in modelling the definitions used here, taken from systems science, are extremely useful. *Figure 1* shows the parallels and differences between the two sets of definitions. Structure, in the systems jargon, is the abstract organizational plan of the system, whereas function is provided by the actual occupants of the compartments plus their rules of interaction and fluxes of matter/energy. For example, one could describe the political system of one's home country, naming the offices and the chains-of-command, without any reference whatsoever to the current occupants and the ways in which they actually interact when conducting the business of government. This is the abstract political 'structure' of the system. The occupants bring to it the functional aspect, just as the compartment occupants in a biological system bring to the system its unique dynamic characteristics.

Clearly, structure is both a more general and more conservative attribute of systems and their models than is function.

2.1 Compartments and flows

Figure 2 shows a diagram of a compartment model. For ecological models, compartments are represented using the 'energy' notation of Odum (6). A

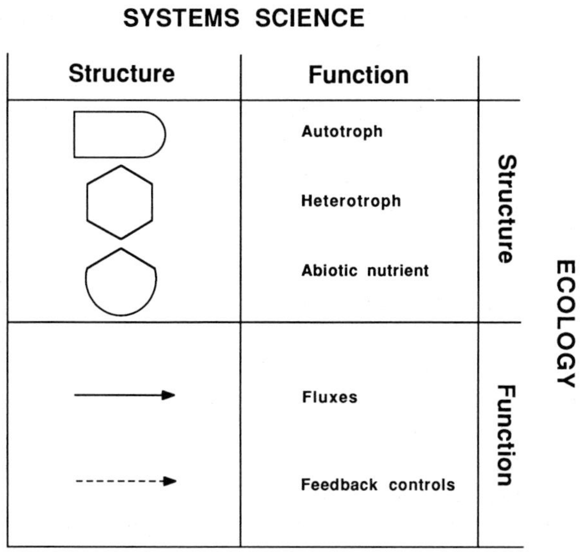

SYSTEMS SCIENCE

Structure	Function	
	Autotroph	Structure
	Heterotroph	
	Abiotic nutrient	
	Fluxes	Function
	Feedback controls	

ECOLOGY

Figure 1. Differences in the definitions of structure and function used in systems science vs. those applied commonly in ecology. Anticlockwise from upper left are: abstract compartments, flows of information and matter/energy, fluxes of matter/energy with controls, and the occupants of the compartments. Redrawn from Wiegert *et al.* (23).

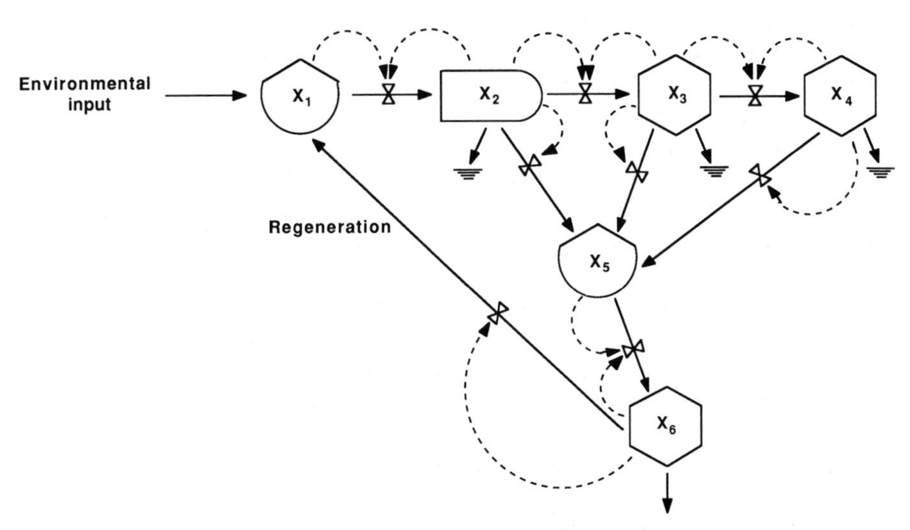

Figure 2. A compartment model, showing the autotrophs (bullet shapes), consumers (hexagons) and abiotic storages (tanks), connected by pathways of flow (solid lines) and regulated by control gates receiving informational flows (dotted lines).

bullet shape represents an autotrophic compartment, the hexagon represents a heterotrophic compartment, and a tank is an abiotic storage compartment (*Figure 1*). This useful notation imparts at a glance information about the biological make-up of the ecosystem. Sources and sinks outside the model are represented by clouds, following Forrester (7). For non-ecological models, i.e. those involving organisms and organ systems or cells and cell organelles, the rectangular box compartments of Forrester would be more appropriate.

Solid arrows represent flows of energy/matter. The unit of flow (the 'book-keeping' unit) of the model should if possible be a conserved entity, such as energy, or an element to keep the difficulties of conversion and maintaining mass balance to a minimum.

2.2 Information transfer and rules of behaviour

In addition to the abstract structure of a model, *Figure 2* shows some of the functional attributes as well. Control of flows of energy/matter between compartments is potentially a function of any other compartment or any factor outside the model boundaries (the surroundings). The convention adopted in this chapter is to represent the action of controlling functions on flows with a 'gate' following Forrester (7). Pathways of transfer for control information are indicated by dotted lines. Such information comes either from compartments or from outside sources indicated by a small circle.

The concept of exponential growth of a population was introduced (Chapter 8) together with several ways in which controlling factors could be represented by mathematical equations. In this section those ideas are extended to cover multi-compartmental models. A general approach to flow equations is developed that permits inclusion of *any* functional form, yet avoids exceeding known biological constraints.

All populations have the capacity to increase autocatalytically, i.e. exponentially, when free of all constraints. The genetic makeup of each population places an upper limit on the specific rate of this exponential increase. Thus if X is the population size (a variable of state, cf. Chapter 8), a mathematical model of such growth is:

$$dX/dt = r_m X, \qquad (1)$$

where r_m is the maximum specific rate of population growth, often called intrinsic rate of population increase. Each biotic compartment has an r_m that cannot be exceeded (for a given optimum environment), barring evolutionary change. If simulated evolutionary change in r_m is part of the goal of the model, then r_m itself must become a variable.

Since the growth of a compartment is the difference between energy/matter taken in and that which is lost, the specific rate of intake must also have a maximum value, here represented by the Greek letter τ. Terms for losses are also required. Mortality (non-predatory since the unrestrained growth of a single compartment is being modelled) is represented by the Greek letter μ. For energy and some materials (carbon for instance) there are losses due to respiration. These are represented in the equations by the Greek letter ρ. Similarly, organisms lose energy/matter via excretion and this is indicated with the Greek letter η.

Note that these rates are all specific rates with dimensions of 1/time, i.e. $time^{-1}$. The egestion rate, Greek letter ε, in contrast to the other basic losses, is not a rate but a dimensionless fraction of the material ingested.

Equation 1, the unrestrained growth of a population (X), can be rewritten in terms of the input and output of energy/matter, i.e. as a flow equation (also called a mass balance equation in Chapter 8):

$$dX/dt = [\{\tau(1 - \varepsilon) - \rho - \mu - \eta\}]X \quad (2)$$

Equation 2 is, of course, a representation of unrestrained growth, something rarely, if ever, seen in real systems and then for only brief periods. Generally one or more restraining factors operate to reduce the intake rate from the maximum (τ) or increase the losses from their minimal values. Furthermore, Equation 2 is a differential equation representing the net change as a result of flows into and out of a compartment. To construct a compartmental flow model the components of Equation 2 must be separated into equations describing the individual flows between compartments. To facilitate this process three flow categories are defined and the terms *determine* and *control* are introduced.

2.3 Model flows and control functions

2.3.1 Classification of flows

Flows between compartments can be named according to the type of donor versus the recipient compartments.

- biotic or abiotic to abiotic
- abiotic to biotic
- biotic to biotic

This categorization shows differences in the types of restraints on flows and in the effects of the losses on the donor dynamics. The words *determine* and *control* are used in the sense of their common dictionary definitions. *Determine* means to set limits (range) to parameter values and flow rates. *Control* means to restrain the values within these limits or ranges.

Abiotic (tank) compartments have no inherent dynamics; as recipients they are passive sinks receiving flows from other biotic or abiotic compartments. They exert no control on these flows, nor do they determine their maximum or minimum values. Thus flows to tanks are, by definition, donor-determined and donor-controlled. They are the simplest to model, usually represented adequately by linear equations. For example, excretion is the product of the specific rate of excretion and the compartment size (x_j). The recipient compartment is designated X_k, a passive abiotic compartment. Then:

$$F_{jk} = \eta_j X_j, \tag{3}$$

where F_{jk} is the flow from X_j to X_k and η_j is the specific rate of excretion.

Abiotic to biotic flows are usually recipient-determined, because it is the recipient that has the dynamic capability to grow exponentially. The flow is controlled within the limits $0 <= \tau_r <= \tau$, where τ_r stands for the realized rate of ingestion. This flow is labelled donor/recipient-controlled because ingestion can be restrained either by scarcity of the resource or by factors related to the density of the recipient. The latter are generally regarded as space-related.

The third category, biotic to biotic flows, is identical to the second in so far as the flow equations, determination, and control are concerned. The distinction is made only to illustrate the differences in potential effect of ingestion on the rate of supply of the resource. An abiotic tank, because it is a passive storage compartment, passes nothing back up the trophic (feeding) chain to its own donors. Specifically, taking material from the tank does not directly affect the rates at which it is supplied. Decomposers utilizing the leaves of the forest floor do not directly affect the rate at which the trees produce and drop leaves; their effects are only indirect (time-delayed), through mechanisms such as nutrient regeneration, etc. Feeding from a living compartment, however, directly changes its standing crop and thus affects its rate of productivity. This is a fundamental and important difference between consumers of living material (biophages) and those which utilize dead material (saprophages; 8).

2.3.2 Control functions

A final addition to our arsenal of terms permits the construction of a full functional compartmental simulation model. A method is needed to incorporate the mechanisms of control. This can be done very simply, in a manner that does not restrict the form of the control function that can be used. The following examples use the ingestion rate (τ). But the method can be used for increasing or decreasing any other rate of flow in the model.

The procedure is to insert the control function(s) as a multiplier of the rate to be controlled and constrain its value between 0 (no ingestion) and 1 (maximum rate). The controls may be functions of any variable in the model. In Equation 4 the function is that of a material resource, X_i. The convention adopted in Equation 4 is that egestion, which passes through the recipient without being available for maintenance or growth, is subtracted from total ingestion, since the models considered here are too simple to separately represent abiotic tanks as sinks for egested material. Thus, Equation 4 represents the net ingestion.

$$F_{ij} = X_j \tau_{ij}(1 - \varepsilon_{ij}) f(X_i), \tag{4}$$

where $f(X_i)$ is a control function of X_i and $0 <= f(X_i) <= 1$.

One accepted mathematical convention for indicating the latter constraint is to write the function as $[f(X_i)]_+$: the subscript + indicates that the value of the expression within the brackets is always ≥ 0. In programming the model this constraint can be implemented by defining and calling a function in the program. The function should add the value in brackets to its absolute value and divide the sum by 2. This will constrain the expression to ≥ 0. In most computer languages it will be faster, if not as compact, to use IF comparator statements to achieve the same goal. To implement the other part of the constraint, namely that the function not exceed 1, requires that the function be written in the proper form, as in the examples in the following two sections.

2.3.3 Linear functions

Control functions may be either linear or non-linear. If they are linear, the unit response of the function to a unit change in the controlling state variable is a constant. Control functions are also categorized, according to the responsible state variable, as either donor or recipient. In the former, the permitted fraction of the maximum rate is zero for standing stocks of the donor (resource) compartment that are unavailable, i.e. below the refuge level. The fraction then rises linearly to the maximum for levels at or above some satiation threshold. In recipient control just the opposite occurs. Realized rates are at the maximum for standing stock of recipient equal to or less than a response threshold, and decrease as the recipient compartment approaches the carrying capacity. Note that, at this latter level, the ingestion rate does not go to zero but is equal to the irreducible losses, i.e. intake just balances outflow. The function must provide for such requirements. In the zone between the two sets of threshold levels the function can take any form required by the rules of interaction between donor or recipient and the realized rate of ingestion. The simplest functions are linear, and these are the forms of choice in the absence of data to the contrary; hence the popularity of controls like the logistic equation, a generalized version of which is given as the first example.

$$f(X_j) = [1 - c\{(X_{jj} - \alpha_{jj})/(\gamma_{jj} - \alpha_{jj})\}_+]_+, \quad (5)$$

where α_{jj} is the lower response threshold, γ_{jj} is the carrying capacity, and $c = [1 - \lambda_j/\{\tau_{ij}\,(1 - \varepsilon_{ij})\}]$

The correction term c includes a term (λ) for the summed minimal losses, i.e. those such as respiration, excretion, etc. In Equation 5, when $X_j \leq \alpha_{jj}$ the term within parentheses disappears (it becomes zero or negative and thus is set to zero because of the subscript + convention). At that point $f(X_j) = 1.0$ and ingestion is maximum. When $\alpha_{jj} < X_j$, the realized rate of ingestion is reduced from the maximum in a linear manner. When $X_j = \gamma_{jj}$, Equation 5 becomes

$$f(X_j) = \lambda_j/\{\tau_{ij}(1 - \varepsilon_{ij})\}. \quad (6)$$

The logistic control function as it is commonly used in the ecological literature has no lower (response) threshold. Thus if α_{jj} is set to zero, Equation 5 becomes identical with the control function in the flow form of the common logistic equation.

The overall flow equation is written in differential form (from Equations 2 and 4):

$$dX_j/dt = \{\tau_{ij}(1 - \varepsilon_{ij}) f(X_j) - \lambda_j\}X_j. \tag{7}$$

Whenever $f(X_j)$ is replaced with $\lambda_j/\{\tau_{ij}(1 - \varepsilon_{ij})\}$, as it is when X_j equals the carrying capacity (γ_{jj}), the realized net rate of ingestion is λ_j and $dX_j/dt = 0$.

If the controlling factor is the amount of resource, then

$$f(X_i) = [1 - \{(\gamma_{ij} - X_i)/(\gamma_{ij} - \alpha_{ij})\}_+]_+, \tag{8}$$

where α_{ij} is the refuge level or minimum concentration available and γ_{ij} is the satiation level.

This has essentially the same properties as $f(X_j)$ except that the function goes to zero as the resource decreases to the refuge threshold; one might think of this function as the resource equivalent of the space-related logistic control.

In practice both these potential control sources, donor and recipient, need to be in the flow equations of the model, along with many other potential controlling factors. The utility of the approach developed in this section is that all functions are multiplied by the maximum rate. When all controlling compartments are at optimal levels, i.e. no negative feedbacks, then each function assumes the value unity and the maximum rate is achieved.

2.3.4 Non-linear functions

The linear forms described above are not always adequate to explain the behaviour of the population as thresholds are passed. For example, if a predator increased its effort as prey became scarce, but later had to concentrate on alternative resources, the function of the primary resource would be curvilinear. Sometimes the nature of the function can be inferred from knowledge of the interaction. Most desirable, of course, would be a set of data on ingestion versus resource density. From this a fitted line (an empirical model) could be used to produce the best function directly from the data. There is no restriction on the type or complexity of the control function that may be used, as long as it is written in a form that permits the constraint $0 \leqslant f(X) \leqslant 1$. A few examples of different non-linear forms of the two linear control functions should clarify the procedure. A generalized form of the widely used Michaelis–Menten function is also often useful (9). The shapes of the following forms of $f(X)$ are shown in *Figures 3* and *4*. The exponent a permits the functions to be fitted to a wide variety of non-linear behaviours.

$$f(X_j) = [1 - c\{(X_j - \alpha_{jj})_+/(\gamma_{jj} - \alpha_{jj})\}^a]_+ \tag{9}$$

$$f(X_j) = [1 - c(X_j - \alpha_{jj})_+/(\gamma_{jj} - \alpha_{jj})]^a_+ \tag{10}$$

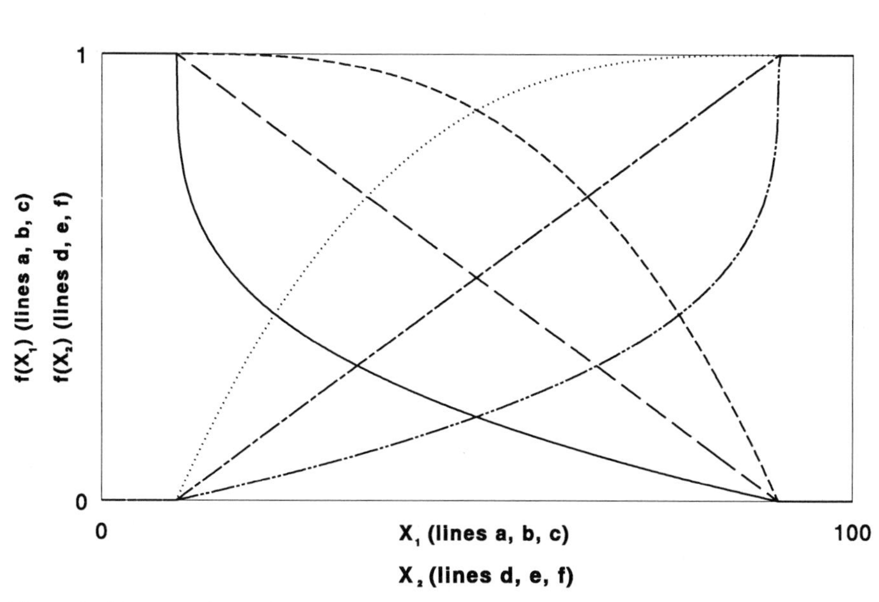

Figure 3. Linear and non-linear controls on ingestion as a function of available space (lines a, b, c (Equation 9)) and as a function of available resource (lines d, e, f (Equation 11)). Values of the exponent *a* are 0.3, 1, and 3.0.

$$f(X_i) = [1 - \{(\gamma_{ij} - X_i)_+/(\gamma_{ij} - \alpha_{ij})\}^a]_+ \tag{11}$$

$$f(X_i) = [1 - (\gamma_{ij} - X_i)_+/(\gamma_{ij} - \alpha_{ij})]^a_+ \tag{12}$$

Most ecological systems can be adequately simulated using one of the above examples of control functions. But occasionally more complicated control functions may be required (10, 11).

2.3.5 Model construction

The actual construction of a multi-compartmental simulation model follows a series of steps that are summarized in *Protocol 1*. The first three steps involve the structure of the model. The boundaries of the system relative to its surroundings are delimited. The purpose(s) of the model must be specified before the amount and type of necessary structure can be decided upon. Finally the abstract structure (boxes and flow arrows) of the model can be set down. Step 4 of the protocol requires the specification of the functional processes that are necessary to the goals of the model. From this verbal description the writing of equations and the computer program itself proceed straightforwardly. Steps 6–10 concern simulations with the model, changes, and the use of the model to guide further research on the system. Examples are discussed in the later sections of this chapter.

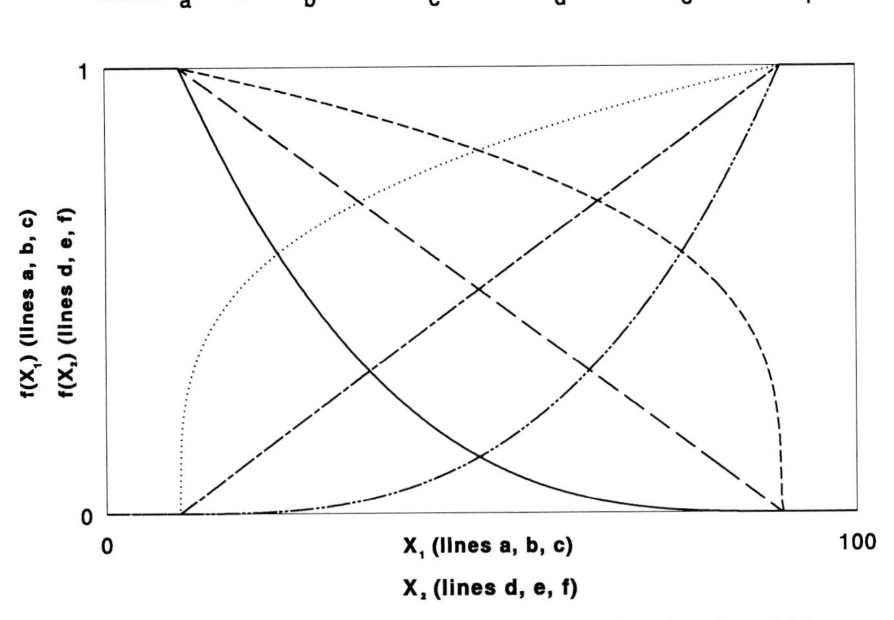

Figure 4. Linear and non-linear controls on ingestion as a function of available space (lines a, b, c (Equation 10)) and as a function of available resource (lines d, e, f (Equation 12)). Values of the exponent (a) are 0.3, 1, and 3.0.

Protocol 1. Compartmental model construction, simulation, and modification [a]

1. Define the system of interest.
2. List the goals of the model.
3. Specify the structure needed to satisfy these goals.
4. Verbalize the functional interactions between the compartments in the model.
5. From the verbalization, construct the mathematical equations, including the control functions.
6. Write a computer program to integrate the equations numerically.
7. Simulate the dynamics of the system by running the model program for specified times.
8. Assess the value of the output by comparisons and tests.
9. Modify structural and/or functional attributes of the model in light of the initial output and the rerun.

10. Use the output to guide research—modify the model with new data and repeat steps 7–10.

[a] See also *Protocol 1*, Chapter 8, from which this protocol differs only in details related to compartmental models.

3. Model behaviour

3.1 Resilience, resistance, and stability

Multi-compartmental simulation models exhibit a number of behavioural attributes, among which three are particularly useful in classification. They are:

- stability
- resilience
- resistance

Unfortunately, the ecological literature abounds with differing definitions of these terms. In the case of the latter two, each has been at times defined as the other! Nevertheless, the utility of the words can be retained without the confusion as long as they are explicitly defined.

Stability is used here in the sense of Smith (12) when he coined the term 'stay-ability' to describe a system's (or model's) ability to persist in time with no compartments becoming extinct. In other words, the structure of the system remains intact. Thus this definition of stability encompasses not only the case of a constant, or steady state, condition of the variables, but also dynamic change in time, providing that it does not lead to extinction. Thus stability can be qualified with a number of modifiers, such as steady state stability or limit cycle stability (where a repeated cycle in time is established). For example, a straight horizontal line with time represents a steady state while a sine curve would be an example of a limit cycle. A special case of system behaviour that is borderline stable, called chaotic behaviour, is discussed in the next section.

Resilience is a measure of the degree and speed with which a model returns to a previous stable configuration following a perturbation or displacement. Clearly, this is a relative and somewhat subjective term, but it is useful in comparing one version of a model with another.

Resistance is the opposite of resilience. It is a measure of the relationship between the magnitude of a perturbation and the degree and rapidity of the response. Again the term is relative and its application to some degree subjective. Furthermore, the evaluation of both resilience and resistance in a model is determined by just what state variables or parameters in the model are to be perturbed. All of the terms here are most useful when making a sensitivity analysis of the model (see Section 3.5.2).

3.2 Chaotic behaviour

Model behaviour that is unpredictable in time is commonly associated with parameter stochasticity (Section 4.2). What is less commonly realized is that totally deterministic compartmental models can, under certain conditions, exhibit temporal behaviour that is indistinguishable from random behaviour. The first demonstration of chaotic behaviour in deterministic models was made by a meteorologist (Lorenz), but it has recently become an active area of research in many scientific fields (4). The relevance of chaotic behaviour (or chaos) to the topic of this chapter is the degree of uncertainty that can be introduced into even the most deterministic model. One of the simplest forms of a model capable of chaotic behaviour is the difference form of the logistic. May's analysis (13) of this showed the onset of chaotic behaviour to be related to the value of r_m chosen. I (14) pointed out the relation of this result to the fixed nature of the logistic with respect to decreases following an overshoot above the carrying capacity. With a different kind of negative feedback, the onset of chaos need not be tied to a certain value of r_m. The differential (non-flow) form of the logistic model is

$$dX_j/dt = r_m X_j(1 - X_j/\gamma_{jj}). \tag{13}$$

In this differential form the model cannot exhibit chaotic behaviour if the time step used in numerical solution is small enough. However, if the equation is written in difference form:

$$X_{j(t+1)} = X_{j(t)} \exp \{r_m (1 - X_{j(t)}/\gamma_{jj})\}, \tag{14}$$

then, for values of $r_m = 2.69$ or larger the model shows chaotic behaviour. This is because of the feedback characteristic of the logistic, wherein the further that X_j exceeds the carrying capacity in any one generation, the further toward zero the population falls in the subsequent generation. Rewriting the logistic model in the difference flow form of Wiegert (14) produces

$$X_{j(t+1)} = X_{j(t)} \exp \{(r_m - r_m X_{j(t)}/\gamma_{jj} + \lambda_j)_+ - \lambda_j\}. \tag{15}$$

This form has the advantage of permitting the loss term, λ_j, to be specified separately from the growth function in the model. Whenever $X_{j(t)} \leqslant \gamma_{jj}$ and $\gamma_j = r_m (X_{j(t)}/\gamma_{jj} - 1)$, then Equation 15 reduces to Equation 14. However, in many, perhaps most, cases, the mortality term, λ_j, should be quite a different function. A more realistic version (1) is given in Equation 16 where the exponent a permits various levels of mortality following an overshoot of the carrying capacity:

$$\lambda_j = \{\log_e(X_{j(t)}/\gamma_{jj})\}^a. \tag{16}$$

Figure 5 shows the result of different values of the exponent a in simulations with a model constructed using Equations 15 and 16. When $a = 1.0$ the density in the generation following as overshoot of the carrying capacity will equal the carrying capacity. For values of a less than 1.0, the approach to the carrying capacity after an overshoot is more gradual the closer a is to zero. For values of a greater than 1.0, the model goes through a series of damped cycles, multi-period cycles, and finally chaotic behaviour. Thus whether a model shows chaotic behaviour or not depends on a sufficiently high potential rate of growth interacting with the necessary mortality function operating once an overshoot of the carrying capacity has occurred.

Multi-compartmental models can exhibit chaotic behaviour, even when constructed in the differential equation form and using small time steps in the numerical integration. Modellers must be on the watch for such behaviour, for it can lead to valuable insight into the mechanisms governing biological systems.

3.3 Small compartmental models

Small compartmental models (those with 2–5 compartments) are seldom useful as simulators with which to guide research programs or as predictors of the behaviour of real systems. They have, however, great utility in developing an understanding of the behaviour of ecological systems with differing attributes and parameter values. As theoretical tools, such models can provide valuable insight into the theory of competition, stability theory, etc. (14, 15).

The organization of these small compartmental models can be specified by two categories:

- linear or chain models
- branched or web models

The linear models are structured as an unbranched chain. Two three-compartment models, combined in one computer program are used as examples (*Appendix 9.1*). The model is written in IBM BASIC Version 3.0 and should be portable to any IBM-compatible DOS computer with little if any modification. The program produces graphic screen output of state variables and also offers the option of printing output, including not only state variables, but also feedback control functions, to a file on virtual disk D:. The graphic output is for a Color Graphics Adapter (CGA) screen in high resolution mode (SCREEN 2). Both the print file destination and the graphic output is easily modified for machines that possess other than a D: virtual disk and/or a CGA screen. To change to a different screen resolution the SCREEN command (statement 1250) must be changed and the width (WW) and height (WH) variables of statement 1250 must be set to the new screen dimensions. To write the ASCII file output to a new disk or to change the filename modify the NAM$ variable in Statement 380, which at present read PREDATE.DAT and COMPETE.DAT.

There are a number of software packages that can construct and run models without requiring literacy in any high level programming language (the ex-

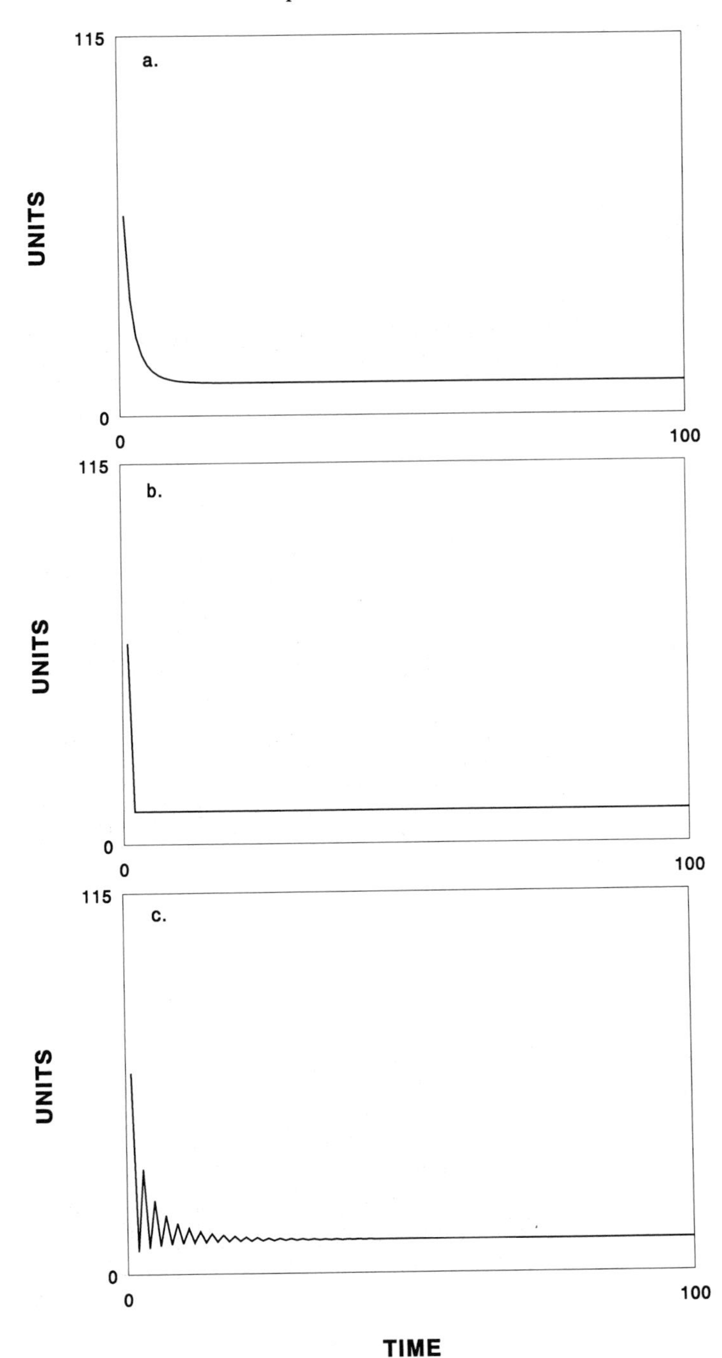

Figure 5. The influence of the mortality function in determining whether a deterministic model shows chaotic behaviour or not. Computed by substituting Equation 16 into

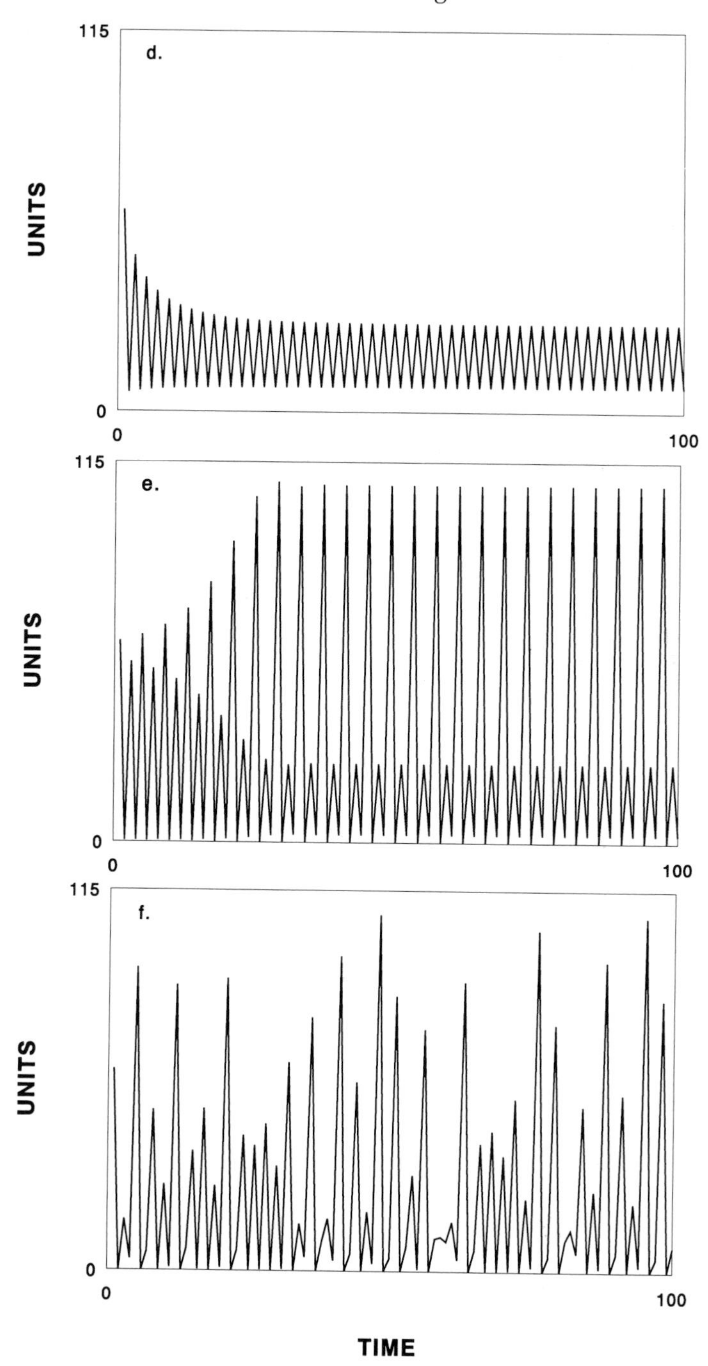

Equation 15 and solving for X with time using different values for exponent a (a, 0.3; b, 1.0; c, 1.2; d, 1.3; e, 2.7; f, 3.5).

ample of *ISIM* was presented in Chapter 8). For casual and/or infrequent modelling efforts, particularly for small compartmental models, these packages are excellent. Often these packages deliver no code that can be modified to run more efficiently with high speed compilers. For serious research work, particularly with systems that require large compartmental models (Section 3.5), the modeller should usually write his or her own programs or collaborate with a good programmer as the time saved when doing dozens or hundreds of runs during sensitivity analyses will more than repay the initial effort at programming.

3.3.1 The linear (chain) model

The two compartment linear model is shown in *Figure 6*; there is an abiotic (constant input) resource compartment used by the autotroph which is in turn

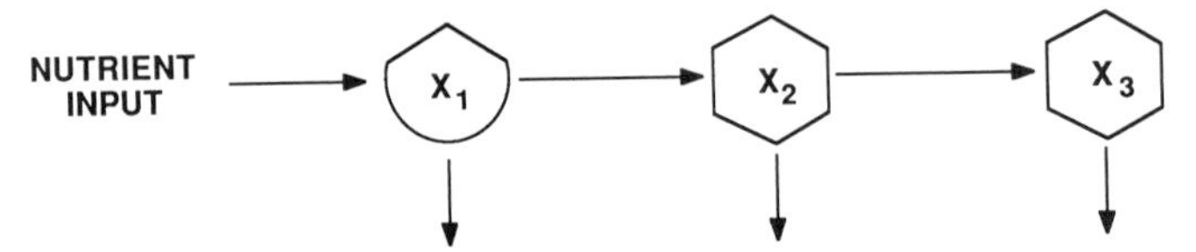

Figure 6. The three-compartment linear predator–prey model given in *Appendix 9.1* (predation model).

preyed upon by the top consumer. The feedback controls used are from Equations 5 (space- or density-related) and 8 (resource-related).

$$\frac{dX_i}{dt} = F1 - X_i\lambda_i - X_j\tau_{ij}f(X_i)f(X_j), \tag{17}$$

$$\frac{dX_j}{dt} = X_j\{\tau_{ij}f(X_i)f(X_j) - \lambda_j\} - X_k\{\tau_{jk}f(X_j)'f(X_k)\}, \tag{18}$$

and

$$\frac{dX_k}{dt} = X_k\{\tau_{jk}f(X_j)'f(X_k) - \lambda_k\}, \tag{19}$$

where $f(X_i)$ is from Equation 8, $f(X_j)$ is from Equation 5, $f(X_j)'$ is from Equation 8, and $f(X_k)$ is from Equation 5.

Equations 17–19 are incorporated in the model program given in *Appendix 9*, and Statements 1590–1610, with V$ = 1, give the differential equations for the linear model. The separate fluxes, F terms, are computed in Statements 1450–1550 using control functions, FB terms, computed in Statements 1340–1440. This model is presented as an example of how one can explore the conditions under which a model, with realistic control functions, will show steady state behaviour or a limit cycle. *Figure 7* shows the output from this model using the state variable and parameter values from *Table 1*. The three

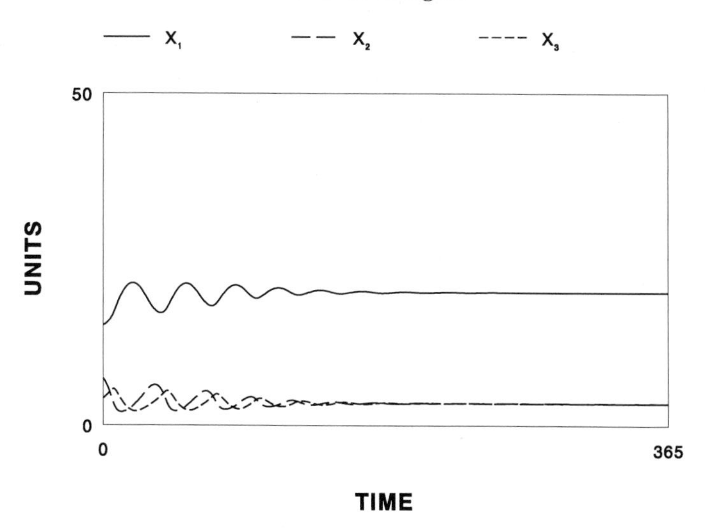

Figure 7. The steady state reached by the linear predator–prey model using the initial conditions and parameter values given in *Table 1*.

Table 1. Parameter values used in the linear population model simulations shown in *Figures 7* and *8*

Parameter	**Symbol in**		**Value used in**	
	text	**program**	***Figure 7***	***Figure 8***
Resource input	f_1	f1	3.0	3.0
Prey ingestion	τ_{12}	t12	0.3	0.3
Predator ingestion	τ_{23}	t23	0.25	0.25
Resource loss	ρ_1	r1	0.1	0.1
Prey loss	ρ_2	r2	0.1	0.1
Predator loss	ρ_3	r3	0.2	0.2
X_1 satiation level	γ_{12}	g12	20.0	20.0
X_1 refuge level	α_{12}	a12	5.0	5.0
Prey satiation level	γ_{23}	g23	4.0	3.5[a]
Prey refuge level	α_{23}	a23	0.6	0.45[a]
Prey carrying capacity	γ_{22}	g22	70.0	70.0
Prey response threshold	α_{22}	a22	20.0	20.0
Predator carrying capacity	γ_{33}	g33	100.0	100.0
Predator response threshold	α_{33}	a33	50.0	50.0
Initial resource	X1	x01	15.0	15.0
Initial competitor 1	X2	x02	7.0	7.0
Initial competitor 2	X3	x03	4.0	4.0

[a] Either change produces a limit cycle—see text

compartments quickly reach a steady state, no matter what initial conditions of the state variables are set. In this example the top consumer has a relatively high tolerance for crowding (γ) and, compared to the autotrophic compartment, a relatively low maximum ingestion rate (τ). The level of enrichment (rate of supply to the initial resource compartment) is relatively high. Under these conditions, the system behaviour is responsive to the range of availability of the prey (autotroph) of the top consumer. If this range is changed by a small amount, for example either by decreasing the refuge (α_{23}) from 0.6 to 0.45 or by decreasing the satiation level (γ_{23}) from 4 to 3.5, the prey is made more available to the top consumer and limit cycle behaviour persists (*Figure 8*) instead of being damped out to the steady state as in *Figure 7*. This example

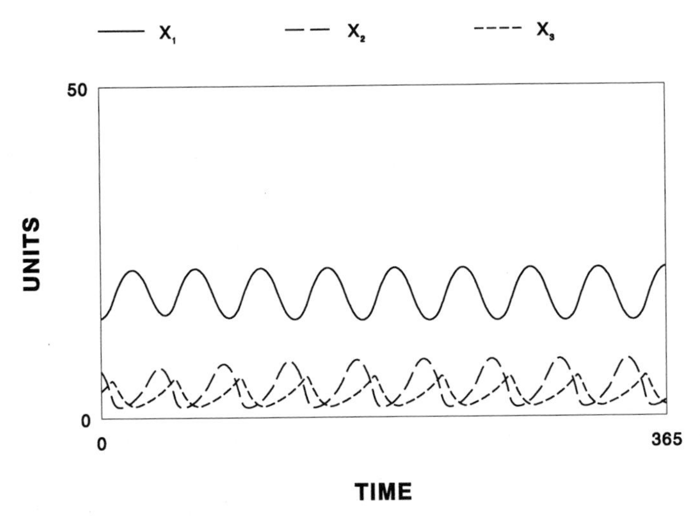

Figure 8. The linear predator–prey model showing the effect of changing only the autotroph satiation level (g23) from 4 to 3.5. A persistent limit cycle emerges. The same effect is also observed if the autotroph refuge level (a23) is decreased from 0.6 to 0.45. All other parameters remain the same (*Table 1*).

shows how small a change need occur in a variable for a major change in the stability attributes of a system to ensue. Because parameter values in real systems are highly unlikely to remain constant, we might expect many systems in nature to be delicately poised between the steady state and limit cycles. Indeed, this simple three-compartment chain model can, with certain parameter values, even exhibit more than one locally stable steady state (14).

3.3.2 The branched (web) model

A three-compartment branched or web model is shown in *Figure 9*. In this configuration the two biotic compartments are in competition for a single

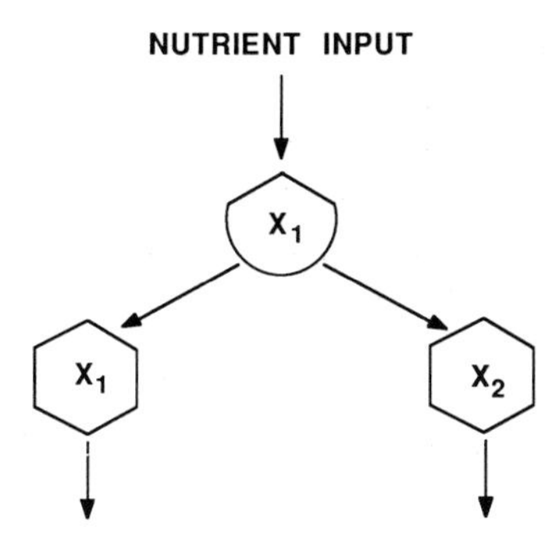

Figure 9. Diagram of three-compartment branched or web competition model given in *Appendix 9.1* (competition model).

shared resource. Here a third potential controlling factor, that of 'interference' competition, can be separated from 'exploitation' competition for a shared resource (16). This is accomplished by rewriting Equation 5 as

$$f(X_j) = [1 - c\{(X_j + \beta_k X_k - \alpha_{jj})/(\gamma_{jj} - \alpha_{jj})\}_+]_+ \qquad (20)$$

and

$$f(X_k) = [1 - c\{(X_t + \beta_j X_j - \alpha_{kk})/(\gamma_{kk} - \alpha_{kk})\}_+]_+. \qquad (21)$$

In Equations 20 and 21, β_k is the effect of a unit of the competitor X_k on the space available to X_j relative to the effect of that unit of X_k on its own space, and β_j is the effect of a unit of the competitor X_j on the space available to X_k, relative to the effect of that unit of X_j on its own space.

The classical analysis of these competition equations is as a modified logistic form with only one feedback control term combining the diverse effects of either limitation by space or material resources, i.e. with no explicit recognition of the effects of exploitative competition in lowering available resources, e.g. Equations 18 and 19. In such cases the dependence of the outcome on the competition coefficients (β values) is easily shown (17). When both β values are greater than unity, i.e. each compartment exerts a greater negative effect of crowding on its competitor than it does on itself, then there is always one winner, determined by the initial densities. If only one β value is greater than 1, that compartment will always win, the other becoming extinct. Conversely, if both coefficients are less than 1, then the system exhibits a stable equilibrium point where both compartments persist.

However, the model presented here has been made more realistic by the inclusion of a control term for available material resources in addition to the logistic-type control related to space (Equation 4). The full equations are written as

$$\frac{dX_i}{dt} = F1 - X_i\lambda_i - X_j\{\tau_{ij}f(X_i)f(X_j)\} - \dot{X}_k\{\tau_{ik}f(X_i)'f(X_k)\}, \qquad (22)$$

$$\frac{dX_j}{dt} = X_j\{\tau_{ij}f(X_i)f(X_j) - \lambda_j\}, \qquad (23)$$

and

$$\frac{dX_k}{dt} = X_k\{\tau_{ik}f(X_i)'f(X_k) - \lambda_k\}, \qquad (24)$$

where $f(X_i)$ and $f(X_i)'$ are from Equation 8, $f(X_j)$ is from Equation 20, and $f(X_k)$ is from Equation 21.

These equations are incorporated into the model program in *Appendix 9.1*. In this case the program variable V$ is 2. Otherwise the earlier comments about statement numbers apply here.

This inclusion of control by either interference or exploitative competition complicates an algebraic demonstration of the conditions under which a stable equilibrium can be achieved. What can be shown easily is that the conditions from the classical analysis hold whenever the resource, X_i, is sufficiently abundant to exceed both of the satiation parameters (γ_{ij} and γ_{ik}), for in that circumstance the resource feedback terms drop out of the equations. However, when one or both of the competitors is limited by both scarcity of resource and crowding, then the outcome of competition can be influenced by the availability of the limiting material resource (exploitative competition) as well as be interference competition for available space. Thus, a compartment that is a poor interference competitor, and would normally be eliminated from the system, could survive (and even eliminate its rival) if its exploitative ability were superior enough, and the limiting resource was scarce enough. The outcome of competition is still determined by the relative position of the zero growth intercepts, but these are now complicated expressions involving the resource compartment as well as both competitor compartments. As an example, consider *Figure 10* (the parameter values for the following examples are given in *Table 2*). In this Case X3 has the interference advantage ($b_3 = 1.2$ and $b_2 = 0.8$). When limitation by resources is not a factor, X3 would always win. But manipulation of the parameters governing the response to resource density can change the outcome, producing, in addition to the one winner case, stable and unstable equilibria. The isocline intercepts can still be used to ascertain which case will be associated with a given set of parameter values. In this example, the intercepts of the X2 growth isocline are X23 (X2 = 0) and X22 (X3 = 0). The corresponding intercepts for the X3 isocline are X32 (X3 = 0) and X33 (X2 = 0). These four

Table 2. Competition parameter values used in the web model simulations shown in *Figure 10*

Parameter	**Symbol in**		**Value used in part of *Figure 10***					
	text	**program**	**a**	**b**	**c**	**d**	**e**	**f**
Resource input	f_1	f1	6.0	6.0	6.0	6.0	6.0	6.0
X_2 ingestion	τ_{12}	t12	0.2	0.2	0.2	0.4	0.4	0.2
X_3 ingestion	τ_{13}	t13	0.2	0.2	0.2	0.2	0.2	0.2
X_1 resource loss	ρ_1	r1	0.1	0.1	0.1	0.1	0.1	0.1
X_2 loss	ρ_2	r2	0.1	0.1	0.1	0.3	0.3	0.1
X_3 loss	ρ_3	r3	0.1	0.1	0.1	0.1	0.1	0.1
X_1–X_2 satiation level	γ_{12}	g12	27.0	27.0	27.0	27.0	27.0	35.0
X_1–X_2 refuge level	α_{12}	a12	5.0	5.0	5.0	5.0	5.0	5.0
X_1–X_3 satiation level	γ_{13}	g13	35.0	32.5	32.5	35.0	35.0	35.0
X_1–X_3 refuge level	α_{13}	a13	5.0	5.0	5.0	5.0	5.0	5.0
X_2 carrying capacity	γ_{22}	g22	40.0	50.0	50.0	40.0	40.0	40.0
X_2 response threshold	α_{22}	a22	10.0	10.0	10.0	10.0	10.0	10.0
X_3 carrying capacity	γ_{33}	g33	40.0	60.0	60.0	40.0	40.0	40.0
X_3 response threshold	α_{33}	a33	10.0	10.0	10.0	10.0	10.0	10.0
Competition coefficient	B_2	b2	0.8	0.8	0.8	0.8	0.8	0.8
Competition coefficient	B_3	b3	1.2	1.2	1.2	1.2	1.2	1.2
Initial resource	X1	X01	20.0	20.0	20.0	20.0	20.0	20.0
Initial competitor 1	X2	X02	5.0	20.0	5.0	30.0	10.0	20.0
Initial competitor 2	X3	X03	20.0	5.0	20.0	10.0	30.0	5.0

intercepts are found by setting Equations 23 and 24 equal to zero, substituting the steady state value of X1 (X1 = (F01 − R2*X2 − R3*X3)R1, and solving each equation for X2 when X3 = 0 and for X3 when X2 = 0, with the constraint that X1 is in all cases less than or equal to the smaller of the two satiation (γ) levels.

In *Figure 10a*, X23 > X33 and X22 > X32; the better exploitative competitor always wins, no matter what the initial densities of X2 and X3. In *Figure 10b* and *10c*, X33 > X23 and X22 > X32. This produces an unstable equilibrium, with the winner dependent on the initial starting densities of X2 and X3. In *Figure 10d* and *10e*, X23 > X33 and X32 < X22. This is a stable equilibrium, with the system converging to a stable point no matter where in positive X2/X3 space the simulation is started. Finally, in *Figure 10f*, X33 > X23 and X32 > X22, producing the case where X3 always wins because the exploitative advantage of X2 has been removed.

The basic functional attributes of compartmental models have now been outlined. A combination of the various flows and functional forms introduced thus far will permit the beginning modeller to simulate a wide variety of real systems. Because the interest will normally not centre on developing theory, but rather on the topic of this book, analysis of biological data, the compartment models will tend to be much larger than those which I have used to

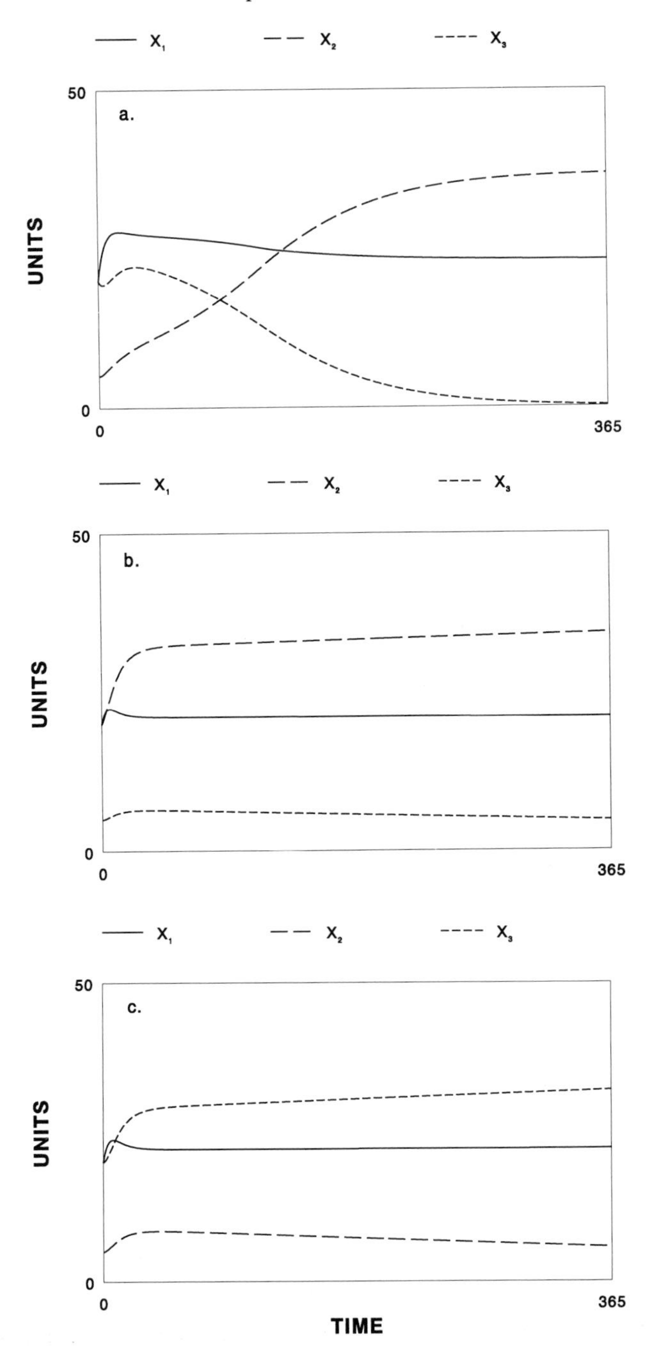

Figure 10. The dynamics of the competitor model for the case where X3 has a permanent advantage with respect to inteference competition (b3 = 1.2 and b2 = 0.8): (a) the better exploitative competitor (X2) always wins; (b) and (c) the unstable equilibrium case where

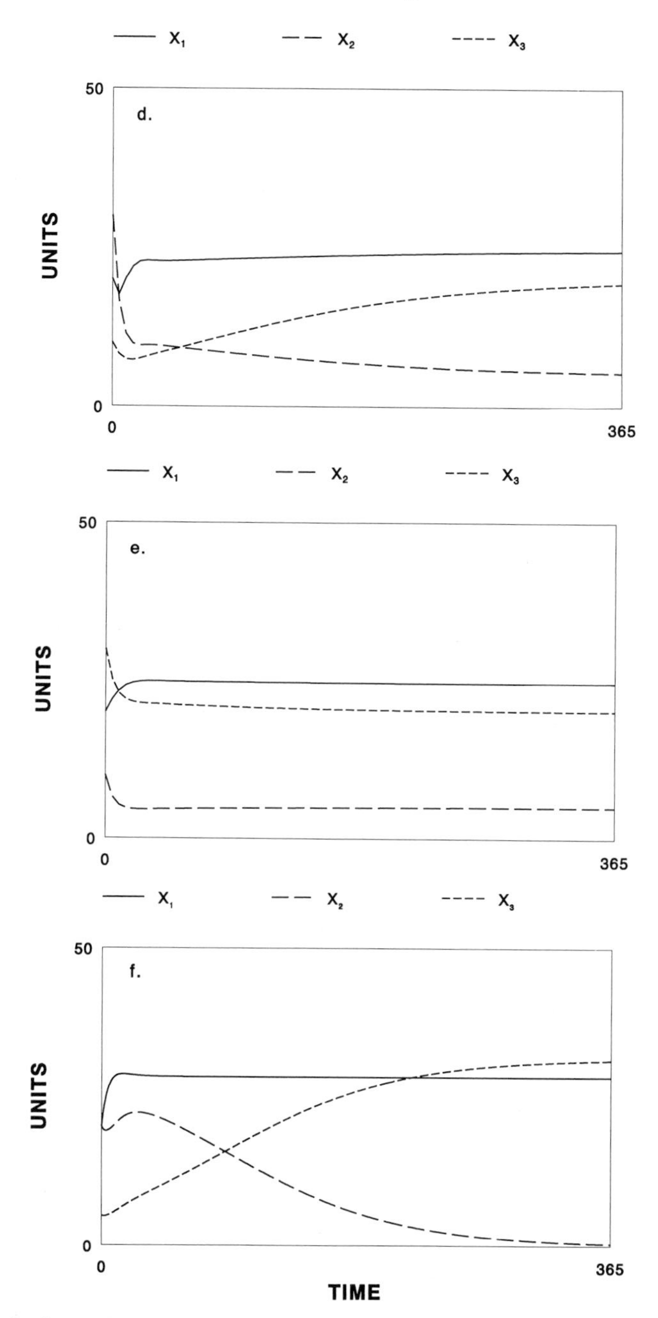

the eventual winner depends on the initial densities; (d) and (e) the stable equilibrium case where the densities converge to the same steady state regardless of the initial densities; and (f) the better interference competitive ability permits X3 to always win. Parameter values for all cases are given in *Table 2*.

illustrate the principles of compartmental modelling. These larger models of existing systems bring with them some inherent problems as well as some new approaches to analysis.

3.4 Large compartmental models

By 'large' compartmental models is meant those with many compartments (commonly ranging from 5–10 up to dozens). There is of course an attendant increase in the pathways of flow and information and in the number of parameters that must be evaluated.

3.4.1 The 'condensation' problem

In even the simplest of common ecosystems, for example a soil/litter community, there will be found hundreds of species and dozens of relevant abiotic candidates for state variable status. In such systems it is impractical to consider compartmentalizing the model in any degree approaching the complexity of nature. Thus to construct a mechanistic model of such a system requires careful reduction of the trophic complexity commensurate with the objectives of the model. This is the so-called 'condensation problem. What species or life-history stages may be lumped together in a compartment? This has always been, and remains, one of the central problems facing modellers of ecosystems.

The desire to seek solutions to this problem led me to the study of thermal spring systems. In Yellowstone National Park these are communities of bacteria, cyanobacteria (blue–green algae), grazing flies, and a few species of predacious and parasitic invertebrate. Despite the trophic diversity, a typical community may contain as few as 20 species. These systems are ideal outdoor laboratories for studying the effects of model condensation.

Given the limited goals that must be set for any mechanistic compartmental models, a considerable amount of simplification can be accomplished before any structural diagrams are produced. For example, if interest centres primarily on the grazing food web, one is justified, at least initially, in eliminating or greatly simplifying the saprophage pathways on the basis that recycling usually has a much longer response time than the grazing components and may thus for quite long periods be virtually decoupled.

To elucidate some rules for condensation a very detailed model of the grazing chain of thermal communities was used (18). Many simulation experiments were run with this model involving various degrees of simplification (compartmental lumping). These are the sorts of decision that have to be made at the outset when modelling the usual complex natural community. From the results of these simulations two major rules were derived that have served well as guides to condensation in compartmental models of complex natural ecosystems:

- components with very different potential rates of increase should not be placed in the same compartment

- the structural complexity of the model needs to be approximately matched by the level of information included in the functional attributes

The first rule is rather obvious with hindsight; it summarizes the difficulty encountered when trying to simulate the dynamics of a compartment containing components with disparate maximum rates of increase or loss. Each compartment can have only one maximum rate of ingestion, for example, for a given material resource. This means that if the relative proportion of any of the species comprising a compartment changes, the weighted maximum rate must change. But there is no way to evaluate these individual species separately; all we have is the standing stock of a conglomerate compartment. When all maximum rates are similar it doesn't matter; if they are vastly different it does. Thus grouping components with vastly different rates should be done only when the compartmental dynamics are not principal parts of the model goals.

The second rule is much less obvious. Indeed, before the results of the simulations with the thermal spring model, I would have intuitively stated the reverse. One would think that an improvement in the complexity of the model in either structure or function would improve both its verification and validity (see Section 4.1). However, experience shows a simple model usually produces better results than a model with a great deal of superficial complexity in the structural part of the model, but leaving the functional information largely to guesswork. The reason behind this observation is that structural complexity (more compartments or pathways of flow) is easy to add to a model based on species lists, whereas functional information requires detailed research. These rules are summarized in *Protocol 2*.

Protocol 2. Simplifying models of complex systems

1. When specifying goals, try to identify parts of the system that may be simplified greatly or omitted, at least initially.
2. When aggregating components of the real system into compartments of the model do not include components with greatly differing maximum rates of growth.
3. When specifying the structural attributes of the model, do not exceed the level of functional information available.
4. A useful rule to observe in initial models of large systems is to aim for functional information equally divided between
   (i) data from the system modelled
   (ii) data from the literature
   (iii) estimates by researchers familiar with the component/system

---

3.4.2 Sensitivity analyses

One of the best ways to use a model is to do a sensitivity analysis, whether the objective is to develop theory or to guide a research program. Sensitivity analysis was introduced in Chapter 8, Section 2.11; here I will discuss only those aspects peculiar to large compartmental models.

The simplest sensitivity analysis is made by changing something in the model and observing the result compared against the earlier, unchanged simulation. We are dealing with deterministic, mechanistic models, so any change has to be the result of the perturbation, whether it was applied to a parameter or a control function. In fact, even models with stochastic processes can be analysed in this manner (see Section 4.2). The problem, particularly with large compartmental models, is the possibility of synergism and antagonism that are so common in these complex interactive models. Changing each of two parameters, one at a time, might produce little change, but changing them simultaneously could produce a major change. Clearly in small models it would be possible to change all parameter pairs and examine the possible results. But even in small models the number of parameters in all possible combinations is far too large to be handled in this manner and in large models even changing all parameters one at a time may be too time-consuming to be worthwhile.

One solution of this problem is to carefully choose only those parameters whose sensitivity may be very important and whose error is appreciable, i.e. the data on which the parameter is based are few or unreliable. Second, the grouping of parameters when changing values is important. Rates that are known to be antagonistic, e.g. ingestion and excretion, should not usually be changed together in the same direction; the increased ingestion is partially or wholly cancelled by the increased losses (but other compartments in the system could well be affected). Sometimes only some subsystems of the larger model are of interest. In such cases the sensitivity analysis problem is greatly simplified.

Another computer-intensive technique that has been proposed is to vary all of the parameters in the model stochastically (see Section 4.2) and store the results, say at selected times during a year. The variation can have a specified mean and standard deviation. When enough simulation runs have been made, the relationships of variation in selected groups of parameters can be compared with state variables and flows in the model. Usually some form of multivariate technique would be chosen for the analysis because many of the parameters to be varied are not independent. The major drawback of this technique is the large number of simulations required to show relationships with any confidence, often in the thousands for models with 100 or more parameters.

4. Special topics

4.1 Verification and validation

Verification (see Chapter 8, Section 2.9) requires comparing the output from the model to a data set, drawn from the system of interest, that was wholly or partially used in the construction of the model. In other words, does the model do adequately what it was constructed to do? Verification can be likened to the process of fitting a regression line in an empirical model; does the line represent the data to the desired degree?

Validation, however, asks how well the model does when asked to match an independent data set. A data set obtained from measurements on the unperturbed system may exist independently of the construction of the model, i.e. the parameter values may have been derived from independent experiment/observation. In such a case verification becomes the initial step in validation. But a fully validated model would have to be tested against a number of independent perturbations. These must be of the type the model was built to address; a model of a tidal marsh for example, may be quite valid to predict the effects of a toxic waste entering estuarine water, but be totally unable to predict the effects of a dike that changes tidal patterns of flow. Unfortunately, data sets adequate for validation are seldom available. When they are available and prediction is the only goal, an empirical model is usually used. Because mechanistic models have other, more important uses than simple prediction, they must be verified but not necessarily validated. Indeed, the initial model(s) constructed to be used with an ongoing research program are almost by definition invalid (in the sense used here) as they are constructed with incomplete data and are designed to be changed, i.e. made more valid, as the research progresses.

4.2 Parameter stochasticity

The majority of mechanistic models are deterministic, i.e. for constant initial conditions they will produce exactly the same behaviour each time they are run. Most of them, except those with multiple steady states or cycles or those exhibiting chaos, will settle into the same behaviour with time despite different initial conditions. This lack of probabilistic behaviour is regarded as a positive attribute. The modeller generally wants to ascertain the model response to perturbations: both acute and long-term and extraneous 'noise' would only confuse the experiment. Sometimes, however, the stochastic element is desired. Modelling the behaviour of individuals almost always requires a large element of probability because it cannot be averaged out using the law of large numbers as is done with models of the growth of entire populations. When modelling the physical changes in part of a system, the data on persistence may themselves consist of averages and error terms, not virtually error-free measurements from a laboratory, or else the mean frequency of perturbations may be known but not the pattern. In all such cases, the model must contain the information requisite for simulation of stochastic events. The steps necessary to implement this requirement are given in *Protocol 3*. The algorithms in the protocol are adapted from (19).

Protocol 3. Modelling stochastic processes

1. Decide whether the process is simulated by a simple uniform distribution of random numbers or requires a normal distribution with specified mean and standard deviation.
2. If the uniform distribution is desired, simply compute a random number in whatever programming language you are using and transform it to fit the magnitude of the stochastic parameter being generated. For example, if the parameter ranges from 0 to 0.25 and your random number generator produces numbers from 0–1, you simply multiply the random number by 0.25.
3. To approximate a normal distribution with specified mean and standard deviation (assuming random numbers range from 0–1), generate and sum 12 random numbers, subtract 6 from the total, then multiply by the specified standard deviation and add the specified mean.[a]

[a] The algorithm in 3 is derived from the fact that the sum of n random numbers is distributed normally, with mean = $n/2$ and standard deviation = $n/12$ as n approaches infinity. This distribution is approximated adequately for an n of 12 and this number is convenient because it gives a standard deviation multiplier of 1. Subtracting 6 from the sum normalizes to a mean of zero, to which the specified mean is then added. Note: if the standard deviation is greater than $1/6$ of the mean, then there is a finite probability that the number generated by this algorithm will be negative. This probability is extremely small unless the standard deviation exceeds $1/4$ of the mean. In such cases one can simply increase the size of n to lower the probability and insert a statement in the program to reject negative values.

Adding stochasticity to a model makes changing and debugging the model very difficult because the output is different each time. It also may not be desirable when doing sensitivity analyses on the model. The stochasticity can be eliminated in most high level programming languages because of the 'seed' requirement. Most of the randomization algorithms require that the initial value used to start the algorithm be a different seed; otherwise the same random series is produced. Usually the seed is taken from the system clock (in BASIC the command is RANDOMIZE TIMER, where TIMER returns the number of seconds that have elapsed since the machine was turned on). If, however, one uses a constant as the seed, the same random sequence is generated and the output remains the same for each simulation.

4.3 Temporal heterogeneity and time delays

The mechanistic compartmental models examined to this point were assumed homogeneous in space and in time, except for the fact of compartmentalization. The latter implies heterogeneity in space, but presents no pattern. Temporal change in the models took place as a series of very small changes over small intervals with rules supplied by the differential equations.

Temporal heterogeneity is used here to represent discontinuous change of considerable magnitude. These can conveniently be referred to as step functions, as opposed to the threshold discontinuities incorporated in the control functions. Examples are:

- harvesting
- abrupt changes in behaviour
- physical events such as storms, mud slides, etc.

Often these are important events in determining system behaviour. They may operate for long (chronic) or short (acute) periods. They may be incorporated into the model within the equations in the same manner as the thresholds in the control functions, i.e. the time counter in the model is a variable in the equation. Alternatively they may be turned on and off by means of comparator statements, i.e. if a certain time has passed or day reached the operator is turned on (off).

Time delays are a different category; they are a measure of the importance of history in the instantaneous dynamics of the system. For example, in the simple control function of Equation 8, the realized rate of ingestion is a function of the standing stock of resource at time t. But suppose this is not the case and some time is necessary for a change in the resource to be reflected in changes in ingestion (or more properly reproduction, since the latter is contained in the ingestion). Then the realized feeding rate at time t might be a function of X_{t-td}, where td is the time delay. This kind of time delay is *discrete* because it uses the value at a discrete time in the past. An alternative is to regard the behaviour at time t as a function of the mean standing stock throughout the time delay. This is an example of a *continuous* time delay. Any weight distribution of the values of X could be substituted in place of the unweighted mean.

Protocol 4. Modelling time delays[a]

1. Assume the unit of time in the model is one (minute, hour, day, etc.). This will be the lag or delay unit.
2. Five parameters need to be set: the initial value of the state variable X (XINIT), the time delay in delay units (TD), the number of iterations in a delay unit (NTS), the sum of all values of X over all delay units in the time delay (SUMX), and the running average of X over the interval TD. SUMX and AVEX are initially set to zero. NTS is equal to 1/(the constant solution interval). If an integration procedure with variable time steps is used, this procedure must be suitably modified.

Protocol 4. *Continued*

3. Dimension a vector (array) with TD cells, X(TD). At the start of a simulation place XINIT in all cells of the vector.
4. Establish two integer counters, say ICOUNT and INDEX, and set them to zero initially. Increment ICOUNT each iteration. Test to see if the counter equals NTS, if not skip the remaining steps and continue the iteration.
5. If the counter equals NTS then change SUMX by subtracting the amount currently in cell X(INDEX) and add the amount currently in X. Replace AVEX with SUMX/TD and X(INDEX) with the value of X.
6. Test to see if INDEX is less than TD; if so then increment INDEX by 1. If not set INDEX to 1.
7. Set ICOUNT to zero and continue with the iteration.

[a] Note that such variable time delays are often difficult or impossible to write into many simulation modelling packages, although straightforward in high level programming languages (e.g. BASIC).

Perusal of *Protocol 4* will show the logic underlying the algorithm. Each time the number of iterations adds to the delay unit the oldest value of X is removed from SUMX and the newest added to both SUMX and X(INDEX). The INDEX pointer is then advanced to point to the oldest remaining value of X.

4.4 Spatial heterogeneity

Spatial heterogeneity is currently at the forefront of concern in biological modelling in general and ecological modelling in particular. Spatial heterogeneity has two attributes:

- scale
- pattern

Scale refers to the dimensinal aspect of the heterogeneity. How large or small are the scales in the model to be? Clearly, spatial heterogeneity at the scale of a model of a large estuary will emphasize very different aspects of the system as compared with a model of ten hectares of tidal salt marsh. Many of these definitional aspects of scale will have been dealt with in the initial description of the system of interest and the modelling goals (see *Protocol 1*).

Pattern refers to arrangement of the heterogeneity. If the goal of the model is simply to simulate the dynamics of two different spatial aspects of a system to arrive at an averaged value, with flows between the different aspects of little consequence, then relative weight is paramount and pattern is of little consequence. In models of landscapes, however, where interaction between the patches is important, then both patch size and placement in the system (pattern) must be incorporated into the model.

In the first case the simulation method is simple. Essentially two models are constructed and designed to run simultaneously. Sometimes it is easiest simply to increase the number of compartments in a single model. For example, assume one wishes to simulate the total production by plants on a field containing patches of three very distinct types of vegetation. Instead of constructing three separate models, a single model with three compartments is sufficient. In such cases, the spatial heterogeneity is fixed, at least over modelling times, and there is relatively little coupling between the compartments.

Where there is strong coupling due to the movement of biotic and/or abiotic components throughout the system, simple compartmentalization, even with flows connecting them, will not suffice. In this case the accumulations of energy/matter actually determine the scale and pattern of all or part of the heterogeneity. Further, the flow patterns are determined by the degree of adjacency of different parts of the system. Examples of such models would be models of breeding birds using various kinds of forest for differential breeding and models of coastal upwelling (these may even be three-dimensional). The way such situations are modelled is to divide the system into cells (rectangular or hexagonal in two-dimensional models and boxes in the case of three-dimensional models). Within each cell a simulation is run, and flow between cells is governed by a separate set of rules. There is nothing particularly difficult in theory about constructing such models. However, they can quickly grow to sizes that tax all but the fastest computers. Many such models are currently designed to take advantage of the latest parallel processing computers.

5. Summary of compartmental modelling

This necessarily brief overview of modelling has emphasized some of the practical aspects of proceeding from single compartment, homogeneous models to *n*-compartment models that may have both temporal and spatial heterogeneity. It gives the beginning modeller some tools with which to begin constructing models. It does not cover all or even a large fraction of the techniques that can be applied to set up a simulation of one or more aspects of a real biological system. Computer modelling of this type is a very young discipline (as is all of computer science) and is advancing rapidly. The modelling literature is widely scattered, partly because models often are embedded in more traditional experimental/observational papers. In Chapter 8, Dr Bowker suggests sources for more advanced techniques. In addition to endorsing his list, I would suggest the journals *Simulation* and *Ecological Modelling* as well as some additional textbooks (20, 21, 22).

Modelling not only aids in doing good science, it can also be a great deal of fun!

Acknowledgements

The data and theoretical constructs on which the majority of this chapter is based were gathered/developed with the support of Grants BSR-8615503, 1987–1991, from NSF, and DE-FG09-89ER60881, 1989–1992, from DOE.

References

1. Miller, J. G. (1965). Living systems. *J. Behav. Sci.* **10**(3), 193–411.
2. Wiegert, R. G. (1975). Simulation models of ecosystems. *Ann. Rev. Ecol. Systematics* **6,** 311–38.
3. Wiegert, R. G. and Penas-Lado, E. (1982). Optimal exploitation, by mussel rafts, of the Ria de Arosa, Spain: Predictions of a first-generation model. In *Marine ecosystem modeling: Proceedings*. US Dept. of Commerce, NOAA, Nat. Environ. Satellite, Date and Info. Service.
4. Gleick, J. (1987). *Chaos: making a new science.* Viking Press, New York.
5. Wiegert, R. G. (1979). Modeling salt marshes and estuaries: Progress and problems. In: *Estuarine and wetland processes* (ed P. Hamilton and K. B. Macdonald), pp. 527–40. Plenum Press, New York.
6. Odum, H. T. (1983). *Systems ecology: an introduction.* John Wiley, New York.
7. Forrester, J. W. (1961). *Industrial dynamics.* MIT Press, Cambridge, Mass.
8. Wiegert, R. G. and Owen, D. F. (1971). Trophic structure, available resources and population density in terrestrial vs. aquatic ecosystems. *J. Theor. Biol.* **30,** 69–81.
9. Wiegert, R. G. (1979). Modeling coastal, estuarine and marsh ecosystems: State-of-the-art. In *Contemporary quantitative ecology and related ecometrics* (ed G. P. Patil and M. L. Rosenzweig), pp. 319–41. International Co-op Publishing House, Fairland, MD.
10. Christian, R. R. and Wetzel, R. L. (1978). Interactions between substrate microbes and consumers of *Spartina* 'detritus' in estuaries. In *Estuarine interactions* (ed M. Wiley), pp. 93–114. Academic Press, New York.
11. Wiegert, R. G., Christian, R. R., Gallagher, J. L., Hall, J. R., Jones, R. D. H., and Wetzel, R. L. (1975). A preliminary ecosystem model of coastal Georgia *Spartina* marsh. In *Estuarine research, Vol. 1: Chemistry, biology and the estuarine ecosystem* (ed L. E. Cronin), pp. 583–601. Academic Press, New York.
12. Smith, F. E. (1972). Spatial heterogeneity, stability, and diversity in ecosystems. *Trans. Conn. Acad. Arts Sci.* **44,** 307–35.
13. May, R. M. (1974). Biological populations with non-overlapping generations: stable points, stable cycles and chaos. *Science* **186,** 645–7.
14. Wiegert, R. G. (1979). Population models: experimental tools for the analysis of ecosystems. In *Analysis of ecological systems* (ed D. J. Horn and D. Mitchell), pp. 233–76. Ohio State University Press, Columbus, OH.
15. May, R. M. (1973). *Stability and complexity in model ecosystems.* Princeton University Press, Princeton.
16. Schoener, T. W. (1973). Population growth regulated by intraspecific competition for energy or time: some simple representations. *Theor. Pop. Biol.* **4,** 56–84.

17. Slobodkin, L. B. (1961). *Growth and regulation of animal populations*. Holt, Reinhart and Winston, New York.
18. Wiegert, R. G. (1977). A model of a thermal spring food chain. In *Ecosystem modeling in theory and practice: an introduction with case histories* (ed. C. A. S. Hall and J. W. Day Jr.), pp. 290–315. John Wiley, New York.
19. Davies, R. G. (1971). *Computer programming in quantitative biology*. Academic Press, New York.
20. Gold, H. J. (1977). *Mathematical modeling of biological systems—an introductory guidebook*. John Wiley, New York.
21. Kitching, R. L. (1983). *Systems ecology: an introduction to ecological modelling*. University of Queensland Press, St Lucia.
22. Swartzman, G. L. and Kaluzny, S. P. (1987). *Ecological simulation primer*. Macmillan, New York.
23. Wiegert, R. G., Christian, R. R., and Wetzel, R. L. (1981). A model view of the marsh. In *The ecology of a salt marsh* (ed L. C. Pomeroy and R. G. Wiegert), pp. 183–218. Springer, New York.

Appendix 9.1. Code for BASIC program PREDCOMP.BAS

```
10   REM :PROGRAM PREDCOMP.BAS
20   REM :PROGRAMMED BY R.G. WIEGERT
30   REM :Program to simulate the dynamics of a three compartment
40   REM :system with two optional structures: 1)linear or 2)web.
50   REM :Option 1 is a resource, prey, predator configuration.
60   REM :Option 2 is a resource with two competing consumers.
70   REM************************************************************************************
80   REM DIMENSION VARIABLES AND DEFINE FUNCTIONS.
90   REM************************************************************************************
100  DIM NAM$(50),VALUE(50)
110  DIM X1(50),X2(50),X3(50)
120  DEF FNP1(X,Y)=(ABS(X-Y)+(X-Y))/2
130  DEFINT I,J,K,L
140  SCREEN 0:CLS:KEY OFF
150  REM************************************************************************************
160  REM READ PARAMETER NAMES AND VALUES INTO ARRAYS.
170  REM************************************************************************************
180  PRINT "What option do you want? Predation(1) or Competition(2)"
190  V$=INKEY$: IF V$=""THEN 190
200  IF V$="1" THEN GOTO 260
210  DATA f1, 6.0 ,t12, .2 ,tl3, .2 ,r1, .1 ,r2, .1 ,r3, .1 ,g12, 27
220  DATA g22, 40 ,g13, 35 ,g33, 40 ,a12, 5 ,a22, 10 ,a13, 5 ,a33, 10
230  DATA b2,.8 ,b3, 1.2 ,delt, .1 ,tlag, 0 ,nul, 0 ,time, 365 ,print1, 5
240  DATA icount, 0 ,x01, 50 ,x02, 5 ,x03, 5 ,factor1, 1 ,factor2,1,factor3,1
250  FOR I=1 TO 28:READ NAM$(I):READ VALUE(I):NEXT I:GOTO 340
260  REM LABEL
270  FOR I=1 TO 28:READ NAM$(I):READ VALUE(I):NEXT I
280  FOR I=1 TO 28:READ NAM$(I):READ VALUE(I):NEXT I:GOTO 340
290  DATA f1,3 ,t12, .3 ,t23, .25 ,r1, .1 ,r2, .1 ,r3, .2 ,g12, 20
300  DATA g22, 70 ,g23, 2 ,g33,100 ,a12, 5 ,a22, 20 ,a23,.5 ,a33, 50
310  DATA b2, 0 ,b3, 0 ,delt, .1 ,tlag, 0 ,nul, 0, time,365 ,print1, 5
320  DATA icount,0,x01,15,x02,7,x03,4,factor1,.25,factor2,.25,factor3,.25
330  FOR I=1 TO 28:READ NAM$(I):READ VALUE(I):NEXT I
340  REM LABEL
350  REM************************************************************************************
360  REM OPEN FILE FOR STORAGE OF STATE VARIABLES AND FEEDBACKS.
370  REM************************************************************************************
380  IF V$="1" THEN NAM$="PREDATE.DAT" ELSE NAM$="COMPETE.DAT"
390  OPEN "O",#1,NAM$
400  PROG$="complag"
410  PRINT#1,PROG$
420  PRINT#1,DATE$,TIME$
430  PRINT#1," ";
440  REM LABEL
450  REM************************************************************************************
460  REM SET INITIAL VALUES OF STATE VARIABLES AND PARAMETERS.
470  REM************************************************************************************
480  F1=VALUE(1)
490  T12=VALUE(2)
500  IF V$="1" THEN T23=VALUE(3) ELSE T13=VALUE(3)
```

Appendix 9.1. *(contd.)*

```
510  R1=VALUE(4)
520  R2=VALUE(5)
530  R3=VALUE(6)
540  G12=VALUE(7)
550  G22=VALUE(8)
560  IF V$="1" THEN G23=VALUE(9) ELSE G13=VALUE(9)
570  G33=VALUE(10)
580  A12=VALUE(11)
590  A22=VALUE(12)
600  IF V$="1" THEN A23=VALUE(13) ELSE A13=VALUE(13)
610  A33=VALUE(14)
620  B2=VALUE(15)
630  B3=VALUE(16)
640  DELT=VALUE(17)
650  TLAG=VALUE(18)
660  LGST=VALUE(19)
670  TIME=VALUE(20)
680  PRINT1=VALUE(21)
690  ICOUNT=VALUE(22)
700  X01=VALUE(23)
710  X02=VALUE(24)
720  X03=VALUE(25)
730  FACTOR1=VALUE(26)
740  FACTOR2=VALUE(27)
750  FACTOR3=VALUE(28)
760  CLS
770  REM******************************************************************************************
780  REM PRINT INITIAL VALUES TO THE SCREEN.
790  REM******************************************************************************************
800  FOR I=1 TO 28 STEP 3
810  FOR J=0 TO 2
820  IF NAM$(I+J)="" THEN PRINT:GOTO 850
830  PRINT TAB(15+J*17)I+J;"";NAM$(I+J);"";VALUE(I+J);
840  NEXT J:PRINT:NEXT I
850  REM LABEL
860  REM******************************************************************************************
870  REM OPTION TO CHANGE INITIAL VALUES.
880  REM******************************************************************************************
890  PRINT"Do you wish to make changes? y/n"
900  X$=INKEY$: IF X$="" THEN 900
910  IF X$<>"Y" THEN IF X$<>"y" THEN GOTO 940
920  GOSUB 2380
930  GOTO 440
940  REM LABEL
950  REM******************************************************************************************
960  REM PRINT PARAMETER VALUES AND INITIAL CONDITIONS TO FILE.
970  REM******************************************************************************************
980  FOR I=1 TO 28 STEP 7
990  FOR J=0 TO 6
1000 PRINT #1,NAM$(I+J);VALUE(I+J);
```

Appendix 9.1. *(contd.)*

```
1010 NEXT J
1020 PRINT #1,
1030 NEXT I
1040 PRINT #1,
1050 PRINT #1,"   ";
1060 PRINT #1,USING"\   \";"DAY","X1","X2","X3","FBR1","FBS1","FBR2","FBS2"
1070 REM LABEL
1080 REM******************************************************************************************
1090 REM INITIALIZE COUNTERS AND TIMELAG ARRAYS.
1100 REM******************************************************************************************
1110 IPRINT=0
1120 JPRINT=PRINT1/DELT
1130 LGST=TLAG/DELT:IF TLAG>1 THEN LGST=LGST/TLAG
1140 IDAY=0
1150 X1=X01:X2=X02:X3=X03
1160 FOR I=1 TO 50:X1(I)=X01:X2(I)=X02:X3(I)=X03:NEXT I
1170 REM******************************************************************************************
1180 REM PRINT INITIAL VALUES TO THE FILE.
1190 REM******************************************************************************************
1200 PRINT#1,USING"####.####";IDAY;X1;X2;X3;FBR1;FBS1;FBR2;FBS2
1210 ITIME=INT(TIME/DELT +.5)
1220 SUMX1=TLAG*X01:SUMX2=TLAG*X02:SUMX3=TLAG*X03
1230 INDEX=1
1240 REM LABEL
1250 CLS:SCREEN2:WW=640:WH=199
1260 LINE(0,0)-(WW-1, WH-1),, B
1270 FACTOR4=640/ITIME
1280 REM******************************************************************************************
1290 REM ENTER THE MAIN PROGRAM LOOP.
1300 REM******************************************************************************************
1310 REM******************************************************************************************
1320 FOR J=1 TO ITIME
1330 REM Compute feedback control functions.
1340 REM******************************************************************************************
1350 FBR1=FNP1(G12,X1(INDEX))/(G12-A12)
1360 FBR1=FNP1(1,FBR1)
1370 FBS1=FNP1(X2(INDEX)+B3*X3(INDEX),A22)/(G22-A22)
1380 FBS1=FNP1(1,(1-R2/T12)*FBS1)
1390 IF V$="2" THEN FBR2=FNP1(G13,X1(INDEX))/(G13-A13)
1400 IF V$="1" THEN FBR2=FNP1(G23,X2(INDEX))/(G23-A23)
1410 FBR2=FNP1(1,FBR2)
1420 FBS2=FNP1(X3(INDEX)+B2*X2(INDEX),A33)/(G33-A33)
1430 IF V$="2" THEN FBS2=FNP1(1,(R3/T13)*FBS2)
1440 IF V$="1" THEN FBS2=FNP1(1,(R3/T23)*FBS2)
1450 REM******************************************************************************************
1460 REM Compute fluxes.
1470 REM******************************************************************************************
1480 F01=F1
1490 F10=R1*X1
1500 F12=T12*X2*FBR1*FBS1
```

Appendix 9.1. (*contd.*)

```
1510 IF V$="1" THEN F23=T23*X3*FBR2*FBS2 ELSE F13=T13*X3*FBR2*FBS2
1520 F20=R2*X2
1530 F30=R3*X3
1540 DEBIT=F01-F10-F12-F13+X1/DELT
1550 IF DEBIT<0 THEN F12=F12-DEBIT*F12/(F12+F13):F13=F13-DEBIT*F13/(F12+F13)
1560 REM********************************************************************************
1570 REM Compute changes in state variables.
1580 REM********************************************************************************
1590 DX1=F01-F10-F12-F13
1600 DX2=F12-F20-F23
1610 IF V$="1" THEN DX3=F23-F30 ELSE DX3=F13-F30
1620 REM********************************************************************************
1630 REM Increment the state variables
1640 REM********************************************************************************
1650 X1=FNP1(X1+DX1*DELT,0)
1660 X2=FNP1(X2+DX2*DELT,0)
1670 X3=FNP1(X3+DX3*DELT,0)
1680 REM********************************************************************************
1690 REM Increment the counters.
1700 REM********************************************************************************
1710 LAG=LAG+1
1720 IPRINT=IPRINT+1
1730 REM********************************************************************************
1740 REM Compute time-delayed values.
1750 REM********************************************************************************
1760 IF LAG<LGST THEN 1830
1770 LAG=0
1780 SUMX1=SUMX1-X1(INDEX)+X1
1790 SUMX2=SUMX2-X2(INDEX)+X2
1800 SUMX3=SUMX3-X3(INDEX)+X3
1810 X1(INDEX)=X1:X2(INDEX)=X2:X3(INDEX)=X3
1820 IF INDEX<TLAG THEN INDEX=INDEX+1 ELSE INDEX=1
1830 REM LABEL
1840 REM********************************************************************************
1850 REM Print data to file.
1860 REM********************************************************************************
1870 IF IPRINT<JPRINT THEN GOTO 1940
1880 IDAY=IDAY+PRINT1
1890 PRINT#1,USING"####.####";IDAY;X1;X2;X3;FBR1;FBS1;FBR2;FBS2
1900 IPRINT=0
1910 REM********************************************************************************
1920 REM Plot state variables.
1930 REM********************************************************************************
1940 REM LABEL
1950 JJ=J*FACTOR4
1960 PSET(JJ,WH-X1/FACTOR1)
1970 PSET(JJ,WH-X2/FACTOR2)
1980 PSET(JJ,WH-X3/FACTOR3)
1990 A$=INKEY$: IF A$<>"" THEN 2180
2000 REM********************************************************************************
```

Appendix 9.1. *(contd.)*

```
2010 REM LEAVE MAIN PROGRAM LOOP.
2020 REM*********************************************************************************
2030 NEXT J
2040 REM*********************************************************************************
2050 REM PRINT VALUES TO SCREEN GRAPH.
2060 REM*********************************************************************************
2070 LOCATE 2,1
2080 PRINT TAB(5);"tlag=";TLAG;
2090 PRINT TAB(20);PROG$;" ";DATE$;" ";TIME$
2100 PRINT TAB(5);"day=";IDAY;TAB(20);"x1=";X1;TAB(36);"x2=";X2;TAB(56);"x3=
     ";X3
2110 IF V$="1" THEN PRINT TAB(5);"b2=";B2;TAB(20);"b3=";B3;TAB(35);"tau12=
     ";T12;TAB(50);"tau13=";T13
2120 IF V$="2" THEN PRINT TAB(5);"b2=";B2;TAB(20);"b3="B3;TAB(35);"tau12=
     ";T12;TAB(50);"tau23=";T23
2130 PRINT TAB(5);"f01=
     ";F01;TAB(20);"fac1=";FACTOR1;TAB(35);"fac2=";FACTOR2;TAB(50);"fac3=";FAC
     TOR3
2140 REM*********************************************************************************
2150 REM PAUSE TO ALLOW SCREEN DUMP TO PRINTER. HIT ANY KEY TO
     RESUME.
2160 A$=INKEY$: IF A$="" THEN 2160
2170 REM*********************************************************************************
2180 REM LABEL
2190 SCREEN 0
2200 LOCATE 23,2
2210 PRINT "Hit any key except CR to continue"
2220 S$=INKEY$:IF S$="" THEN 2220
2230 REM
2240 IF ASC(S$)=13 THEN GOTO 2320
2250 LOCATE 23,2
2260 PRINT "Hit any key except CR to auto. increase time lag"
2270 T$=INKEY$:IF T$="" THEN 2270
2280 IF ASC(T$)=13 THEN GOTO 1240
2290 TLAG=TLAG+1
2300 IF TLAG>10 THEN GOTO 2320
2310 GOTO 1070
2320 REM LABEL
2330 PRINT"Hit CR to exit program:any other key restarts from beginning"
2340 U$=INKEY$:IF U$="" THEN 2340
2350 IF ASC(U$)<>13 THEN CLOSE#1:CLS:GOTO 340
2360 CLS:KEY ON:SCREEN 0:END
2370 REM*********************************************************************************
2380 REM LABEL Subroutine CHANGE
2390 REM*********************************************************************************
2400 PRINT"To change values type#,value or type,CR to exit
2410 INPUT ORD#,VALUE
2420 IF ORD#=0 THEN 2450
2430 VALUE(ORD#)=VALUE
2440 GOTO 2380
2450 REM LABEL
2460 RETURN
```

A

Software packages

A list of the commercially available computer packages that have been used illustratively in the chapters of this book follows. Where possible, one North American and one European supplier has been given for each package. Brief notes about the package are also included. These notes are compilations from those written by the authors contributing to this book who have used the packages concerned.

***CANOCO* version 2.1**
C. F. J. Ter Braak
Agricultural Mathematics Group
Box 100, 6700 AC Wageningen
The Netherlands

A Fortran program for canonical community ordination (see reference 16 in Chapter 5), available for VAX computers and IBM mainframes, as well as the IBM PC-compatible family of computers. *CANOCO* consists of about 5000 lines of code written in standard Fortran77. Includes options for partial, detrended, and canonical correspondence analysis, principal components analysis and redundancy analysis. A plotting program *CANOPLOT* is included. Data input can be as a standard rectangular matrix, or in Cornell compressed data format.

***GLIM* version 3.77**
Numerical Algorithms Group Ltd
Wilkinson House
Jordan Hill Road
Oxford
OX2 8DA
UK
Tel: 44 0865 511245
Fax: 44 0865 310139

Numerical Algorithms Group Inc.
1400 Opus Place, Suite 200
Downer's Grove
IL 60515-1702
USA
Tel: 0101 1708 971 2337
Fax: 0101 1708 971 2706

This is a specialist package solely for fitting the general linear model. Such models include ANOVA and linear and multiple regression. It is available for the IBM PC-compatible family of computers. It is command-based and the syntax of the command language is somewhat different from that used in other statistical packages. It is intended for use by the professional statistician and the output can be difficult to interpret by those not familiar with the statistical theory of the general linear model.

ISIM

ISIM Simulation
Salford Tramways Building
P.O. Box 50
Frederick Road
Salford
M6 6BY
UK
Tel: 44 061 736 8921
Fax: 44 061 737 0880

Crosbie, Hay & Associates
P.O. Box 943
Chico
Ca 95927
USA

ISIM runs under MS-DOS on IBM PC, PC/XT, and PC/AT or compatible computers. There is optional support for machines with an 8087 maths co-processor. *ISIM* supports standard CGA, EGA, and other medium/high resolution screens.

ISIM is a complete simulation environment for the modelling of small- to medium-sized continuous dynamic systems. Its features include the following: a self-contained high-level programming language which incorporates a subset of Fortran functions; a choice of four algorithms for numerical integration; a line-by-line diagnostic editor for entering programs and checking errors; an advanced interpreter providing fast simulation without the delays caused by compilation and linking; a facility to monitor or change any variables before, during, or after the execution of a program, and the display of simulation data on screen or printer in either text or graphics mode.

***Minitab* release 7.1 and 8.2**

Clecom Ltd
The Research Park
Vincent Drive,
Edgbaston
Birmingham
B15 2SQ
UK
Tel: 44 021 471 4199
Fax: 44 021 471 5169

Minitab Inc.
3081 Enterprise Drive
State College
PA 16801-2756
USA
Tel: 0101 814 238 3280
Fax: 0101 814 238 4383

Comprehensive statistical package available for the IBM PC-compatible family and Apple Macintosh computers. Command-based program running fully interactively, with comprehensive data handling and macro facilities. Release 8.2 incorporates a menu-based interface which can be operated by a mouse. This release allows cutting and pasting from the scrollable text output screen to the worksheet. This obviates the need to enter some statistics from the keyboard, as described in the text. The graphics are relatively poor. A very easy package to start to use with lots of supporting literature available. Covers ANOVA, linear, bivariate, and multiple regression, some time series analysis, principal component analysis and exploratory data analysis. Release 7.1 was used by most authors in this book, but all the macros have also been tested on release 8.2.

***SAS* release 6.03**

SAS Software Ltd
Wittington House
Henley Road
Medmenham
Marlow
SL7 2EB
UK
Tel: 44 6284 86933
Fax: 44 6284 83203

SAS Institute Inc.
SAS Campus Drive
Cary
NC 27513
USA
Tel: 0101 919 677 8000
Fax: 0101 919 677 8123

Comprehensive statistical package available for the IBM PC-compatible family of computers. It is a very large program that, in its entirety, takes up a great deal of storage space, but it can be subdivided into modules. It is a command-based package, but a menu-based command system is available and the package can be used interactively. It is a very complex package to use, intended to serve all the needs of the computer user. It includes a programming language and graphics package as well as the statistics package. The base *SAS* and *SAS* STAT modules include ANOVA, linear and multiple regression, principal component analysis, many time series routines, and a range of methods for cluster analysis.

***SPSS/PC+* version 3.0**
SPSS Europe BV
P.O. Box 115
4200 AC Gorinchem
The Netherlands
Tel: 010 31 1830 36711

SPSS Inc.
444 N. Michigan Avenue
Chicago
IL. 60611
USA
Tel: 0101 312 329 3300

Comprehensive statistical package available for IBM PC-compatible computers. This is a very large program that takes up a vast amount of disk space, but can be loaded in modules if space is limited. It is a command-based package, but command lists can be generated from menus and interactive operation is possible. It is a complex program and the high level graphics section only work when linked to *Microsoft Chart.* Covers ANOVA, linear, and multiple regression, a wide range of factor analysis techniques, which include a type of principal component analysis, many time series analysis routines, and a limited variety of cluster analysis techniques.

***Statgraphics* version 2.1**
STSC International Ltd
Royal Albert House
Sheet Street
Windsor
Berkshire
SL4 1BE
Tel: 44 0754 831451
Fax: 44 0753 831541

STSC Inc.
2115 East Jefferson Street
Rockville
MD 20852
USA
Tel: 0101 301 984 5412
Fax: 0101 301 984 5094

Comprehensive statistical package available for the IBM PC-compatible family of computers. Menu-based program. Covers ANOVA, bivariate linear and non-linear regression, multiple regression, a comprehensive range of time series analysis routines, principal component, factor, and cluster analysis. More recent products are *Statgraphics* version 5 and *Statgraphics Plus*; the latter is for computers with 80386/486 processors only and can handle very large numbers of data points.

***Systat* version 5.0**
Eurostat Ltd
Icknield House
Eastcheap
Letchworth
Herts
SG6 3DA
UK
Tel: 44 0462 482822
Fax: 44 0462 482855

Systat, Inc.
1800 Sherman Avenue
Evanston
IL 60201-3793
USA
Tel: 0101 708 864 5670
Fax: 0101 708 492 3568

Comprehensive statistical package available for IBM PC-compatible and Apple Macintosh computers. Command- and menu-based. Comprehensive data handling facilities and high resolution graphics are provided. A relatively hard package to use; expensive. Covers ANOVA, linear, bivariate, and multiple regression, non-linear regression, some time series analysis, principal component and factor analysis, and a limited range of cluster analysis techniques.

B

Statistical tables

JOHN C. FRY and TERENCE C. ILES

In all cases P is the tail area of the distribution.

Appendix B.1. Critical values for the F-distribution
Appendix B.2. Critical values of Hartley's F_{max} at $P = 0.05$
Appendix B.3. Critical values of Cochran's C at $P = 0.05$
Appendix B.4. Critical values for the correlation test for normality at $P = 0.05$
Appendix B.5. Critical values and formulae used for testing outliers by Dixon's test
Appendix B.6. Critical values for the two-tailed Student's t-distribution
Appendix B.7 Critical values for the studentized range statistic at $P = 0.05$
Appendix B.8. Critical values for the χ^2 distribution
Appendix B.9. Critical values for correlation coefficients at $P = 0.05$ for $k = 1$–7 predictor variables
Appendix B.10. Critical values of the Durbin–Watson statistics at $P = 0.05$ for $k = 1$–8 predictor variables
Appendix B.11. Bonferroni-modified Student's t values at $P = 0.05$
Appendix B.12. Multipliers for Scheffé's confidence intervals at $P = 0.05$

Appendix B.1. Critical values for the *F*-distribution

All the values were calculated with *Minitab* release 7.1 for $P = 0.5, 0.05, 0.01$ and 0.001 at df_{num} degrees of freedom in the numerator and df_{denom} degrees of freedom in the denominator

		df_{num}										
df_{denom}	*P*	1	2	3	4	5	6	7	8	9	10	12
1	.5	1.000	1.500	1.709	1.823	1.894	1.942	1.977	2.004	2.025	2.042	2.067
	.05	161.44	199.50	215.70	224.58	230.16	233.98	236.76	238.88	240.54	241.88	243.90
	.01	4052.1	4999.4	5403.3	5624.5	5763.6	5858.9	5928.3	5981.0	6022.4	6055.8	6106.2
	.001	405292.	500008.	540389.	562510.	576415.	585948.	592885.	598156.	602296.	605633.	610680.
2	.5	0.667	1.000	1.135	1.207	1.252	1.282	1.305	1.321	1.334	1.345	1.361
	.05	18.513	19.000	19.164	19.247	19.296	19.329	19.353	19.371	19.385	19.396	19.412
	.01	98.503	99.000	99.166	99.249	99.299	99.333	99.356	99.374	99.388	99.399	99.416
	.001	998.544	999.013	999.179	999.263	999.313	999.346	999.370	999.388	999.402	999.413	999.430
3	.5	0.585	0.881	1.000	1.063	1.102	1.129	1.148	1.163	1.174	1.183	1.197
	.05	10.128	9.552	9.277	9.117	9.013	8.941	8.887	8.845	8.812	8.786	8.745
	.01	34.116	30.817	29.458	28.710	28.237	27.911	27.672	27.489	27.345	27.229	27.052
	.001	167.031	148.504	141.110	137.102	134.581	132.849	131.587	130.620	129.862	129.248	128.318
4	.5	0.549	0.828	0.941	1.000	1.037	1.062	1.080	1.093	1.104	1.113	1.126
	.05	7.709	6.944	6.591	6.388	6.256	6.163	6.094	6.041	5.999	5.964	5.912
	.01	21.198	18.000	16.694	15.977	15.522	15.207	14.976	14.799	14.659	14.546	14.374
	.001	74.138	61.6246	56.178	53.436	51.712	50.526	49.658	48.997	48.475	48.053	47.412
5	.5	0.528	0.799	0.907	0.965	1.00	1.024	1.041	1.055	1.065	1.073	1.085
	.05	6.608	5.786	5.409	5.192	5.050	4.950	4.876	4.818	4.772	4.735	4.678
	.01	16.258	13.274	12.060	11.392	10.967	10.672	10.456	10.289	10.158	10.051	9.888
	.001	47.181	37.123	33.203	31.085	29.753	28.835	28.163	27.650	27.245	26.917	26.418
6	.5	0.515	0.780	0.886	0.942	0.977	1.000	1.017	1.030	1.040	1.048	1.060
	.05	5.987	5.143	4.757	4.534	4.387	4.284	4.207	4.147	4.099	4.060	4.000
	.01	13.745	10.925	9.780	9.148	8.746	8.466	8.260	8.102	7.976	7.874	7.718
	.001	35.508	27.000	23.703	21.924	20.803	20.030	19.463	19.030	18.688	18.411	17.989

7	**.5**	0.506	0.767	0.871	0.926	0.960	0.983	1.000	1.013	1.022	1.030	1.042
	.05	5.591	4.737	4.347	4.120	3.972	3.866	3.787	3.726	3.677	3.637	3.575
	.01	12.246	9.547	8.451	7.847	7.461	7.191	6.993	6.840	6.719	6.620	6.469
	.001	29.245	21.689	18.772	17.198	16.206	15.521	15.019	14.634	14.330	14.083	13.707
8	**.5**	0.499	0.757	0.860	0.915	0.948	0.971	0.988	1.000	1.010	1.018	1.029
	.05	5.318	4.459	4.066	3.838	3.687	3.581	3.500	3.438	3.388	3.347	3.284
	.01	11.259	8.649	7.591	7.006	6.632	6.371	6.178	6.029	5.911	5.814	5.667
	.001	25.415	18.494	15.830	14.392	13.485	12.858	12.398	12.046	11.767	11.540	11.195
9	**.5**	0.494	0.749	0.852	0.906	0.939	0.962	0.978	0.990	1.000	1.008	1.019
	.05	5.117	4.256	3.863	3.633	3.482	3.374	3.293	3.230	3.179	3.137	3.073
	.01	10.562	8.022	6.992	6.422	6.057	5.802	5.613	5.467	5.351	5.257	5.111
	.001	22.857	16.387	13.902	12.560	11.714	11.128	10.698	10.368	10.107	9.894	9.570
10	**.5**	0.490	0.743	0.845	0.899	0.932	0.954	0.971	0.983	0.992	1.000	1.012
	.05	4.965	4.103	3.708	3.478	3.326	3.217	3.135	3.072	3.020	2.978	2.913
	.01	10.044	7.559	6.552	5.994	5.636	5.386	5.200	5.057	4.942	4.849	4.706
	.001	21.040	14.905	12.553	11.283	10.481	9.926	9.517	9.204	8.956	8.754	8.445
12	**.5**	0.484	0.735	0.835	0.888	0.921	0.943	0.959	0.972	0.981	0.989	1.000
	.05	4.747	3.885	3.490	3.259	3.106	2.996	2.913	2.849	2.796	2.753	2.687
	.01	9.330	6.927	5.953	5.412	5.064	4.821	4.640	4.499	4.388	4.296	4.155
	.001	18.643	12.974	10.804	9.633	8.892	8.379	8.001	7.710	7.480	7.292	7.005
14	**.5**	0.479	0.729	0.828	0.881	0.914	0.936	0.952	0.964	0.973	0.981	0.992
	.05	4.600	3.739	3.344	3.112	2.958	2.848	2.764	2.699	2.646	2.602	2.534
	.01	8.862	6.515	5.564	5.035	4.695	4.456	4.278	4.140	4.030	3.939	3.800
	.001	17.143	11.779	9.729	8.622	7.922	7.436	7.077	6.802	6.583	6.404	6.130
16	**.5**	0.476	0.724	0.823	0.876	0.908	0.930	0.946	0.958	0.967	0.975	0.986
	.05	4.494	3.634	3.239	3.007	2.852	2.741	2.657	2.591	2.538	2.494	2.425
	.01	8.531	6.226	5.292	4.773	4.437	4.202	4.026	3.890	3.780	3.691	3.553
	.001	16.120	10.971	9.006	7.944	7.272	6.805	6.460	6.195	5.984	5.812	5.547
18	**.5**	0.474	0.721	0.819	0.872	0.904	0.926	0.941	0.953	0.962	0.970	0.981
	.05	4.414	3.555	3.160	2.928	2.773	2.661	2.577	2.510	2.456	2.412	2.342
	.01	8.285	6.013	5.092	4.579	4.248	4.015	3.841	3.705	3.597	3.508	3.371
	.001	15.379	10.390	8.488	7.459	6.808	6.355	6.021	5.763	5.558	5.390	5.132

Appendix B.1. *contd.)*

df_{denom}	*P*	df_{num} 1	2	3	4	5	6	7	8	9	10	12
20	**.5**	0.472	0.718	0.816	0.868	0.900	0.922	0.938	0.950	0.959	0.966	0.977
	.05	4.351	3.493	3.098	2.866	2.711	2.599	2.514	2.447	2.393	2.348	2.278
	.01	8.096	5.849	4.938	4.431	4.103	3.871	3.699	3.564	3.457	3.368	3.231
	.001	14.819	9.953	8.098	7.096	6.461	6.019	5.692	5.440	5.239	5.075	4.823
22	**.5**	0.470	0.715	0.814	0.866	0.898	0.919	0.935	0.947	0.956	0.963	0.974
	.05	4.301	3.443	3.049	2.817	2.661	2.549	2.464	2.397	2.342	2.297	2.226
	.01	7.945	5.719	4.817	4.313	3.988	3.758	3.587	3.453	3.346	3.258	3.121
	.001	14.380	9.612	7.796	6.814	6.191	5.758	5.438	5.190	4.993	4.832	4.583
24	**.5**	0.469	0.714	0.812	0.863	0.895	0.917	0.932	0.944	0.953	0.961	0.972
	.05	4.260	3.403	3.009	2.776	2.621	2.508	2.423	2.355	2.300	2.255	2.183
	.01	7.823	5.614	4.718	4.218	3.895	3.667	3.496	3.363	3.256	3.168	3.032
	.001	14.028	9.339	7.554	6.589	5.977	5.550	5.235	4.991	4.797	4.638	4.393
26	**.5**	0.468	0.712	0.810	0.861	0.893	0.915	0.930	0.942	0.951	0.959	0.970
	.05	4.225	3.369	2.975	2.743	2.587	2.474	2.388	2.321	2.265	2.220	2.148
	.01	7.721	5.526	4.637	4.140	3.818	3.591	3.421	3.288	3.182	3.094	2.958
	.001	13.739	9.116	7.357	6.406	5.802	5.381	5.070	4.829	4.637	4.480	4.238
28	**.5**	0.467	0.711	0.808	0.860	0.892	0.913	0.929	0.940	0.950	0.957	0.968
	.05	4.196	3.340	2.947	2.714	2.558	2.445	2.359	2.291	2.236	2.190	2.118
	.01	7.636	5.453	4.568	4.074	3.754	3.528	3.358	3.226	3.120	3.032	2.896
	.001	13.498	8.931	7.193	6.253	5.657	5.241	4.933	4.695	4.505	4.349	4.109
30	**.5**	0.466	0.709	0.807	0.858	0.890	0.912	0.927	0.939	0.948	0.955	0.966
	.05	4.171	3.316	2.922	2.690	2.534	2.421	2.334	2.266	2.211	2.165	2.092
	.01	7.562	5.390	4.510	4.018	3.699	3.473	3.305	3.173	3.067	2.979	2.843
	.001	13.293	8.773	7.054	6.125	5.534	5.122	4.817	4.581	4.393	4.239	4.001
40	**.5**	0.463	0.705	0.802	0.854	0.885	0.907	0.922	0.934	0.943	0.950	0.961
	.05	4.085	3.232	2.839	2.606	2.449	2.336	2.249	2.180	2.124	2.077	2.003
	.01	7.314	5.179	4.313	3.828	3.514	3.291	3.124	2.993	2.888	2.801	2.665
	.001	12.609	8.251	6.595	5.698	5.128	4.731	4.436	4.207	4.024	3.874	3.642

60	**.5**	0.461	0.701	0.798	0.849	0.880	0.901	0.917	0.928	0.937	0.945	0.956
	.05	4.001	3.150	2.758	2.525	2.368	2.254	2.167	2.097	2.040	1.993	1.917
	.01	7.077	4.977	4.126	3.649	3.339	3.119	2.953	2.823	2.718	2.632	2.496
	.001	11.973	7.768	6.171	5.307	4.757	4.372	4.086	3.865	3.687	3.541	3.315
120	**.5**	0.458	0.697	0.793	0.844	0.875	0.896	0.912	0.923	0.932	0.939	0.950
	.05	3.920	3.072	2.680	2.447	2.290	2.175	2.087	2.016	1.959	1.910	1.834
	.01	6.851	4.787	3.949	3.480	3.174	2.956	2.792	2.663	2.559	2.472	2.336
	.001	11.380	7.321	5.781	4.947	4.416	4.044	3.767	3.552	3.379	3.237	3.016
1000	**.5**	0.455	0.694	0.789	0.840	0.871	0.892	0.907	0.919	0.928	0.935	0.946
	.05	3.851	3.005	2.614	2.381	2.223	2.108	2.019	1.948	1.889	1.840	1.762
	.01	6.660	4.626	3.801	3.338	3.035	2.820	2.657	2.529	2.425	2.339	2.202
	.001	10.892	6.956	5.464	4.655	4.139	3.778	3.508	3.299	3.130	2.991	2.774

						df_{num}						
df_{denom}	P	**14**	**16**	**18**	**20**	**25**	**30**	**40**	**50**	**80**	**120**	**1000**
1	**.5**	2.086	2.100	2.110	2.119	2.135	2.145	2.158	2.166	2.178	2.185	2.196
	.05	245.36	246.46	247.32	248.01	249.25	250.09	251.14	251.77	252.72	253.25	254.12
	.01	6142.6	6170.0	6191.4	6208.7	6239.7	6260.6	6286.7	6302.4	6326.2	6339.3	6361.0
	.001	614316.	617057.	619201.	620922.	624031.	626114.	628725.	630301.	632671.	633963.	636164.
2	**.5**	1.372	1.381	1.388	1.393	1.403	1.410	1.418	1.423	1.430	1.434	1.442
	.05	19.424	19.433	19.440	19.446	19.456	19.462	19.470	19.475	19.483	19.487	19.495
	.01	99.428	99.436	99.443	99.449	99.458	99.464	99.471	99.479	99.487	99.491	99.496
	.001	999.44	999.45	999.45	999.46	999.47	999.47	999.48	999.49	999.50	999.50	999.46
3	**.5**	1.207	1.215	1.220	1.225	1.234	1.239	1.246	1.251	1.257	1.261	1.267
	.05	8.715	8.692	8.675	8.660	8.634	8.617	8.594	8.581	8.561	8.549	8.529
	.01	26.924	26.827	26.751	26.690	26.579	26.505	26.411	26.355	26.269	26.221	26.134
	.001	127.64	127.13	126.73	126.42	125.83	125.45	124.96	124.66	124.22	123.97	123.52
4	**.5**	1.135	1.142	1.147	1.152	1.160	1.165	1.172	1.176	1.182	1.185	1.191
	.05	5.873	5.844	5.821	5.803	5.769	5.746	5.717	5.699	5.673	5.658	5.632
	.01	14.249	14.153	14.080	14.020	13.911	13.838	13.745	13.690	13.606	13.558	13.474
	.001	46.948	46.597	46.322	46.101	45.699	45.429	45.089	44.884	44.573	44.400	44.092

Appendix B.1. *contd.*)

df_{denom}	*P*	df_{num} 14	16	18	20	25	30	40	50	80	120	1000
5	**.5**	1.094	1.101	1.106	1.111	1.118	1.123	1.130	1.134	1.139	1.143	1.148
	.05	4.636	4.604	4.579	4.558	4.521	4.496	4.464	4.444	4.415	4.398	4.369
	.01	9.770	9.680	9.610	9.553	9.449	9.379	9.291	9.238	9.157	9.112	9.031
	.001	26.057	25.783	25.568	25.395	25.080	24.869	24.602	24.441	24.197	24.061	23.816
6	**.5**	1.069	1.075	1.080	1.084	1.092	1.097	1.103	1.107	1.112	1.116	1.121
	.05	3.956	3.922	3.896	3.874	3.835	3.808	3.774	3.754	3.722	3.705	3.673
	.01	7.605	7.519	7.451	7.396	7.296	7.229	7.143	7.091	7.013	6.969	6.890
	.001	17.683	17.450	17.267	17.120	16.853	16.673	16.445	16.307	16.098	15.981	15.773
7	**.5**	1.051	1.057	1.062	1.066	1.074	1.079	1.085	1.088	1.094	1.097	1.102
	.05	3.529	3.494	3.467	3.445	3.404	3.376	3.340	3.319	3.286	3.267	3.234
	.01	6.359	6.275	6.209	6.155	6.058	5.992	5.908	5.858	5.781	5.737	5.660
	.001	13.434	13.227	13.063	12.932	12.692	12.530	12.326	12.202	12.014	11.909	11.721
8	**.5**	1.038	1.044	1.049	1.053	1.060	1.065	1.071	1.075	1.080	1.083	1.089
	.05	3.237	3.202	3.173	3.150	3.108	3.079	3.043	3.020	2.986	2.967	2.932
	.01	5.559	5.477	5.412	5.359	5.263	5.198	5.116	5.065	4.989	4.946	4.869
	.001	10.943	10.752	10.601	10.480	10.258	10.109	9.919	9.804	9.630	9.532	9.358
9	**.5**	1.028	1.034	1.039	1.043	1.050	1.055	1.061	1.064	1.070	1.073	1.078
	.05	3.025	2.989	2.960	2.936	2.893	2.864	2.826	2.803	2.768	2.748	2.712
	.01	5.005	4.924	4.860	4.808	4.713	4.649	4.567	4.517	4.441	4.398	4.321
	.001	9.334	9.154	9.012	8.898	8.689	8.548	8.369	8.260	8.094	8.001	7.836
10	**.5**	1.020	1.026	1.031	1.035	1.042	1.047	1.053	1.056	1.062	1.064	1.070
	.05	2.865	2.828	2.798	2.774	2.730	2.700	2.661	2.637	2.601	2.580	2.543
	.01	4.601	4.520	4.457	4.405	4.311	4.247	4.165	4.115	4.039	3.996	3.919
	.001	8.220	8.048	7.913	7.804	7.604	7.469	7.297	7.193	7.034	6.944	6.784
12	**.5**	1.008	1.014	1.019	1.023	1.030	1.035	1.041	1.044	1.049	1.052	1.057
	.05	2.637	2.599	2.568	2.544	2.498	2.466	2.426	2.401	2.363	2.341	2.302
	.01	4.052	3.972	3.909	3.858	3.765	3.701	3.619	3.569	3.493	3.449	3.371
	.001	6.794	6.634	6.507	6.405	6.217	6.090	5.928	5.829	5.678	5.593	5.440

14	**.5**	1.000	1.006	1.011	1.015	1.022	1.026	1.032	1.036	1.041	1.044	1.049
	.05	2.484	2.445	2.413	2.388	2.341	2.308	2.266	2.241	2.201	2.178	2.136
	.01	3.698	3.619	3.556	3.505	3.412	3.348	3.266	3.215	3.138	3.094	3.015
	.001	5.930	5.776	5.655	5.557	5.377	5.254	5.098	5.002	4.856	4.773	4.625
16	**.5**	0.994	1.000	1.005	1.009	1.015	1.020	1.026	1.029	1.034	1.037	1.042
	.05	2.373	2.334	2.302	2.276	2.227	2.194	2.151	2.124	2.083	2.059	2.016
	.01	3.451	3.372	3.310	3.259	3.165	3.101	3.018	2.968	2.889	2.845	2.764
	.001	5.353	5.205	5.087	4.992	4.817	4.697	4.545	4.451	4.308	4.226	4.080
18	**.5**	0.989	0.995	1.000	1.004	1.011	1.015	1.021	1.024	1.030	1.032	1.037
	.05	2.290	2.250	2.217	2.191	2.141	2.107	2.063	2.035	1.993	1.968	1.923
	.01	3.269	3.190	3.128	3.077	2.983	2.919	2.835	2.784	2.705	2.660	2.577
	.001	4.943	4.798	4.683	4.590	4.418	4.301	4.151	4.058	3.917	3.836	3.690
20	**.5**	0.985	0.992	0.996	1.000	1.007	1.011	1.017	1.020	1.026	1.029	1.034
	.05	2.225	2.184	2.151	2.124	2.074	2.039	1.994	1.966	1.922	1.896	1.850
	.01	3.130	3.051	2.989	2.938	2.843	2.778	2.695	2.643	2.563	2.517	2.433
	.001	4.637	4.495	4.382	4.290	4.121	4.005	3.856	3.765	3.624	3.544	3.398
22	**.5**	0.982	0.988	0.993	0.997	1.004	1.008	1.014	1.017	1.022	1.025	1.030
	.05	2.173	2.131	2.098	2.071	2.020	1.984	1.938	1.909	1.864	1.838	1.790
	.01	3.019	2.941	2.879	2.827	2.733	2.667	2.583	2.531	2.450	2.403	2.317
	.001	4.401	4.260	4.149	4.058	3.891	3.776	3.629	3.538	3.397	3.317	3.171
24	**.5**	0.980	0.986	0.991	0.994	1.001	1.006	1.011	1.015	1.020	1.023	1.028
	.05	2.130	2.088	2.054	2.027	1.975	1.939	1.892	1.863	1.816	1.790	1.740
	.01	2.930	2.852	2.789	2.738	2.643	2.577	2.492	2.440	2.357	2.310	2.223
	.001	4.212	4.074	3.963	3.873	3.707	3.593	3.447	3.356	3.216	3.136	2.989
26	**.5**	0.978	0.984	0.988	0.992	0.999	1.003	1.009	1.013	1.018	1.020	1.025
	.05	2.094	2.052	2.018	1.990	1.938	1.901	1.853	1.823	1.776	1.749	1.698
	.01	2.857	2.778	2.715	2.664	2.569	2.503	2.417	2.364	2.281	2.233	2.144
	.001	4.059	3.921	3.812	3.723	3.558	3.445	3.299	3.208	3.068	2.988	2.840
28	**.5**	0.976	0.982	0.987	0.990	0.997	1.002	1.007	1.011	1.016	1.019	1.024
	.05	2.064	2.021	1.987	1.959	1.906	1.869	1.820	1.790	1.742	1.714	1.662
	.01	2.795	2.716	2.653	2.602	2.506	2.440	2.354	2.300	2.216	2.167	2.077
	.001	3.932	3.795	3.687	3.598	3.434	3.321	3.176	3.085	2.945	2.864	2.716

Appendix B.1. *contd.)*

df_{denom}	*P*	14	16	18	20	25	df_{num} 30	40	50	80	120	1000
30	**.5**	0.974	0.980	0.985	0.989	0.996	1.000	1.006	1.009	1.014	1.017	1.022
	.05	2.037	1.995	1.960	1.932	1.878	1.841	1.792	1.761	1.712	1.683	1.630
	.01	2.742	2.663	2.600	2.549	2.453	2.386	2.299	2.245	2.160	2.111	2.019
	.001	3.825	3.689	3.581	3.493	3.330	3.217	3.072	2.981	2.841	2.760	2.610
40	**.5**	0.969	0.975	0.980	0.983	0.990	0.994	1.000	1.003	1.008	1.011	1.016
	.05	1.948	1.904	1.868	1.839	1.783	1.744	1.693	1.660	1.608	1.577	1.517
	.01	2.563	2.484	2.421	2.369	2.271	2.203	2.114	2.058	1.969	1.917	1.819
	.001	3.471	3.338	3.232	3.145	2.984	2.872	2.727	2.636	2.493	2.410	2.255
60	**.5**	0.964	0.969	0.974	0.978	0.984	0.989	0.994	0.998	1.003	1.006	1.011
	.05	1.860	1.815	1.778	1.748	1.690	1.649	1.594	1.559	1.502	1.467	1.399
	.01	2.394	2.315	2.251	2.198	2.098	2.028	1.936	1.877	1.783	1.726	1.617
	.001	3.147	3.017	2.912	2.827	2.667	2.555	2.409	2.316	2.169	2.082	1.915
120	**.5**	0.958	0.964	0.969	0.972	0.979	0.983	0.989	0.992	0.997	1.000	1.005
	.05	1.775	1.728	1.690	1.659	1.598	1.554	1.495	1.457	1.392	1.352	1.267
	.01	2.234	2.154	2.089	2.035	1.932	1.860	1.763	1.700	1.597	1.533	1.401
	.001	2.851	2.723	2.620	2.534	2.375	2.262	2.113	2.017	1.862	1.767	1.574
1000	**.5**	0.954	0.959	0.964	0.968	0.974	0.979	0.984	0.987	0.992	0.995	1.000
	.05	1.702	1.654	1.614	1.581	1.517	1.471	1.406	1.363	1.289	1.239	1.110
	.01	2.099	2.018	1.952	1.897	1.791	1.716	1.613	1.544	1.428	1.351	1.159
	.001	2.611	2.484	2.382	2.297	2.136	2.022	1.868	1.767	1.597	1.487	1.216

Appendix B.2. Critical values of Hartley's F_{max} at $P = 0.05$.

When calculated F_{max} < critical $F_{max(a,n-1)}$ the variances are homogenous, where n is the group size and a is the number of groups

	a										
***n*-1**	**2**	**3**	**4**	**5**	**6**	**7**	**8**	**9**	**10**	**11**	**12**
2	39.0	87.5	142.	202.	266.	333.	403.	475.	550.	626.	704.
3	15.4	27.8	39.2	50.7	62.0	72.9	83.5	93.9	104.	114.	124.
4	9.60	15.5	20.6	25.2	29.5	33.6	37.5	41.1	44.6	48.0	51.4
5	7.15	10.8	13.7	16.3	18.7	20.8	22.9	24.7	26.5	28.2	29.9
6	5.82	8.38	10.4	12.1	13.7	15.0	16.3	17.5	18.6	19.7	20.7
7	4.99	6.94	8.44	9.70	10.8	11.8	12.7	13.5	14.3	15.1	15.8
8	4.43	6.0	7.18	8.12	9.03	9.78	10.5	11.1	11.7	12.2	12.7
9	4.03	5.34	6.31	7.11	7.80	8.41	8.95	9.45	9.91	10.3	10.7
10	3.72	4.85	5.67	6.34	6.92	7.42	7.87	8.28	8.66	9.01	9.34
12	3.28	4.16	4.79	5.30	5.72	6.09	6.42	6.72	7.00	7.25	7.48
15	2.86	3.54	4.01	4.37	4.68	4.95	5.19	5.40	5.59	5.77	5.93
20	2.46	2.95	3.29	3.54	3.76	3.94	4.10	4.24	4.37	4.49	4.59
30	2.07	2.40	2.61	2.78	2.91	3.02	3.12	3.21	3.29	3.36	3.39
60	1.67	1.85	1.96	2.04	2.11	2.17	2.22	2.26	2.30	2.33	2.36
∞	1.00	1.00	1.00	1.00	1.00	1.00	1.00	1.00	1.00	1.00	1.00

Extracted with permission from David, H.A. (1952). *Biometrika* **39**, 422–4

Appendix B.3. Critical values[a] of Cochran's C at $P = 0.05$

When the calculated $C < C_{(a,n-1)}$ the variances are homogeneous

	a														
***n*-1**	**2**	**3**	**4**	**5**	**6**	**7**	**8**	**9**	**10**	**15**	**20**	**30**	**40**	**60**	**120**
1	0.999	0.967	0.907	0.841	0.781	0.727	0.680	0.639	0.602	0.471	0.389	0.293	0.237	0.174	0.010
2	0.975	0.871	0.768	0.684	0.616	0.561	0.516	0.478	0.445	0.335	0.271	0.198	0.158	0.113	0.063
3	0.939	0.798	0.684	0.598	0.532	0.480	0.437	0.403	0.373	0.276	0.221	0.159	0.126	0.090	0.050
4	0.906	0.746	0.629	0.544	0.480	0.431	0.391	0.358	0.331	0.242	0.192	0.138	0.108	0.077	0.042
5	0.877	0.707	0.590	0.507	0.445	0.397	0.360	0.329	0.303	0.220	0.174	0.124	0.097	0.068	0.037
6	0.853	0.677	0.560	0.478	0.418	0.373	0.336	0.307	0.282	0.203	0.160	0.114	0.089	0.062	0.034
7	0.833	0.653	0.537	0.456	0.398	0.354	0.319	0.290	0.267	0.191	0.150	0.106	0.083	0.058	0.031
8	0.816	0.633	0.518	0.439	0.382	0.338	0.304	0.277	0.254	0.182	0.142	0.100	0.078	0.055	0.029
9	0.801	0.617	0.502	0.424	0.368	0.326	0.293	0.266	0.244	0.174	0.136	0.096	0.075	0.052	0.028
10	0.788	0.603	0.488	0.412	0.357	0.315	0.283	0.257	0.235	0.167	0.130	0.092	0.071	0.050	0.027
16	0.734	0.547	0.437	0.365	0.314	0.276	0.246	0.223	0.203	0.143	0.111	0.077	0.060	0.041	0.022
36	0.660	0.475	0.372	0.307	0.261	0.228	0.202	0.182	0.166	0.114	0.088	0.060	0.046	0.032	0.017
144	0.581	0.403	0.309	0.251	0.212	0.183	0.162	0.145	0.131	0.089	0.068	0.046	0.035	0.023	0.012
∞	0.500	0.333	0.250	0.200	0.167	0.143	0.125	0.111	0.100	0.067	0.050	0.033	0.025	0.017	0.008

[a] Extracted with permission from a longer table from Eisenhart, C., Hastay, M. W., and Wallis, W. A. (1947). *Selected techniques of statistical analysis for scientific and industrial research and production and management engineering*. McGraw-Hill, New York

Appendix B.4. Critical[a] values for the correlation test for normality at $P = 0.05$

When the correlation between the normal scores and the residuals > critical value the residuals are normally distributed. N is the number of residuals

N	Critical value
4	0.873
6	0.892
8	0.907
10	0.918
12	0.927
14	0.934
16	0.940
18	0.945
20	0.950
22	0.953
24	0.956
26	0.959
28	0.961
30	0.964
35	0.968
40	0.972
45	0.974
50	0.976
55	0.978
60	0.980
65	0.982
70	0.983
75	0.984
100	0.988
125	0.990
150	0.991

[a] Calculated from a shorter table from the *Minitab* reference manual Release 7 (1989), Minitab Incorporated, State College

Appendix B.5. Critical values[a] and formulae used for testing outliers by Dixon's test

The formula is selected according to the group size (n) to which the outlier to be tested belongs. When $r_n >$ critical value the outlier is significantly different from the other values in the group. Critical values at $P = 0.1$, 0.05, and 0.01 are provided

	P			
n	**0.10**	**0.05**	**0.01**	**Formula**
3	0.886	0.941	0.988	
4	0.679	0.765	0.889	
5	0.557	0.642	0.780	$r_{10} = \frac{x_2 - x_1}{x_n - x_1}$
6	0.482	0.560	0.698	
7	0.434	0.507	0.637	
8	0.479	0.554	0.683	
9	0.441	0.512	0.635	$r_{11} = \frac{x_2 - x_1}{x_{n-1} - x_1}$
10	0.409	0.477	0.597	
11	0.517	0.576	0.679	
12	0.490	0.546	0.642	$r_{21} = \frac{x_3 - x_1}{x_{n-1} - x_1}$
13	0.467	0.521	0.615	
14	0.492	0.546	0.641	
15	0.472	0.525	0.616	
16	0.454	0.507	0.595	
17	0.438	0.490	0.577	
18	0.424	0.475	0.561	
19	0.412	0.462	0.547	$r_{22} = \frac{x_3 - x_1}{x_{n-2} - x_1}$
20	0.401	0.450	0.535	
21	0.391	0.440	0.524	
22	0.382	0.430	0.514	
23	0.374	0.421	0.505	
24	0.367	0.413	0.497	
25	0.360	0.406	0.489	

[a] Modified slightly from Rohlf, F. J. and Sokal, R. R. (1981). *Statistical tables*, W. H. Freeman, San Francisco; printed with permission

Appendix B.6. Critical values for the two-tailed Student's *t*-distribution

All the values were calculated with *Minitab* release 7.1 for $P = 0.9, 0.5, 0.3, 0.1, 0.05, 0.01$, and 0.001 at df degrees of freedom

	P						
df	**0.9**	**0.5**	**0.3**	**0.1**	**0.05**	**0.01**	**0.001**
1	0.158	1.000	1.963	6.314	12.70	63.65	636.6
2	0.142	0.816	1.386	2.920	4.303	9.925	31.59
3	0.137	0.765	1.250	2.353	3.182	5.841	12.92
4	0.134	0.741	1.190	2.132	2.776	4.604	8.610
5	0.132	0.727	1.156	2.015	2.571	4.032	6.869
6	0.131	0.718	1.134	1.943	2.447	3.707	5.959
7	0.130	0.711	1.119	1.895	2.365	3.499	5.408
8	0.130	0.706	1.108	1.860	2.306	3.355	5.041
9	0.129	0.703	1.100	1.833	2.262	3.250	4.781
10	0.129	0.700	1.093	1.812	2.228	3.169	4.587
11	0.129	0.697	1.088	1.796	2.201	3.106	4.437
12	0.128	0.695	1.083	1.782	2.179	3.055	4.318
13	0.128	0.694	1.079	1.771	2.160	3.012	4.221
14	0.128	0.692	1.076	1.761	2.145	2.977	4.140
15	0.128	0.691	1.074	1.753	2.131	2.947	4.073
16	0.128	0.690	1.071	1.746	2.120	2.921	4.015
17	0.128	0.689	1.069	1.740	2.110	2.898	3.965
18	0.127	0.688	1.067	1.734	2.101	2.878	3.922
19	0.127	0.688	1.066	1.729	2.093	2.861	3.883
20	0.127	0.687	1.064	1.725	2.086	2.845	3.850
21	0.127	0.686	1.063	1.721	2.080	2.831	3.819
22	0.127	0.686	1.061	1.717	2.074	2.819	3.792
23	0.127	0.685	1.060	1.714	2.069	2.807	3.768
24	0.127	0.685	1.059	1.711	2.064	2.797	3.745
25	0.127	0.684	1.058	1.708	2.060	2.787	3.725
26	0.127	0.684	1.058	1.706	2.056	2.779	3.707
27	0.127	0.684	1.057	1.703	2.052	2.771	3.690
28	0.127	0.683	1.056	1.701	2.048	2.763	3.674
29	0.127	0.683	1.055	1.699	2.045	2.756	3.659
30	0.127	0.683	1.055	1.697	2.042	2.750	3.646
35	0.127	0.682	1.052	1.690	2.030	2.724	3.591
40	0.126	0.681	1.050	1.684	2.021	2.704	3.551
45	0.126	0.680	1.049	1.679	2.014	2.690	3.520
50	0.126	0.679	1.047	1.676	2.009	2.678	3.496
75	0.126	0.678	1.044	1.665	1.992	2.643	3.425
100	0.126	0.677	1.042	1.660	1.984	2.626	3.391
150	0.126	0.676	1.040	1.655	1.976	2.609	3.357
200	0.126	0.676	1.039	1.653	1.972	2.601	3.340
1000	0.126	0.675	1.037	1.646	1.962	2.581	3.300
∞	0.126	0.674	1.036	1.644	1.960	2.576	3.291

Appendix B.7. Critical values[a] for the studentized range statistic at $P = 0.05$

The values are tabulated for *a* groups at df degrees of freedom; for the multiple range tests df is normally df_{error}

	a								
df	**2**	**3**	**4**	**5**	**6**	**7**	**8**	**9**	**10**
1	17.97	26.98	32.82	37.08	40.41	43.12	45.40	47.36	49.07
2	6.085	8.331	9.798	10.88	11.75	12.44	13.03	13.54	13.99
3	4.501	5.910	6.825	7.502	8.037	8.478	8.853	9.177	9.462
4	3.927	5.040	5.757	6.287	6.707	7.053	7.347	7.602	7.826
5	3.635	4.602	5.218	5.673	6.033	6.330	6.582	6.802	6.995
6	3.461	4.339	4.896	5.305	5.628	5.895	6.122	6.319	6.493
7	3.344	4.165	4.681	5.060	5.359	5.606	5.815	5.998	6.158
8	3.261	4.041	4.529	4.886	5.167	5.399	5.597	5.767	5.918
9	3.199	3.949	4.415	4.756	5.024	5.244	5.432	5.595	5.739
10	3.151	3.877	4.327	4.654	4.912	5.124	5.305	5.461	5.599
11	3.113	3.820	4.256	4.574	4.823	5.028	5.202	5.353	5.487
12	3.082	3.773	4.199	4.508	4.751	4.950	5.119	5.265	5.395
13	3.055	3.735	4.151	4.453	4.690	4.885	5.049	5.192	5.318
14	3.033	3.702	4.111	4.407	4.639	4.829	4.990	5.131	5.254
15	3.014	3.674	4.076	4.367	4.595	4.782	4.940	5.077	5.198
16	2.998	3.649	4.046	4.333	4.557	4.741	4.897	5.031	5.150
17	2.984	3.628	4.020	4.303	4.524	4.705	4.858	4.991	5.108
18	2.971	3.609	3.997	4.277	4.495	4.673	4.824	4.956	5.071
19	2.960	3.593	3.977	4.253	4.469	4.645	4.794	4.924	5.038
20	2.950	3.578	3.958	4.232	4.445	4.620	4.768	4.896	5.008
24	2.919	3.532	3.901	4.166	4.373	4.541	4.684	4.807	4.915
30	2.888	3.486	3.845	4.102	4.302	4.464	4.602	4.720	4.824
40	2.858	3.442	3.791	4.039	4.232	4.389	4.521	4.635	4.735
60	2.829	3.399	3.737	3.977	4.163	4.314	4.441	4.550	4.646
120	2.800	3.356	3.685	3.917	4.096	4.241	4.363	4.468	4.560
∞	2.772	3.314	3.633	3.858	4.030	4.170	4.286	4.387	4.474

	a								
df	**11**	**12**	**13**	**14**	**15**	**16**	**17**	**18**	**19**
1	50.59	51.96	53.20	54.33	55.36	56.32	57.22	58.04	58.83
2	14.39	14.75	15.08	15.38	15.65	15.91	16.14	16.37	16.57
3	9.717	9.946	10.15	10.35	10.53	10.69	10.84	10.98	11.11
4	8.027	8.208	8.373	8.525	8.664	8.794	8.914	9.028	9.134
5	7.168	7.324	7.466	7.596	7.717	7.828	7.932	8.030	8.122
6	6.649	6.789	6.917	7.034	7.143	7.244	7.338	7.426	7.508
7	6.302	6.431	6.550	6.658	6.759	6.852	6.939	7.020	7.097
8	6.054	6.175	6.287	6.389	6.483	6.571	6.653	6.729	6.802
9	5.867	5.983	6.089	6.186	6.276	6.359	6.437	6.510	6.579
10	5.722	5.833	5.935	6.028	6.114	6.194	6.269	6.339	6.405

Appendix B.7. (*contd.*)

df	*a* 11	12	13	14	15	16	17	18	19
11	5.605	5.713	5.811	5.901	5.984	6.062	6.134	6.202	6.265
12	5.511	5.615	5.710	5.798	5.878	5.953	6.023	6.089	6.151
13	5.431	5.533	5.625	5.711	5.789	5.862	5.931	5.995	6.055
14	5.364	5.463	5.554	5.637	5.714	5.786	5.852	5.915	5.974
15	5.306	5.404	5.493	5.574	5.649	5.720	5.785	5.846	5.904
16	5.256	5.352	5.439	5.520	5.593	5.662	5.727	5.786	5.843
17	5.212	5.307	5.392	5.471	5.544	5.612	5.675	5.734	5.790
18	5.174	5.267	5.352	5.429	5.501	5.568	5.630	5.688	5.743
19	5.140	5.231	5.315	5.391	5.462	5.528	5.589	5.647	5.701
20	5.108	5.199	5.282	5.357	5.427	5.493	5.553	5.610	5.663
24	5.012	5.099	5.179	5.251	5.319	5.381	5.439	5.494	5.545
30	4.917	5.001	5.077	5.147	5.211	5.271	5.327	5.379	5.429
40	4.824	4.904	4.977	5.044	5.106	5.163	5.216	5.266	5.313
60	4.732	4.808	4.878	4.942	5.001	5.056	5.107	5.154	5.199
120	4.641	4.714	4.781	4.842	4.898	4.950	4.998	5.044	5.086
∞	4.552	4.622	4.685	4.743	4.796	4.845	4.891	4.934	4.974

df	*a* 20	22	24	26	28	30	32	34	36
1	59.56	60.91	62.12	63.22	64.23	65.15	66.01	66.81	67.56
2	16.77	17.13	17.45	17.75	18.02	18.27	18.50	18.72	18.92
3	11.24	11.47	11.68	11.87	12.05	12.21	12.36	12.50	12.63
4	9.233	9.418	9.584	9.736	9.875	10.00	10.12	10.23	10.34
5	8.208	8.368	8.512	8.643	8.764	8.875	8.979	9.075	9.165
6	7.587	7.730	7.861	7.979	8.088	8.189	8.283	8.370	8.452
7	7.170	7.303	7.423	7.533	7.634	7.728	7.814	7.895	7.972
8	6.870	6.995	7.109	7.212	7.307	7.395	7.477	7.554	7.625
9	6.644	6.763	6.871	6.970	7.061	7.145	7.222	7.295	7.363
10	6.467	6.582	6.686	6.781	6.868	6.948	7.023	7.093	7.159
11	6.326	6.436	6.536	6.628	6.712	6.790	6.863	6.930	6.994
12	6.209	6.317	6.414	6.503	6.585	6.660	6.731	6.796	6.858
13	6.112	6.217	6.312	6.398	6.478	6.551	6.620	6.684	6.744
14	6.029	6.132	6.224	6.309	6.387	6.459	6.526	6.588	6.647
15	5.958	6.059	6.149	6.233	6.309	6.379	6.445	6.506	6.564
16	5.897	5.995	6.084	6.166	6.241	6.310	6.374	6.434	6.491
17	5.842	5.940	6.027	6.107	6.181	6.249	6.313	6.372	6.427
18	5.794	5.890	5.977	6.055	6.128	6.195	6.258	6.316	6.371
19	5.752	5.846	5.932	6.009	6.081	6.147	6.209	6.267	6.321
20	5.714	5.807	5.891	5.968	6.039	6.104	6.165	6.222	6.275
24	5.594	5.683	5.764	5.838	5.906	5.968	6.027	6.081	6.132
30	5.475	5.561	5.638	5.709	5.774	5.833	5.889	5.941	5.990
40	5.358	5.439	5.513	5.581	5.642	5.700	5.753	5.803	5.849
60	5.241	5.319	5.389	5.453	5.512	5.566	5.617	5.664	5.708
120	5.126	5.200	5.266	5.327	5.382	5.434	5.481	5.526	5.568
∞	5.012	5.081	5.144	5.201	5.253	5.301	5.346	5.388	5.427

Appendix B.7. *(contd.)*

df	*a* 38	40	50	60	70	80	90	100
1	68.26	68.92	71.73	73.97	75.82	77.40	78.77	79.98
2	19.11	19.28	20.05	20.66	21.16	21.59	21.96	22.29
3	12.75	12.87	13.36	13.76	14.08	14.36	14.61	14.82
4	10.44	10.53	10.93	11.24	11.51	11.73	11.92	12.09
5	9.250	9.330	9.674	9.949	10.18	10.38	10.54	10.69
6	8.529	8.601	8.913	9.163	9.370	9.548	9.702	9.839
7	8.043	8.110	8.400	8.632	8.824	8.989	9.133	9.261
8	7.693	7.756	8.029	8.248	8.430	8.586	8.722	8.843
9	7.428	7.488	7.749	7.958	8.132	8.281	8.410	8.526
10	7.220	7.279	7.529	7.730	7.897	8.041	8.166	8.276
11	7.053	7.110	7.352	7.546	7.708	7.847	7.968	8.075
12	6.916	6.970	7.205	7.394	7.552	7.687	7.804	7.909
13	6.800	6.854	7.083	7.267	7.421	7.552	7.667	7.769
14	6.702	6.754	6.979	7.159	7.309	7.438	7.550	7.650
15	6.618	6.669	6.888	7.065	7.212	7.339	7.449	7.546
16	6.544	6.594	6.810	6.984	7.128	7.252	7.360	7.457
17	6.479	6.529	6.741	6.912	7.054	7.176	7.283	7.377
18	6.422	6.471	6.680	6.848	6.989	7.109	7.213	7.307
19	6.371	6.419	6.626	6.792	6.930	7.048	7.152	7.244
20	6.325	6.373	6.576	6.740	6.877	6.994	7.097	7.187
24	6.181	6.226	6.421	6.579	6.710	6.822	6.920	7.008
30	6.037	6.080	6.267	6.417	6.543	6.650	6.744	6.827
40	5.893	5.934	6.112	6.255	6.375	6.477	6.566	6.645
60	5.750	5.789	5.958	6.093	6.206	6.303	6.387	6.462
120	5.607	5.644	5.802	5.929	6.035	6.126	6.205	6.275
∞	5.463	5.498	5.646	5.764	5.863	5.947	6.020	6.085

[a] Extracted from a larger table from Rohlf, F. J. and Sokal, R. R. (1981). *Statistical Tables*, W. H. Freeman, San Francisco; printed with permission

Appendix B.8. Critical values for the χ^2 distribution

All values were calculated with *Minitab* release 8.2 for $P = 0.9, 0.7, 0.5, 0.3, 0.1, 0.05, 0.01$, and 0.001 at df degrees of freedom

df	*P* 0.9	0.7	0.5	0.3	0.1	0.05	0.01	0.001
1	0.016	0.148	0.455	1.074	2.706	3.841	6.635	10.828
2	0.211	0.713	1.386	2.408	4.605	5.991	9.210	13.816
3	0.584	1.424	2.366	3.665	6.251	7.815	11.345	16.266
4	1.064	2.195	3.357	4.878	7.779	9.488	13.277	18.467
5	1.610	3.000	4.351	6.064	9.236	11.070	15.086	20.515
6	2.204	3.828	5.348	7.231	10.645	12.592	16.812	22.458
7	2.833	4.671	6.346	8.383	12.017	14.067	18.475	24.322

Appendix B.8. (*contd.*)

df	*P* 0.9	0.7	0.5	0.3	0.1	0.05	0.01	0.001
8	3.490	5.527	7.344	9.524	13.362	15.507	20.090	26.125
9	4.168	6.393	8.343	10.656	14.684	16.919	21.666	27.877
10	4.865	7.267	9.342	11.781	15.987	18.307	23.209	29.588
11	5.578	8.148	10.341	12.899	17.275	19.675	24.725	31.264
12	6.304	9.034	11.340	14.011	18.549	21.026	26.217	32.910
13	7.042	9.926	12.340	15.119	19.812	22.362	27.688	34.528
14	7.790	10.821	13.339	16.222	21.064	23.685	29.141	36.124
15	8.547	11.721	14.339	17.322	22.307	24.996	30.578	37.697
16	9.312	12.624	15.339	18.418	23.542	26.296	32.000	39.254
17	10.085	13.531	16.338	19.511	24.769	27.587	33.409	40.789
18	10.865	14.440	17.338	20.601	25.989	28.869	34.805	42.312
19	11.651	15.352	18.338	21.689	27.204	30.143	36.191	43.819
20	12.443	16.266	19.337	22.775	28.412	31.410	37.566	45.315
21	13.240	17.182	20.337	23.858	29.615	32.671	38.932	46.797
22	14.041	18.101	21.337	24.939	30.813	33.924	40.290	48.270
23	14.848	19.021	22.337	26.018	32.007	35.172	41.638	49.726
24	15.659	19.943	23.337	27.096	33.196	36.415	42.980	51.179
25	16.473	20.867	24.337	28.172	34.382	37.653	44.314	52.622
26	17.292	21.792	25.336	29.246	35.563	38.885	45.642	54.054
27	18.114	22.719	26.336	30.319	36.741	40.113	46.963	55.477
28	18.939	23.647	27.336	31.391	37.916	41.337	48.278	56.893
29	19.768	24.577	28.336	32.461	39.087	42.557	49.588	58.303
30	20.599	25.508	29.336	33.530	40.256	43.773	50.892	59.703
31	21.434	26.440	30.336	34.598	41.422	44.985	52.192	61.100
32	22.271	27.373	31.336	35.665	42.585	46.194	53.486	62.486
33	23.110	28.307	32.336	36.731	43.745	47.400	54.775	63.868
34	23.952	29.242	33.336	37.795	44.903	48.602	56.061	65.246
35	24.797	30.178	34.336	38.859	46.059	49.802	57.342	66.622
36	25.643	31.115	35.336	39.922	47.212	50.998	58.619	67.986
37	26.492	32.053	36.336	40.984	48.363	52.192	59.893	69.353
38	27.343	32.992	37.335	42.045	49.513	53.384	61.163	70.709
39	28.196	33.932	38.335	43.105	50.660	54.572	62.429	72.060
40	29.051	34.872	39.335	44.165	51.805	55.759	63.691	73.408
45	33.350	39.585	44.335	49.452	57.505	61.656	69.957	80.078
50	37.689	44.313	49.335	54.723	63.167	67.505	76.154	86.659
55	42.060	49.055	54.335	59.980	68.796	73.312	82.292	93.169
60	46.459	53.809	59.335	65.227	74.397	79.082	88.381	99.621
65	50.883	58.573	64.335	70.462	79.973	84.820	94.420	105.974
70	55.329	63.346	69.334	75.689	85.527	90.531	100.424	112.309
75	59.795	68.127	74.334	80.908	91.061	96.217	106.392	118.595
80	64.278	72.915	79.334	86.120	96.578	101.879	112.328	124.836
85	68.777	77.710	84.334	91.325	102.079	107.522	118.236	131.040
90	73.291	82.511	89.334	96.524	107.565	113.145	124.115	137.194
95	77.818	87.317	94.334	101.717	113.037	118.751	129.970	143.319
100	82.358	92.129	99.334	106.906	118.499	124.343	135.811	149.483
200	174.835	189.049	199.334	209.986	226.022	233.997	249.455	267.620

Appendix B.9. Critical values[a] for correlation coefficients at $P = 0.05$ for $k = 1–7$ predictor variables

When the calculated linear (r; $k = 1$) or multiple (R; $k = 2–7$) correlation coefficient > critical r or R the coefficient is significant; n is the number of data points used to calculate the coefficient

	k						
n	**1**	**2**	**3**	**4**	**5**	**6**	**7**
3	0.997						
4	0.950	0.999					
5	0.878	0.975	0.999				
6	0.811	0.930	0.983	0.999			
7	0.754	0.881	0.950	0.987	1.000		
8	0.707	0.836	0.912	0.961	0.990	1.000	
9	0.666	0.795	0.874	0.930	0.968	0.991	1.000
10	0.632	0.758	0.839	0.898	0.942	0.973	0.993
11	0.602	0.726	0.807	0.867	0.914	0.950	0.977
12	0.576	0.697	0.777	0.838	0.886	0.925	0.956
13	0.553	0.671	0.750	0.811	0.860	0.900	0.934
14	0.532	0.648	0.726	0.786	0.835	0.876	0.911
15	0.514	0.627	0.703	0.763	0.812	0.854	0.889
16	0.497	0.608	0.683	0.741	0.790	0.832	0.868
17	0.482	0.590	0.664	0.722	0.770	0.812	0.848
18	0.468	0.574	0.646	0.703	0.751	0.792	0.829
19	0.456	0.559	0.630	0.686	0.733	0.774	0.811
20	0.444	0.545	0.615	0.670	0.717	0.757	0.793
21	0.433	0.532	0.601	0.655	0.701	0.741	0.777
22	0.423	0.520	0.587	0.641	0.687	0.726	0.762
23	0.413	0.509	0.575	0.628	0.673	0.712	0.747
24	0.404	0.498	0.563	0.615	0.660	0.698	0.733
25	0.396	0.488	0.552	0.604	0.647	0.686	0.720
26	0.388	0.479	0.542	0.593	0.636	0.673	0.707
27	0.381	0.470	0.532	0.582	0.624	0.662	0.696
28	0.374	0.462	0.523	0.572	0.614	0.651	0.684
29	0.367	0.454	0.514	0.562	0.604	0.640	0.673
30	0.361	0.446	0.506	0.553	0.594	0.640	0.663
32	0.349	0.432	0.490	0.536	0.576	0.612	0.643
34	0.339	0.419	0.476	0.521	0.560	0.594	0.626
36	0.329	0.407	0.462	0.507	0.545	0.579	0.609
38	0.320	0.397	0.450	0.494	0.531	0.564	0.594
40	0.312	0.387	0.439	0.482	0.518	0.550	0.580
42	0.304	0.377	0.429	0.470	0.506	0.538	0.566
44	0.279	0.369	0.419	0.460	0.495	0.526	0.554
46	0.291	0.361	0.410	0.450	0.484	0.515	0.542
48	0.285	0.353	0.401	0.441	0.474	0.504	0.531
50	0.297	0.346	0.393	0.432	0.465	0.494	0.521
55	0.266	0.330	0.375	0.412	0.444	0.472	0.498
60	0.254	0.316	0.359	0.395	0.425	0.453	0.477
65	0.244	0.304	0.345	0.380	0.409	0.435	0.459
70	0.235	0.292	0.333	0.366	0.394	0.420	0.443

Appendix B.9. (*contd.*)

	k						
n	**1**	**2**	**3**	**4**	**5**	**6**	**7**
75	0.227	0.283	0.322	0.354	0.381	0.406	0.428
80	0.220	0.274	0.312	0.343	0.369	0.393	0.415
85	0.213	0.265	0.302	0.332	0.359	0.382	0.403
90	0.207	0.258	0.294	0.323	0.349	0.371	0.392
95	0.202	0.251	0.286	0.315	0.339	0.361	0.381
100	0.197	0.245	0.279	0.307	0.331	0.352	0.372
120	0.179	0.223	0.255	0.280	0.302	0.322	0.340
140	0.166	0.207	0.236	0.260	0.280	0.298	0.315
160	0.155	0.194	0.221	0.243	0.262	0.279	0.295
180	0.146	0.182	0.208	0.229	0.247	0.263	0.278
200	0.139	0.173	0.197	0.217	0.235	0.250	0.264

[a] Extracted with permission from Tables 6.2 and 6.6 from Neave, H. R. (1978). *Statistical Tables*, George Allen & Unwin, London

Appendix B.10. Critical values[a] of the Durbin–Watson statistic at $P = 0.05$ for $k = 1$–8 predictor variables

When the calculated Durbin–Watson statistic (DW) $< d_U$ autocorrelation is not significant, when DW $< d_L$ autocorrelation is significant and when DW is between d_L and d_U the result is uncertain; n is the number of residuals

n	$k = 1$		$k = 2$		$k = 3$		$k = 4$		$k = 5$		$k = 6$		$k = 7$		$k = 8$	
	d_L	d_U	d_L	d_U	d_L	d_U	d_L	d_U	d_L	d_U	d_L	d_U	d_L	d_U	d_L	d_U
6	0.610	1.400														
7	0.700	1.356	0.467	1.896												
8	0.763	1.332	0.559	1.777	0.368	2.287										
9	0.824	1.320	0.629	1.699	0.455	2.128	0.296	2.588								
10	0.879	1.320	0.697	1.641	0.525	2.016	0.376	2.414	0.243	2.822						
11	0.927	1.324	0.758	1.604	0.595	1.928	0.444	2.283	0.316	2.645	0.203	3.005				
12	0.971	1.331	0.812	1.579	0.658	1.864	0.512	2.177	0.379	2.506	0.268	2.832	0.171	3.149		
13	0.010	1.340	0.861	1.562	0.715	1.816	0.574	2.094	0.445	2.390	0.328	2.692	0.230	2.985	0.147	3.266
14	1.045	1.350	0.905	1.551	0.767	1.779	0.632	2.030	0.505	2.296	0.389	2.572	0.286	2.848	0.200	3.111
15	1.077	1.361	0.946	1.543	0.814	1.750	0.685	1.977	0.562	2.220	0.447	2.472	0.343	2.727	0.251	2.979
16	1.106	1.371	0.982	1.539	0.857	1.728	0.734	1.935	0.615	2.157	0.502	2.388	0.398	2.624	0.304	2.860
17	1.133	1.381	1.015	1.536	0.897	1.710	0.779	1.900	0.664	2.104	0.554	2.318	0.451	2.537	0.356	2.757
18	1.158	1.391	1.046	1.535	0.933	1.696	0.820	1.872	0.710	2.060	0.603	2.257	0.502	2.461	0.407	2.667
19	1.180	1.401	1.074	1.536	0.967	1.685	0.859	1.848	0.752	2.023	0.649	2.206	0.459	2.396	0.456	2.589
20	1.201	1.411	1.100	1.537	0.998	1.676	0.894	1.828	0.792	1.991	0.692	2.162	0.595	2.339	0.502	2.521
21	1.221	1.420	1.125	1.538	1.026	1.669	0.927	1.812	0.829	1.964	0.732	2.124	0.637	2.290	0.547	2.460
22	1.239	1.429	1.147	1.541	1.053	1.664	0.958	1.797	0.863	1.940	0.769	2.090	0.677	2.246	0.588	2.407
23	1.257	1.437	1.168	1.543	1.078	1.660	0.986	1.785	0.895	1.920	0.804	2.061	0.715	2.208	0.628	2.360
24	1.273	1.446	1.188	1.546	1.101	1.656	1.013	1.775	0.925	1.902	0.837	2.035	0.751	2.174	0.666	2.318
25	1.288	1.454	1.206	1.550	1.123	1.654	1.038	1.767	0.953	1.886	0.868	2.012	0.784	2.144	0.702	2.280
26	1.302	1.461	1.224	1.553	1.143	1.652	1.062	1.759	0.979	1.873	0.897	1.992	0.816	2.117	0.735	2.246
27	1.316	1.469	1.240	1.556	1.162	1.651	1.084	1.753	1.004	1.861	0.925	1.974	0.845	2.093	0.767	2.216

28	1.328	1.476	1.255	1.560	1.181	1.650	1.104	1.747	1.028	1.850	0.951	1.958	0.874	2.071	0.798	2.188
29	1.341	1.483	1.270	1.563	1.198	1.650	1.124	1.743	1.050	1.841	0.975	1.944	0.900	2.052	0.826	2.164
30	1.352	1.489	1.284	1.567	1.214	1.650	1.143	1.739	1.071	1.833	0.998	1.931	0.926	2.034	0.854	2.141
31	1.363	1.496	1.297	1.570	1.229	1.650	1.160	1.735	1.090	1.825	1.020	1.920	0.950	2.018	0.879	2.120
32	1.373	1.502	1.309	1.574	1.244	1.650	1.177	1.732	1.109	1.819	1.041	1.909	0.972	2.004	0.904	2.102
33	1.383	1.508	1.321	1.577	1.258	1.651	1.193	1.730	1.127	1.813	1.061	1.900	0.994	1.991	0.927	2.085
34	1.393	1.514	1.333	1.580	1.271	1.652	1.208	1.728	1.144	1.808	1.080	1.891	1.015	1.979	0.950	2.069
35	1.402	1.519	1.343	1.584	1.283	1.653	1.222	1.726	1.160	1.803	1.097	1.884	1.034	1.967	0.971	2.054
36	1.411	1.525	1.354	1.587	1.295	1.654	1.236	1.724	1.175	1.799	1.114	1.877	1.053	1.957	0.991	2.041
37	1.419	1.530	1.364	1.590	1.307	1.655	1.249	1.723	1.190	1.795	1.131	1.870	1.071	1.948	1.011	2.029
38	1.427	1.535	1.373	1.594	1.318	1.656	1.261	1.722	1.204	1.792	1.146	1.864	1.088	1.939	1.029	2.017
39	1.435	1.540	1.382	1.597	1.328	1.658	1.273	1.722	1.218	1.789	1.161	1.859	1.104	1.932	1.047	2.007
40	1.442	1.544	1.391	1.600	1.338	1.659	1.285	1.721	1.230	1.786	1.175	1.854	1.120	1.924	1.064	1.997
45	1.475	1.566	1.430	1.615	1.383	1.666	1.336	1.720	1.287	1.776	1.238	1.835	1.189	1.895	1.139	1.958
50	1.503	1.585	1.462	1.628	1.421	1.674	1.378	1.721	1.335	1.771	1.291	1.822	1.246	1.875	1.201	1.930
55	1.528	1.601	1.490	1.641	1.452	1.681	1.414	1.724	1.374	1.768	1.334	1.814	1.294	1.861	1.253	1.909
60	1.549	1.616	1.514	1.652	1.480	1.689	1.444	1.727	1.408	1.767	1.372	1.808	1.335	1.850	1.298	1.894
65	1.567	1.629	1.536	1.662	1.503	1.696	1.471	1.731	1.438	1.767	1.404	1.805	1.370	1.843	1.336	1.882
70	1.583	1.641	1.554	1.672	1.525	1.703	1.494	1.735	1.464	1.768	1.433	1.802	1.401	1.837	1.369	1.873
75	1.598	1.652	1.571	1.680	1.543	1.709	1.515	1.739	1.487	1.770	1.458	1.801	1.428	1.834	1.399	1.867
80	1.611	1.662	1.586	1.688	1.560	1.715	1.534	1.743	1.507	1.772	1.480	1.801	1.453	1.831	1.425	1.861
85	1.624	1.671	1.600	1.696	1.575	1.721	1.550	1.747	1.525	1.774	1.500	1.801	1.474	1.829	1.448	1.857
90	1.635	1.679	1.612	1.703	1.589	1.726	1.566	1.751	1.542	1.776	1.518	1.801	1.494	1.827	1.469	1.854
95	1.645	1.687	1.623	1.709	1.602	1.732	1.579	1.755	1.557	1.778	1.535	1.802	1.512	1.827	1.489	1.852
100	1.654	1.694	1.634	1.715	1.613	1.736	1.592	1.758	1.571	1.780	1.550	1.803	1.528	1.826	1.506	1.850
150	1.720	1.746	1.706	1.760	1.693	1.774	1.679	1.788	1.665	1.802	1.651	1.817	1.637	1.832	1.622	1.847
200	1.758	1.778	1.748	1.789	1.738	1.799	1.728	1.810	1.718	1.820	1.707	1.831	1.697	1.841	1.686	1.852

[a] Extracted with permission from a larger table (k = 1–20, P = 0.05 and 0.01) from Savin, N. E. and White, K. J. (1977). *Econometrica* **45,** 1992–5

Appendix B.11. Bonferroni-modified Student's t values at $P = 0.05$

These are used to calculate multiple confidence and prediction intervals for regression, where the number of intervals calculated, c, must be less than the number of constants, p'. The t values provided are for $n - p'$ degrees of freedom, df, with n observations used to calculate the regression equation

	df						
c	**5**	**10**	**15**	**20**	**30**	**40**	**50**
1	2.570 58	2.228 14	2.131 45	2.085 98	2.042 27	2.021 08	2.008 56
2	3.163 38	2.633 77	2.489 88	2.423 12	2.359 57	2.328 93	2.310 93
3	3.534 12	2.870 07	2.693 74	2.612 59	2.535 74	2.498 86	2.477 20
4	3.810 00	3.038 25	2.836 63	2.744 37	2.657 35	2.615 70	2.591 28
5	4.032 15	3.169 28	2.946 72	2.845 34	2.750 00	2.704 46	2.677 80
6	4.219 31	3.276 85	3.036 28	2.927 14	2.824 70	2.775 88	2.747 30
7	4.381 75	3.368 22	3.111 80	2.995 81	2.887 21	2.835 53	2.805 29
8	4.525 72	3.447 72	3.177 10	3.055 02	2.940 91	2.886 67	2.854 98
9	4.655 31	3.518 18	3.234 64	3.107 04	2.987 96	2.931 43	2.898 42
10	4.773 35	3.581 41	3.286 04	3.153 41	3.029 80	2.971 17	2.936 96

Appendix B.12. Multipliers for Scheffé's confidence intervals at $P = 0.05$

These are used to calculate any number of multiple confidence and prediction intervals for regression for k predictor variables and $n - p'$ degrees of freedom, df, with n observations used to calculate the regression equation and p' constants in the equation

	df						
k	**5**	**10**	**15**	**20**	**30**	**40**	**50**
1	3.4018	2.8646	2.7138	2.6430	2.5752	2.5423	2.5229
2	4.0285	3.3354	3.1404	3.0488	2.9609	2.9182	2.8931
3	4.5573	3.7299	3.4961	3.3859	3.2800	3.2286	3.1983
4	5.0251	4.0779	3.8087	3.6816	3.5592	3.4996	3.4644
5	5.4499	4.3935	4.0918	3.9489	3.8109	3.7437	3.7038
6	5.8422	4.6849	4.3527	4.1950	4.0423	3.9677	3.9236
7	6.2086	4.9572	4.5963	4.4246	4.2579	4.1763	4.1279
8	6.5538	5.2138	4.8258	4.6406	4.4605	4.3722	4.3198
9	6.8812	5.4573	5.0435	4.8455	4.6525	4.5576	4.5012

Index

Index